Nutrition and Exercise: An Integrated Study

Nutrition and Exercise: An Integrated Study

Edited by Dephne Rowland

SYRAWOOD
PUBLISHING HOUSE
New York

Published by Syrawood Publishing House,
750 Third Avenue, 9th Floor,
New York, NY 10017, USA
www.syrawoodpublishinghouse.com

Nutrition and Exercise: An Integrated Study
Edited by Dephne Rowland

International Standard Book Number: 978-1-68286-693-1 (Hardback)

Cataloging-in-Publication Data

Nutrition and exercise : an integrated study / edited by Dephne Rowland.
p. cm.
Includes bibliographical references and index.
ISBN 978-1-68286-693-1
1. Nutrition. 2. Exercise. 3. Food. 4. Physical education and training. 5. Health.
I. Rowland, Dephne.
RA784 .N88 2019
613.2--dc23

Printed in China.

TABLE OF CONTENTS

PREFACE

Obesity, poor health and health-related disorders are a growing problem in the developing world. Nutrition is the science that studies the contribution of nutrients in the overall growth, development and maintenance of the human body. An unhealthy diet that lacks the essential nutrients in the right proportions can cause several deficiency diseases such as anemia, blindness, scurvy, etc. Excessive intake of nutrients can also cause health conditions and chronic diseases such as metabolic syndrome, cardiovascular disease and diabetes. Appropriate exercise and diet regimes can mitigate these conditions. Research in dietary science and nutrition has modernized the approach towards health management. This book is a compilation of chapters that discuss the most vital concepts and emerging trends in the field of health science especially in the sub-disciplines of nutrition and exercise. It strives to provide a fair idea about this discipline and to help develop a better understanding of the latest advances in this field. Food scientists, nutritionists, physical instructors, researchers and students will find this book helpful.

This book is a comprehensive compilation of works of different researchers from varied parts of the world. It includes valuable experiences of the researchers with the sole objective of providing the readers (learners) with a proper knowledge of the concerned field. This book will be beneficial in evoking inspiration and enhancing the knowledge of the interested readers.

In the end, I would like to extend my heartiest thanks to the authors who worked with great determination on their chapters. I also appreciate the publisher's support in the course of the book. I would also like to deeply acknowledge my family who stood by me as a source of inspiration during the project.

Editor

1

The weight of work: the association between maternal employment and overweight in low- and middle-income countries

Vanessa M. Oddo[1,6*], Sara N. Bleich[2], Keshia M. Pollack[3], Pamela J. Surkan[4], Noel T. Mueller[5] and Jessica C. Jones-Smith[1,6]

Abstract

Background: Maternal employment has increased in low-and middle-income countries (LMIC) and is a hypothesized risk factor for maternal overweight due to increased income and behavioral changes related to time allocation. However, few studies have investigated this relationship in LMIC.

Methods: Using cross-sectional samples from Demographic and Health Surveys, we investigated the association between maternal employment and overweight (body mass index [BMI] ≥ 25 kg/m^2) among women in 38 LMIC (N = 162,768). We categorized mothers as formally employed, informally employed, or non-employed based on 4 indicators: employment status in the last 12 months; aggregate occupation category (skilled, unskilled); type of earnings (cash only, cash and in-kind, in-kind only, unpaid); and seasonality of employment (all year, seasonal/occasional employment). Formally employed women were largely employed year-round in skilled occupations and earned a wage (e.g. professional), whereas informally employed women were often irregularly employed in unskilled occupations and in some cases, were paid in-kind (e.g. domestic work). For within-country analyses, we used adjusted logistic regression models and included an interaction term to assess heterogeneity in the association by maternal education level. We then used meta-analysis and meta-regression to explore differences in the associations pooled across countries.

Results: Compared to non-employed mothers, formally employed mothers had higher odds of overweight (pooled odds ratio [POR] = 1.3; 95% Confidence Interval [CI] 1.2, 1.4) whereas informally employed mothers, compared to non-employed mothers, had lower odds of overweight (POR = 0.72; 95% CI: 0.64, 0.81). In 14 LMIC, the association varied by education. In these countries, the magnitude of the formal employment-overweight association was larger for women with low education (POR = 1.5; 95% CI: 1.1, 1.9) compared to those with high education (POR = 1.2; 95% CI: 1.0, 1.3).

Conclusions: Formally employed mothers in LMIC have higher odds of overweight and the association varies by educational attainment in 14 countries. This knowledge highlights the importance of workplace initiatives to reduce the risk of overweight among working women in LMIC.

Keywords: Maternal employment, Overweight, Low- and middle-income countries, Nutrition transition

* Correspondence: voddo@uw.edu
[1]Department of International Health, Center for Human Nutrition, Johns Hopkins Bloomberg School of Public Health, 615 N. Wolfe St, Baltimore, MD 21205, USA
[6]Nutrition Sciences Program & Department of Health Services, University of Washington School of Public Health, Raitt Hall, Seattle, WA 98195, USA
Full list of author information is available at the end of the article

Background

The launch of the Millennium Development Goals (MDG) raised global interest, awareness, and attention to women's employment as several MDG targets identified promoting women's employment as an intervention strategy to improve health and alleviate poverty. Subsequently, over the past two decades, there have been vast increases in employment and shifts from part-time to full-time work among women in low- and middle-income countries (LMIC) [1, 2]. These increases are paralleled by increases in the prevalence of overweight and a changing nutritional landscape, characterized by shifts in diet (e.g. increases in consumption of processed foods) and physical activity (e.g. decreases in energy expenditure) [3–9]. Higher rates of maternal employment may provide greater exposure to these changes of modernity and adversely impact bodyweight. As environments change, a better understanding of the relationship between maternal employment and overweight in LMIC is critical given that overweight further threatens the health and economic stability of LMIC and the possible need for additional policies and programs designed to support women in the workplace [10].

Only two prior studies have begun to examine the association between maternal employment and overweight in LMIC. Goryakin and Suhrcke found that that being employed, compared to non-employed, was associated with a higher probability of women being overweight in middle-income countries, but a lower probability of being overweight in low-income countries [11]. A second study found that mothers working in professional occupations had higher odds of overweight compared to those working in agriculture [2]. Key limitations of these studies include using a dichotomous indicator of employment and only reporting regional-level trends.

The primary aim of this study is to address key gaps in the literature about the maternal employment-overweight relationship by using the most recent data available from 38 LMIC to explore country-specific estimates, with mothers categorized as formally employed, informally employed, or non-employed. This unique feature of this investigation allowed for a thorough characterization of employment in LMIC settings, and for a novel investigation of the relationship between maternal employment and maternal overweight. The secondary aims of this paper are to assess heterogeneity in the maternal employment-overweight relationship by maternal education level and countries' stage in the nutrition transition, as indicated by gross domestic product (GDP) and urbanization. We hypothesize that maternal employment is associated with higher odds of overweight through several mechanisms, including increased income and behavioral changes related to time allocation.

Methods

Data source and study population

Data were obtained from the Demographic and Health Surveys (DHS), which are cross-sectional household surveys administered in LMIC. DHS employ a multistage cluster sample design and are nationally representative [12]. The surveys are standardized allowing for cross-country comparisons.

This study specifically focused on mothers, rather than all women more broadly, based on several factors. First, we aimed to keep our sample consistent to prior related studies and earlier years of the DHS only collected anthropometrics among women with children under 5 years old. Second, our a priori hypothesis was that mothers' time would be more constrained than that of women without children.

Our analyses utilized one survey per country. We retained surveys from 38 LMIC that met the following criteria for inclusion: 1) it was the most recent survey administered from 2010 to the time of analysis (May 2016), 2) women were queried on their employment status and 3) at least 85% of the women surveyed had anthropometric data collected. Our final analytic sample (n = 162,768) included non-pregnant women, aged 18 to 49 years, who had children between ages 0–5 years since most DHS surveys collected anthropometrics only among this subgroup. Women whose children resided outside the household surveyed were also excluded (n = 173). The Johns Hopkins Institutional Review Board deemed that this analysis of de-identified secondary data was not human subjects research.

Primary dependent variable

Overweight or obese, defined as body mass index (BMI) $\geq$ 25 kg/m^2 (henceforth referred to as overweight), served as our primary dependent variable [13]. Height (in centimeters [cm] to the nearest 0.1 cm) and weight (in kilograms [kg] to the nearest 0.1 kg) were measured by trained technicians using standard techniques [14, 15].

Independent variable

Maternal employment was modeled as a 3-category variable: formally employed, informally employed, and non-employed. Informal employment refers to activities (e.g. domestic work, street vendors, homestead agriculture) and income that are outside regulation and may help woman capitalize on desirable non-wage features of the informal sector, such as flexible hours [16–18]. We separately categorized formal and informal employment based on research indicating that: 1) 60% of women employed in LMIC are engaged in informal employment, 2) factors driving labor force participation differ across labor market sectors, 3) wages are 60–77% lower in the informal sector and 4) the employment-overweight relationship and dietary patterns may vary by the number of hours women work and occupation type [2, 11, 16, 19–24]. Notably, this investigation categorized women as formally employed, informally employed or non-employed, rather than focusing specifically on occupation type, based on qualitative work which suggested that occupation type alone may not capture both the changes in income and time allocation that occur with employment [25]. Additionally, prior literature has focused on the relationship between occupation type (i.e. professional versus agriculture-based occupations) and overweight risk in LMIC [2].

Employment status was defined based on 4 indicators guided by the International Labor Organization's definitions of formal and informal employment [16, 26]: 1) employment status in the last 12 months (employed, non-employed); 2) aggregate occupation category (skilled, unskilled); 3) type of earnings (cash only, cash and in-kind, in-kind only, unpaid); and 4) seasonality of employment (all year, seasonal/occasional employment). Formal employment included three combinations: 1) employed, skilled occupation, cash only earnings, employed all year; 2) employed, skilled occupation, cash only earnings, seasonal/occasional employment; and 3) employed, unskilled occupation, cash only earnings, employed all year. All other employed women were categorized as informally employed (e.g. employed, unskilled occupation, cash only earnings, seasonal/occasional employment) (see Additional file 1: Table S1).

Confounders and effect measure modifiers

We identified confounding factors a priori using a directed acyclic graph, which is a causal diagram used to characterize the relationship between the exposure and outcome based on theorized relationships and relationships documented in the literature [27–29]. Confounders included maternal age (years), marital status (married or living together versus single, widowed, divorced), parity, number of household members, child age (months) and childcare support. Living with ones' mother, mother-in-law, or sister served a proxy for childcare support (a binary variable).

We tested for heterogeneity in the employment-overweight association by maternal education level because prior literature suggests that the employment-nutritional status relationship may vary by educational attainment [30]. Research also shows that women with higher educational attainment more often participate in formal sector employment [16, 19]. We modeled education as a binary variable (< primary school completed versus ≥ primary school completed) based on the distribution of educational attainment across countries.

We additionally explored differences in the country-level associations by log-GDP per capita, adjusted for purchasing power parity (or the financial ability to buy products and services with a sum of money) and percent urban, both theorized drivers of the nutrition transition [8, 31, 32]. GDP-per capita was log transformed due to convention and to reflect the expected influence of a percent increase (e.g. 10%), rather than an absolute dollar increase (e.g. $10 U.S. dollars). We utilized log-GDP and percent urban from the World Development Indicators database, corresponding to the year the survey was administered [33, 34]. Percent urban was defined as the number of people living in urban areas divided by the total population.

Statistical analysis

We used separate multivariable logistic regression models for each country to test the association between maternal employment and overweight. We utilized sampling weights provided by the DHS, which account for differential probability of selection and response. Analyses additionally accounted for the clustered design through the use of Taylor series linearized standard errors. In our primary models, we tested for heterogeneity in the association between maternal employment and overweight by maternal education level using a post-hoc Wald test and retained the interaction term only if statistically significant. If the association between employment and overweight was homogenous by maternal education level, then education was included in the model as a confounder. Because we retained interaction terms in select countries (n = 14), we estimated pooled odds ratios (POR), using random effects meta-analysis, separately for the associations between formal and informal employment and overweight for three subgroups: women in countries where the association did not vary education, women with low educational attainment (< primary) in countries where the association varied by education, and women with high educational attainment (≥ primary) in countries where the association varied by education. Random effects meta-analysis, used to generate pooled odds ratios is the statistical combination of the estimates from separate countries (i.e. it utilizes the country-specific beta coefficient) and assumes that the magnitude of the association between employment and overweight may differ by country. We then assessed differences in the association between countries by log-GDP and urbanization using random-effects meta-regression, which utilized the country-specific effect estimates to statistically test for differences in the employment-overweight effect size by country-level factors (e.g. log-GDP) [35–37]. Alpha was set to 0.05 for main effects and to 0.10 for interaction terms. Analyses were performed using Stata 14.1 (StataCorp LP, College Station, Texas).

As sensitivity analyses, we modeled underweight (BMI < 18.5) and normal weight (BMI ≥ 18.5 to BMI < 25) as outcomes to assess whether the results were consistent with the outcome of overweight. We assessed the robustness of our results when modeling obesity (BMI ≥ 30) and BMI (measured continuously) as outcomes and when controlling for within country residence (urban/rural status). We re-ran our primary models across the full sample of women, which included mothers with children older than 5 years and women without children. Finally, we estimated the difference in the probability of being overweight between formally employed versus non-employed mothers and between informally employed versus non-employed mothers.

Results

Data were analyzed for 162,768 women from 38 LMIC. Selected sample characteristics by country are detailed in Table 1 and by employment type in Additional file 1: Table S2. The percent of mothers formally (3.7% to 54%) and informally (2.1% to 80%) employed was wide-ranging. Approximately 29% of women were overweight, but prevalence rates across countries were wide-ranging (4.3% to 80%).

Being formally employed, compared to non-employed, was associated with 30% higher odds of maternal overweight when pooling estimates across 38 LMIC (POR = 1.3; 95% Confidence Interval [CI] 1.2, 1.4) (Table 2). On the contrary, informal employment was associated with lower odds of being overweight in 18 LMIC and when pooling estimates across all countries (POR = 0.72; 95% CI: 0.64, 0.81).

Heterogeneity in the employment-overweight association by maternal education

Figure 1 details the country-specific relationships between formal and informal employment and overweight in the 24 countries where the association did not vary by maternal level of education. Formally employed mothers, compared to non-employed mothers, had higher odds of overweight in 10 of 24 LMIC (Fig. 1). Informally employed mothers, compared to non-employed mothers, had lower odds of overweight in 13 of 24 LMIC (Fig. 1). When pooling estimates across countries where the association did not vary by maternal education, formally employed women had higher odds of overweight compared to those who were non-employed (POR = 1.2; 95% CI: 1.1, 1.4) (Table 2). In countries where the association did not vary by education, informally employed women had lower odds of overweight compared to non-employed women (POR = 0.71; 95% CI: 0.60, 0.83).

In 14 LMIC, the association between employment and overweight varied by maternal education level (Fig. 2 and Table 2). In countries where the association varied by education, the formal employment-overweight association was larger for women with low education (POR = 1.5; 95% CI: 1.1, 1.9) as compared to the association among those with high education (POR = 1.2; 95% CI: 1.0, 1.3) (POR for the difference [high vs. low] = 0.78; 95% CI: 0.62, 0.98) (Table 2). However, the association was positive in both cases. Both informally employed women with low education (POR = 0.74; 95% CI: 0.62, 0.88) and high education (POR = 0.63; 95% CI: 0.50, 0.79) had lower odds of overweight compared to non-employed women. But the magnitude of the employment-overweight association was not different for informally employed women with high education as compared to the analogous association among informally employed women with low education (POR for the difference [high vs. low] = 0.81; 95% CI: 0.58, 1.1) (Table 2).

Meta-regression

The meta-regression results indicated that neither the formal employment-, nor informal employment-overweight associations were statistically significantly different by log-GDP or urbanization (Additional file 1: Table S3, Figure. S1 and S2).

Sensitivity analyses

Consistent with our results for overweight, formal employment was associated with lower odds of underweight (POR = 0.75; 95% CI: 0.67, 0.83) (Additional file 1: Table S4) and lower odds of normal weight (POR = 0.89; 95% CI: 0.83, 0.95). Informal employment was not associated with underweight (POR = 0.99; 95% CI: 0.89, 1.1), but results indicated that informal employment was associated with higher odds of normal weight (POR = 1.2; 95% CI: 1.1, 1.3).

The direction of the country-specific and pooled associations between both formal and informal employment were robust to modeling obesity as the outcome (Additional file 1: Table S5) and modeling continuous BMI as the outcome (Additional file 1: Table S6). The associations between employment and overweight were also similar in direction and magnitude for the full sample of women (formal POR = 1.4; 95% CI: 1.3, 1.5; informal POR = 0.76; 95% CI: 0.68, 0.85) (Additional file 1: Table S7) and when controlling for within country residence (urban versus rural) (formal POR = 1.2; 95% CI: 1.1, 1.3; informal POR = 0.80; 95% CI: 0.72, 0.88) (Additional file 1: Table S8). Consistent with our primary results, formally employed mothers, compared to non-employed mothers, have a higher probability of being overweight

Table 1 Descriptive characteristics of mothers participating in selected Demographic and Health Surveys

Country	Year	N[b]	N (%)[a] Formally Employed (n = 40,723)[b,c]	Informally Employed (n = 46,970)[b,c]	≥ Primary Education (n = 81,477)[b]	Overweight (n = 48,421)[b,d]
Bangladesh	2011	6224	564 (9.0%)	130 (2.1%)	3929 (63%)	776 (12%)
Benin	2011–12	6372	2658 (42%)	1738 (28%)	999 (16%)	1672 (27%)
Burkina Faso	2010	4204	659 (16%)	2802 (66%)	348 (8.2%)	381 (9.0%)
Cambodia	2014	3477	1527 (43%)	1165 (33%)	1578 (44%)	610 (17%)
Cameroon	2011	2965	962 (32%)	1301 (44%)	1530 (51%)	928 (31%)
Colombia[e]	2010	11,809	4071 (38%)	2734 (25%)	9386 (87%)	4832 (45%)
Comoros	2012	1468	341 (23%)	286 (19%)	584 (39%)	703 (47%)
Cote d'Ivoire	2011–12	2017	544 (28%)	900 (47%)	355 (19%)	444 (23%)
DRC	2013–14	4293	697 (16%)	2753 (65%)	2014 (48%)	638 (15%)
Dominican Republic	2013	2385	1147 (48%)	227 (10%)	1846 (78%)	1202 (51%)
Egypt	2014	9765	1090 (11%)	238 (2.4%)	7517 (77%)	7762 (80%)
Ethiopia	2011	6095	874 (14%)	2659 (42%)	434 (6.8%)	276 (4.3%)
Ghana	2014	1760	807 (47%)	612 (36%)	998 (59%)	703 (41%)
Guinea	2012	1978	470 (24%)	1120 (57%)	239 (12%)	347 (18%)
Haiti	2012	2879	879 (32%)	845 (30%)	1259 (45%)	734 (26%)
Honduras	2011–12	7368	2262 (32%)	1219 (17%)	4786 (68%)	3684 (53%)
Kyrgyz Republic[f]	2012	2686	559 (22%)	86 (3.4%)	2261 (89%)	858 (34%)
Lesotho	2014	1034	248 (25%)	153 (15%)	814 (81%)	463 (46%)
Liberia	2013	2110	562 (30%)	610 (32%)	640 (34%)	464 (24%)
Malawi	2010	3026	508 (17%)	1750 (57%)	789 (26%)	502 (16%)
Mali	2012–13	2308	301 (13%)	658 (28%)	220 (9.4%)	382 (16%)
Mozambique	2011	5848	601 (10%)	2296 (38%)	1157 (19%)	812 (13%)
Namibia	2013	1376	440 (34%)	126 (10%)	1012 (79%)	416 (32%)
Nepal	2011	1681	182 (11%)	1073 (62%)	738 (43%)	173 (10%)
Niger	2012	2771	316 (11%)	413 (15%)	172 (6.1%)	504 (18%)
Nigeria	2013	15,052	8243 (54%)	2598 (17%)	7288 (48%)	3772 (25%)
Pakistan	2012–13	2106	292 (14%)	303 (14%)	815 (38%)	711 (33%)
Peru[g]	2012	7202	3267 (49%)	1341 (20%)	5542 (82%)	4041 (60%)
Rwanda	2010	2721	277 (10%)	2210 (80%)	649 (24%)	439 (16%)
Sierra Leone	2013	3194	583 (18%)	2071 (64%)	706 (22%)	520 (16%)
Tajikistan	2012	2957	334 (11%)	496 (16%)	2902 (95%)	845 (28%)
Tanzania	2010	4269	750 (17%)	3103 (71%)	2772 (63%)	821 (19%)
Timor-Leste	2009–10	4724	317 (6.7%)	1478 (31%)	2431 (51%)	281 (5.9%)
Togo	2013–14	2073	1046 (53%)	633 (32%)	638 (32%)	559 (28%)
Uganda	2011	1187	372 (32%)	540 (47%)	419 (36%)	203 (18%)
Yemen	2013	8476	312 (3.7%)	512 (6.1%)	3961 (48%)	2217 (27%)

Table 1 Descriptive characteristics of mothers participating in selected Demographic and Health Surveys *(Continued)*

Zambia	2013–14	7520	1414 (19%)	2915 (39%)	4001 (53%)	1652 (22%)
Zimbabwe	2010–11	3388	522 (15%)	876 (26%)	2931 (87%)	1003 (30%)
Total	162,768		40,998 (25%)	46,970 (29%)	80,659 (50%)	47,330 (29%)

DRC Democratic Republic of Congo
[a]Number of observations (percentage) were estimated using the country sample weight
[b]Total sample size in each country and by subgroup (e.g. total formally employed) are unweighted
[c]Type of employment was based on 4 following indicators: employment during the last 12 months (yes, no); aggregate occupation category (skilled, unskilled); type of earnings (cash only, cash and in-kind, in-kind only, unpaid); and seasonality of employment (all year, seasonally/occasionally)
[d]Overweight was defined as BMI ≥ 25 kg/m^2
[e]Employment type was based on employment status, occupation category and earnings only because seasonality of employment was not queried in this survey
[f]Maternal education level was dichotomized as < secondary level of education complete and ≥ secondary level of education complete
[g]Employment type was based on employment status, type of earnings, and seasonality only because occupation type was not queried in this survey

(predicted probability: 0.043; 95% CI: 0.026, 0.060) (Additional file 1: Table S9 and Figure. S3 and S4). On the contrary, but also consistent with our primary models, informally employed mothers have a lower probability of being overweight compared to non-employed mothers (predicted probability: -0.045; 95% CI: -0.064, −0.026).

Discussion

This study utilizes nationally representative data from 38 LMIC to investigate the within- and between-country associations between maternal employment and overweight. It is important to better understand the benefits, as well as the potential unintended consequences, of maternal employment on weight status in order to inform intervention approaches that both support women's participation in the labor force and address increasing overweight prevalence in LMIC. Formally employed mothers had higher odds of overweight, while informally employed mothers had lower odds of overweight. The employment-overweight association varied by maternal education level in several countries. The magnitude of the association between employment and overweight was smaller among formally employed mothers with higher education, compared to lower education. Our results also suggested that the employment-overweight relationship did not vary by GDP or urbanization.

Our results for formal employment are largely consistent with previous studies from middle-income countries and high-income countries (where formal employment is predominant), which find that maternal employment is associated with higher odds of overweight [2, 22–24]. Formal employment could result in a positive energy balance and subsequently, higher odds of overweight,

Table 2 Pooled odds ratio for the relationship between formal and informal maternal employment and overweight[a]

	N = 162,768[b] Pooled Odds Ratio (95% Confidence Interval)
Formal Employment[c]	
All low- and middle-income countries	1.3 (1.2, 1.4)
Countries where the association did not vary by education	1.2 (1.1, 1.4)
Countries where the association varied by education: low education[d]	1.5 (1.1, 1.9)
Countries where the association varied by education: high education[d]	1.2 (1.0, 1.3)
Informal Employment[c]	
All low- and middle-income countries	0.72 (0.64, 0.81)
Countries where the association did not vary by education	0.71 (0.60, 0.83)
Countries where the association varied by education: low education[d]	0.74 (0.62, 0.88)
Countries where the association varied by education: high education[d]	0.63 (0.50, 0.79)

[a]Pooled odds ratios (POR) were generated using meta-analysis and pool estimates across country subgroups. Overweight was defined as BMI ≥ 25 kg/m^2. All models were adjusted for maternal age (years), parity, marital status (married, not married), number of household members, child age (months), and substitute childcare provider (yes, no). Models which did not retain the employmentXeducation interaction term were also adjusted for maternal education (< primary education, ≥ primary education completed)
[b]Total sample size is unweighted
[c]Type of employment was based on 4 indicators: 1) employment during the last 12 months (yes, no); 2) aggregate occupation category (skilled, unskilled); 3) type of earnings (cash only, cash and in-kind, in-kind only, unpaid); and 4) seasonality of employment (all year, seasonally/occasionally)
[d]The employmentXeducation interaction term was retained in the following countries: Bangladesh, Benin, Burkina Faso, Democratic Republic of Congo, Ethiopia, Honduras, Kyrgyz Republic, Mozambique, Nigeria, Peru, Rwanda, Tanzania, Uganda, Zimbabwe. The relative difference in the employment-overweight association, comparing mothers with high to low education for formal employment was: POR = 0.78 (95% CI: 0.62, 0.98) and for informal employment was: POR = 0.81 (95% CI: 0.58, 1.1)

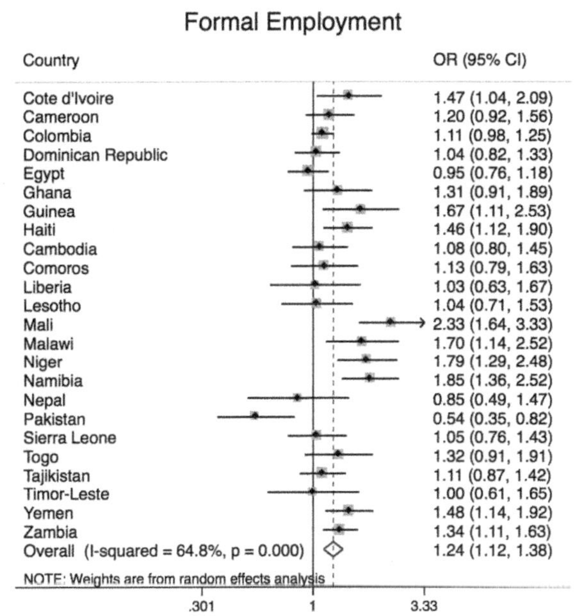

Fig. 1 Adjusted logistic regression for the relationship between maternal employment and overweight, in countries where the association did not vary by education[1, 2]. [1]Country-specific odds ratios were estimated using logistic regression to test the relationship between employment and overweight (BMI ≥ 25 kg/m^2). Overall odds ratios were generated using meta-analysis and pool estimates across countries.[2] Models were adjusted for maternal age (years), parity, marital status (married, not married), number of household members, child age (months), substitute childcare provider (yes, no) and maternal education (< primary education, ≥ primary education)

through several mechanisms. Increased economic resources, stemming from maternal employment, are associated with changes in food procurement behaviors, including increasing household food expenditures and increasing the purchase of energy-dense foods as they become more affordable, which could lead to an over-consumption of energy [38, 39]. Evidence finds an association between labor force participation and consumption of alcohol and meat in LMIC [4]. Behavioral changes related to mother's time allocation may also play a role. Data from the United States indicate that women working full-time spend less time cooking [40]. This is consistent with evidence from LMIC which suggests increases in work hours is associated with significantly lower energy intakes from home and higher intakes from commercially prepared foods [41]. Labor-related physical activity may also decrease as jobs emerging in the formal labor sector are more sedentary and shifting patterns of employment from agriculture into the service sector are associated with overweight among women in LMIC [42]. Maternal mental health may also play a role. Dual parental and employment responsibilities may induce stress among mothers and modest evidence suggests that adverse mental health (e.g. depression) is associated with increased overweight among women [43–46]. It is possible that the rapid transformation of the food and built environment in LMIC, such as the spread of supermarkets and availability of ultra-processed foods, provides an enabling environment for the aforementioned hypothesized changes among formally employed women [47–49].

Limited prior evidence, which pools formal and informal employment, suggests that women's employment is associated with a lower probability of being overweight in low-income countries, where informal employment is predominate [11]. This is consistent with our finding which indicates that informal employment is associated with lower odds of overweight. One explanation for this finding could be that the smaller increases in income and more active occupations associated with informal work may act to prevent women from becoming overweight. Wages in the informal sector employment are 60–77% lower than wages in the formal sector and we hypothesize that more nominal increases in income may illicit different food purchasing behaviors as compared to formally employed women [16]. For example nominal increases in income may allow women to somewhat increase their food expenditures, but not enable them to 'trade up' to energy-dense foods [50]. Substantive dietary changes may not occur until income increases beyond 15% of household expenditures; in a predominantly informally employed sample in Guatemala, for example, employed women reported that some higher-fat, animal source foods largely remained unaffordable [25, 51]. The informal sector includes mothers who voluntarily engage in employment due to part-time hours, which may afford women more flexibility in balancing domestic and employment responsibilities, rendering them less reliant on prepared foods with fewer time constraints [16–18]. Informally employed women are also likely to be engaged in occupational physical activity, particularly those employed in agriculture-based occupations.

Our results suggested heterogeneity in the employment-overweight associations by education in some contexts. It is likely that the combination of higher educational-attainment, increased income, and exposure to more prosocial ideas stemming from interactions with educated, skilled co-workers make formally employed mothers (with relatively high-education) more inclined to allocate resources in ways that are less conducive to weight gain, compared to their lower education, formally employed counterparts. These women may have improved decision-making power, increased efficiency of time use, and be somewhat less inclined to purchase energy-dense foods. Another explanation for the employment-overweight association being larger in magnitude among formally employed mothers with

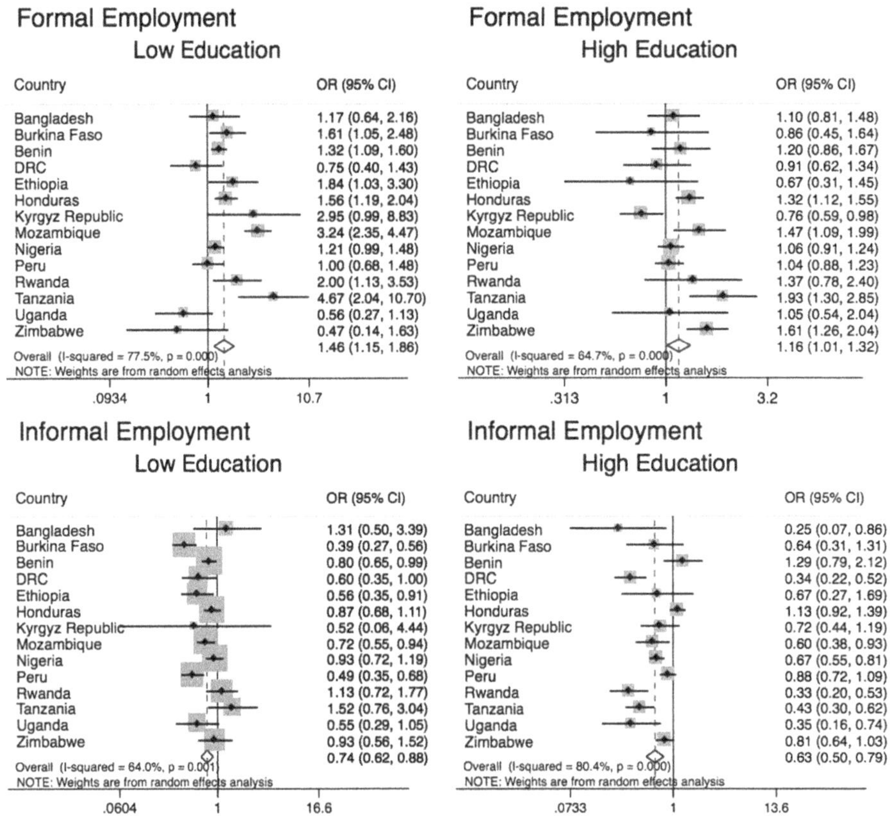

Fig. 2 Adjusted logistic regression for the relationship between maternal employment and overweight, in countries where the association varied by education[1, 2]. DRC = Democratic Republic of Congo.[1] Country-specific odds ratios were estimated using logistic regression to test the relationship employment and overweight (BMI ≥ 25 kg/m^2). Overall odds ratios were generated using meta-analysis and pool estimates across countries.[2] All models were adjusted for maternal age (years), parity, marital status (married, not married), number of household members, child age (months), and substitute childcare provider (yes, no). Models included an employmentXeducation interaction term (< primary education, ≥ primary education completed)

lower education derives from the mismatch of early life with later life environment. Mothers with low educational attainment may have had fewer resources early in life, but now these women have ubiquitous access to calories, increasing their propensity for being overweight [52]. Nevertheless, some aspects of formal employment seem to be associated with a positive energy balance among all formally employed mothers, irrespective of education-level.

Currently, there is a gap in knowledge on how to effectively develop and implement obesity-prevention and control strategies in LMIC. However, there is a consensus that multi-sectoral approaches should be implemented and one such component includes behavioral settings such as the workplace. These results suggest that employers in LMIC should consider implementing workplace strategies that promote healthy eating and physical activity and reduce overweight. For example, employers could consider offering individual-level nutrition education, in combination with environmental approaches to spur behavior change, such as increasing the availability of healthier food and beverage choices in the workplace.

Our study is not without limitations. Due to our study design, we cannot establish temporality or rule out unmeasured or residual confounding. The generalizability of our findings may be limited to women who have children under 5 years of age; however, the results were largely unchanged when we examined women with older children. Moreover, our results can only be generalized to countries that DHS fielded from 2010 to 2016. Our proxy measure of childcare support, which was included as a confounder, was limited in that we do not know if the potential substitute childcare provider was also employed. Finally, evidence suggested that there are two segments of the informal employment sector (voluntary and forced), but we were unable to distinguish between these sectors using the DHS [16].

Despite these limitations, this study has two key strengths which improve upon the existing evidence: 1) we estimate both within- and between-country associations among 38 countries and 2) we distinguish non-employed women from formally and informally employed women.

Conclusions

This study enhances our understanding of the association between maternal employment and overweight in LMIC. We provide evidence that mothers engaged in the formal workforce in LMIC have higher odds of overweight and that the employment-overweight association varies by educational attainment in several contexts. A better understanding of this area is critical given the expected increases in women's labor force participation in LMIC in coming decades. This new knowledge may also be helpful for the development of policies and programs to reduce the risk of overweight among working women in LMIC. Future research exploring the mechanisms of the employment-overweight association and the workplace will help inform potential environmental and contextual interventions (e.g. food offerings at work, transportation to work, and programs to decrease sedentary activity at work) that may mitigate this association.

Acknowledgments
None.

Funding
This work was supported by the National Institutes of Health, Clinical Research and Endocrinology Training Grant in Epidemiology in Diabetes (T32DK062707).

Authors' contributions
The authors contributed as follows: VMO and JCJ-S conceptualized the research question and analysis plan. VMO analyzed the data; VMO drafted the manuscript with critical input from KMP, NTM, SNB, PJS, and JCJ-S. All authors reviewed and approved the final manuscript.

Competing interests
The authors declare that they have no competing interests.

Author details
[1]Department of International Health, Center for Human Nutrition, Johns Hopkins Bloomberg School of Public Health, 615 N. Wolfe St, Baltimore, MD 21205, USA. [2]Department of Health Policy and Management, Harvard T.H. Chan School of Public Health, 677 Huntington Avenue, Boston, MA 02115, USA. [3]Department of Health Policy and Management, Johns Hopkins Bloomberg School of Public Health, 624 N. Broadway, Baltimore, MD 21205, USA. [4]Department of International Health, Social and Behavioral Interventions Program, Johns Hopkins Bloomberg School of Public Health, 615 N. Wolfe St, Baltimore, MD 21205, USA. [5]Department of Epidemiology, Johns Hopkins Bloomberg School of Public Health, 615 N. Wolfe St, Baltimore, MD 21205, USA. [6]Nutrition Sciences Program & Department of Health Services, University of Washington School of Public Health, Raitt Hall, Seattle, WA 98195, USA.

References

1. Adair L, Guilkey D, Bisgrove E, Gultiano S. Effect of childbearing on Filipino women's work hours and earnings. J Popul Econ. 2002;15(4):625–45.
2. Lopez-Arana S, Avendano M, van Lenthe FJ, Burdorf A. Trends in overweight among women differ by occupational class: results from 33 low-and middle-income countries in the period 1992–2009. Int J Obes. 2013;38(1):97–105.
3. NCD Risk Factor Collaboration. Trends in adult body-mass index in 200 countries from 1975 to 2014: a pooled analysis of 1698 population-based measurement studies with 19.2 million participants. Lancet. 2016; 387(10026):1377–96.
4. Dave D, Doytch N, Kelly IR. Nutrient intake: a cross-national analysis of trends and economic correlates. Soc Sci Med. 2016;158:158–67.
5. Du S, Mroz TA, Zhai F, Popkin BM. Rapid income growth adversely affects diet quality in China—particularly for the poor! Soc Sci Med. 2004;59(7):1505–15.
6. Wiggins S, Keats S, Han E, Shimokawa S, Hernández J, Claro R. The rising cost of a healthy diet. London: Overseas Development Institute; 2015. https://www.odi.org/sites/odi.org.uk/files/odi-assets/publications-opinion-files/9580.pdf. Accessed 28 May 2016.
7. Popkin BM. The nutrition transition and obesity in the developing world. J Nutr. 2001;131(3):871S–3S.
8. Popkin BM, Du S. Dynamics of the nutrition transition toward the animal foods sector in China and its implications: a worried perspective. J Nutr. 2003;133(11 Suppl 2):3898S–906S.
9. Dodzin S, Vamvakidis A. Trade and industrialization in developing economies. J Dev Econ. 2004;75(1):319–28.
10. Raymond SU, Leeder S, Greenberg HM. Obesity and cardiovascular disease in developing countries: a growing problem and an economic threat. Curr Opin Clin Nutr Metab Care. 2006;9(2):111–6.
11. Goryakin Y, Suhrcke M. Economic development, urbanization, technological change and overweight: what do we learn from 244 demographic and health surveys? Econ Hum Biol. 2014;14:109–27.
12. Macro ICF. Demographic and health surveys: DHS model questionnaires. Calverton: ICF Macro; 2008.
13. Nishida C, Uauy R, Kumanyika S, Shetty P. The joint WHO/FAO expert consultation on diet, nutrition and the prevention of chronic diseases: process, product and policy implications. Public Health Nutr. 2004;7(1a):245–50.
14. ICF Macro. Training Field Staff for DHS Surveys. Calverton; 2009.
15. Gibson RS. Principles of nutritional assessment. London: Oxford University Press; 2005.
16. Günther I, Launov A. Informal employment in developing countries: opportunity or last resort? J Dev Econ. 2012;97(1):88–98.
17. Magnac T. Segmented or competitive labor markets. Econometrica. 1991: 165–87.
18. Pratap S, Quintin E. Are labor markets segmented in developing countries? A semiparametric approach. Eur Econ Rev. 2006;50(7):1817–41.
19. Fields G. A guide to multisector labor market models. 2005. http://siteresources.worldbank.org/SOCIALPROTECTION/Resources/SP-Discussion-papers/Labor-Market-DP/0505.pdf. Accessed 28 May 2016.
20. Cunningham W, Maloney WF. Heterogeneity among Mexico's micro-enterprises: an application of factor and cluster analysis. World Bank Policy Working Paper. 1999. http://siteresources.worldbank.org/DEC/Resources/Heterogeneity01and0Cluster0Analysis.pdf. Accessed 28 May 2016.
21. Chen MA. The informal economy: definitions, theories and policies. WIEGO Working Paper: Women in informal economy globalizing and organizing; 2012.
22. Courtemanche C. Working yourself to death? The relationship between work hours and obesity. 2008. https://mpra.ub.uni-muenchen.de/25324/1/MPRA_paper_25324.pdf. Accessed 28 May 2016.
23. Au N, Hauck K, Hollingsworth B. Employment, work hours and weight gain among middle-aged women. Int J Obes. 2013;37(5):718–24.
24. Au N, Hollingsworth B. Employment patterns and changes in body weight among young women. Prev Med. 2011;52(5):310–6.
25. Oddo VM, Surkan PJ, Hurley KM, Lowery C, de Ponce S, Jones-Smith JC. Pathways of the Association Between Maternal Employment and Weight Status among Women and Children: Qualitative Findings from Guatemala. Matern Child Nutr. 2017;e12455. https://doi.org/10.1111/mcn.12455.
26. Hussmanns R. Measuring the informal economy: From employment in the informal sector to informal employment. Integration Working Paper. 2004. http://www.ilo.org/wcmsp5/groups/public/—dgreports/—integration/documents/publication/wcms_079142.pdf. Accessed 28 May 2016.
27. Textor J, Hardt J, Knuppel S. DAGitty: a graphical tool for analyzing causal diagrams. Epidemiology. 2011;22(5):745.
28. Greenland S, Pearl J, Robins JM. Causal diagrams for epidemiologic research. Epidemiology. 1999:37–48.
29. Pearl J. Causality: models, reasoning and inference. Economic Theory. 2003; 19:675–85.
30. Galobardes B, Morabia A, Bernstein MS. The differential effect of education

and occupation on body mass and overweight in a sample of working people of the general population. Ann Epidemiol. 2000;10(8):532–7.
31. Nandi A, Sweet E, Kawachi I, Heymann J, Galea S. Associations between Macrolevel economic factors and weight distributions in low-and middle-income Countries: a multilevel analysis of 200 000 adults in 40 Countries. Am J Public Health. 2014;104(2):e162–e71.
32. Ezzati M, Hoorn SV, Lawes CMM, Leach R, James WPT, Lopez AD, et al. Rethinking the" diseases of affluence" paradigm: global patterns of nutritional risks in relation to economic development. PLoS Med. 2005;2(5): 404.
33. The World Bank. World Development Indicators: Gross Domestic Product per capita, based on purchasing power parity. 2016 http://data.worldbank.org/indicator/NY.GDP.PCAP.PP.CD. Accessed 28 May 2016.
34. The World Bank. World Development Indicators: Percent Urban. 2016. http://data.worldbank.org/indicator/SP.URB.TOTL.IN.ZS?view=chart Accessed 28 May 2016.
35. Baker W, Michael White C, Cappelleri J, Kluger J, Coleman C. Understanding heterogeneity in meta-analysis: the role of meta-regression. Int J Clin Pract. 2009;63(10):1426–34.
36. Thompson SG, Higgins J. How should meta-regression analyses be undertaken and interpreted? Stat Med. 2002;21(11):1559–73.
37. Benton T. Using meta-regression to explore moderating effects in surveys of international achievement. Pract Assessment Res Eval. 2014;19(3):2.
38. Popkin BM. Time allocation of the mother and child nutrition. Ecol Food Nutr. 1980;9(1):1–13.
39. Engle PL. Influences of mothers' and fathers' income on children's nutritional status in Guatemala. Soc Sci Med. 1993;37(11):1303–12.
40. Cawley J, Liu F. Maternal employment and childhood obesity: a search for mechanisms in time use data. Econ Hum Biol. 2012;10(4):352–64.
41. Bisgrove EZ, Popkin BM. Does women's work improve their nutrition: evidence from the urban Philippines. Soc Sci Med. 1996;43(10):1475–88.
42. Goldin C. The U-shaped female labor force function in economic development and economic history. In: Schultz TP Investment in Women's human capital and economic Development. Chicago: University of Chicago Press; 1995. p. 61–90.
43. Slater J, Sevenhuysen G, Edginton B, O'Neil J. 'trying to make it all come together': structuration and employed mothers' experience of family food provisioning in Canada. Health Promot Int. 2011;27(3):405–15.
44. de Wit L, Luppino F, van Straten A, Penninx B, Zitman F, Cuijpers P. Depression and obesity: a meta-analysis of community-based studies. Psychiatry Res. 2010;178(2):230–5.
45. Scott KM, Bruffaerts R, Simon GE, Alonso J, Angermeyer M, de Girolamo G, et al. Obesity and mental disorders in the general population: results from the world mental health surveys. Int J Obes. 2008;32(1):192–200.
46. Simon GE, Ludman EJ, Linde JA, Operskalski BH, Ichikawa L, Rohde P, et al. Association between obesity and depression in middle-aged women. Gen Hosp Psychiatry. 2008;30(1):32–9.
47. Reardon T, Berdegue JA. The rapid rise of supermarkets in Latin America: challenges and opportunities for development. Dev Policy Rev. 2002; 20(4):371–88.
48. Reardon T, Timmer CP, Barrett CB, Berdegué J. The rise of supermarkets in Africa, Asia, and Latin America. Am J Agric Econ. 2003;85(5):1140–6.
49. Monteiro CA, Moubarac JC, Cannon G, Ng SW, Popkin B. Ultra-processed products are becoming dominant in the global food system. Obes Rev. 2013;14(S2):21–8.
50. Popkin BM, Du S. Dynamics of the nutrition transition toward the animal foods sector in China and its implications: a worried perspective. J Nutr. 2003;133:3898S–906S.
51. Leroy JL, Ruel M, Verhofstadt E. The impact of conditional cash transfer programmes on child nutrition: a review of evidence using a programme theory framework. J J Dev Effect. 2009;1(2):103–29.
52. Bateson P, Gluckman P, Hanson M. The biology of developmental plasticity and the predictive adaptive response hypothesis. J Physiol. 2014;592(11): 2357–68.

2

The effect of a weight gain prevention intervention on moderate-vigorous physical activity among black women: the Shape Program

Mary L. Greaney[1*], Sandy Askew[2], Sherrie F. Wallington[3], Perry B. Foley[2], Lisa M. Quintiliani[4] and Gary G. Bennett[2,5]

Abstract

Background: Rates of physical inactivity are high among Black women living in the United States with overweight or obesity, especially those living in the rural South. This study was conducted to determine if an efficacious weight gain prevention intervention increased moderate-vigorous physical activity (MVPA).

Methods: The Shape Program, a weight gain prevention intervention implemented in community health centers in rural North Carolina, was designed for socioeconomically disadvantaged Black women with overweight or obesity. MVPA was measured using accelerometers, and summarized into 1- and 10-min bouts. We employed analyses of covariance (ANCOVA) to assess the relationship between changes in MVPA over 12 months, calculated as a change score, and intervention assignment (intervention versus usual care).

Results: Participants completing both baseline and 12-month accelerometer assessments (n = 121) had a mean age of 36.1 (SD = 5.43) years and a mean body mass index of 30.24 kg/m^2 (SD = 2.60). At baseline, 38% met the physical activity recommendation (150 min of MVPA/week) when assessed using 10-min bouts, and 76% met the recommendation when assessed using 1-min bouts. There were no significant differences in change in MVPA participation among participants randomized to the intervention from baseline to 12-months using 1-min bouts (adjusted intervention mean [95% CI]: 20.50 [−109.09 to 150.10] vs. adjusted usual care mean [95% CI]: -80.04 [−209.21 to 49.13], P = .29), or 10-min bouts (adjusted intervention mean [95% CI]: 7.39 [−83.57 to 98.35] vs. adjusted usual care mean [95% CI]: -17.26 [−107.93 to 73.40], P = .70).

Conclusions: Although prior research determined that the Shape intervention promoted weight gain prevention, MVPA did not increase significantly among intervention participants from baseline to 12 months. The classification of bouts had a marked effect on the prevalence estimates of those meeting physical activity recommendations. More research is needed to understand how to promote increased MVPA in weight gain prevention interventions.

Trial registration: This study is registered at www.clinicaltrials.gov database (No. NCT00938535. Retrospectively Registered 7/10/2009).

Keywords: Accelerometers, Black women, Exercise, Accelerometers, Obesity

* Correspondence: mgreaney@uri.edu
[1]Department of Kinesiology and Health Studies, 25 West Independence Way, University of Rhode Island, Kingston, RI 02881, USA
Full list of author information is available at the end of the article

Background

Black women in the United States are disproportionately affected by the obesity epidemic [1–3] with four out of every five Black women having overweight or obesity [2]. Obesity rates are greater among Black adults living in rural areas of the United States than in urban areas (56% versus 43%) [4]. Black women have low levels of physical activity and high rates of sedentary behavior compared to women in other racial/ethnic groups [5, 6], which increases their risk of negative health outcomes associated with obesity, physical inactivity, and sedentary behaviors [7–11].

Adults often gain an average of 0.5–1 kg per year throughout middle age [12, 13], with Black women gaining weight at a greater rate than White women. Weight loss approaches often have only modest impacts; only about 20% of people sustain their weight loss [14]. Therefore, a new paradigm may be useful [15]. Weight gain prevention interventions that focus on weight maintenance and not weight loss may be a valuable new approach to ameliorate or reduce obesity. This approach may be particularly salient for Black women with overweight or obesity, since they have a greater tolerance of a heavier body size [16].

Participation in moderate-vigorous physical activity (MVPA) may be an important strategy for preventing weight gain [17–20]. However, only a limited number of weight gain prevention interventions have focused on and/or have assessed the impact of the intervention on participants' physical activity [21]. Research in this area is needed because physical activity is a weight maintenance strategy that may have important spillover health benefits. In order to address this gap, we examined the impact of The Shape Program, a weight gain prevention program designed for Black women living in the rural South with overweight or obesity [15, 22], on MVPA.

Methods

The Shape Program

The Shape Program (henceforth referred to as Shape) was a randomized controlled trial of a 12-month weight gain prevention intervention implemented in rural North Carolina community health centers between 2009 and 2012. The intervention prevented weight gain at 12 and 18 months [22] and has been described in detail elsewhere [15]. Participants were Black female patients aged 25–44 with a body mass index (BMI) of 25–34.9 kg/m^2 who had made at least one visit to the participating health care system in the previous 24 months, and were fluent in English.

Ethics, consent, and permission

Participants provided signed informed consents and completed baseline assessments. Next, they were fitted with accelerometers, and then randomized to either the intervention arm or usual care. Participants completed additional assessments at 12 months post-enrollment and were again fitted with accelerometers. The study was approved by the Institutional Review Board at Duke University.

The Shape intervention

The Shape intervention was developed using social cognitive theory [23], with self-efficacy selected as the primary mediator [15]. The intervention utilized the interactive obesity treatment approach (iOTA), where individuals self-monitor concise and easy to comprehend tailored behavior change goals. iOTA reduces literacy and numeracy issues that may occur in traditional lifestyle interventions for weight management [15, 22]. Individuals randomized to the intervention arm received: (a) tailored behavior change goals to promote the prevention of weight gain; (b) skills training materials; (c) weekly interactive voice response (IVR) telephone calls for self-monitoring behaviors; (d) monthly telephone coaching from a registered dietitian trained in motivational interviewing; and (e) a no-cost 12-month membership to a YMCA facility of their choice. Based on our prior work [24, 25], participants were assigned goals (versus selecting their own) to maximize the likelihood of success. Goals were tailored to the individual using an algorithm accounting for the participant's need for change, self-efficacy, and readiness for change. Goals were updated every 8 weeks based on output from the original algorithm, with one goal always focused on physical activity. For example, one goal was to walk 7000 steps per day, which increased to 8000 and then 10,000 steps when the goal was regularly met. For the first 8 weeks, individuals were assigned three goals, and for the rest of the intervention period individuals were assigned four goals for each 8-week interval.

Printed skills training materials, tailored to participants' assigned behavior change goals, were designed for low-literacy audiences [26] and included information (e.g., overcoming barriers to physical activity, portion sizes, food shopping tips, healthy recipes) and tracking logs specific to each assigned goals. The training materials also included information useful for behavior change regardless of the behavior (e.g., implementing social environmental change, managing time). Participants received their first set of skills training materials at the baseline assessment and were mailed additional materials every 8 weeks throughout the intervention period when new goals were assigned.

During the coaching calls, health coaches utilized principles of motivational interviewing when reviewing self-monitoring data and when assisting participants in their change efforts. They also offered participants information on a range of topics such as negotiating barriers, engaging social support, identifying ways to be physically active throughout the day, and maintaining motivation.

Although the intervention was implemented in the primary care setting, with the exception of a 12-month YMCA membership provided at no cost, intervention components were designed to be completed at participants' homes. Participants randomized to usual care arm were mailed semi-annual newsletters during the intervention period. These newsletters covered general wellness topics but did not address physical activity, nutrition or weight.

Measures

Physical activity

At the baseline and 12-month assessments, participants were fitted with accelerometers (Actical, Philips Respironics, Inc., Bend, OR, USA). Accelerometers were placed on participants' non-dominant wrists using plastic locking wrist straps (like a wristwatch) that could only be removed by being cut off. Participants were asked to wear the accelerometers continuously until their return visit approximately 14 days later and were informed that the device could be worn while showering and sleeping and only needed to be removed if swimming for more than 30 min. The accelerometer data were screened and processed using procedures consistent with recent recommendations [27, 28]. Complete files were defined as those in which participants wore the monitor for seven or more days for at least 10 h of valid wear time per day. The raw data files were converted into minute-by-minute values of activity energy expenditure (AEE; kcal/kg/min) using a previously published calibration algorithm [29], and summarized into 1- and 10-min bouts of MVPA. We calculated 10-min bouts to align with current physical activity recommendations [30] and, given the low rates of Black women meeting physical activity recommendations [5, 6], we wanted to explore whether participants increased their MVPA if shorter bouts of MVPA were taken into account. Both 1-min and 10-min bouts were used to determine whether participants met current physical activity recommendations (150+ minutes of MVPA/week).

Health-related measures

Trained study staff measured weight to the nearest 0.1 kg using a portable electronic scale (Seca Model 876) and measured height using a calibrated wall-mounted stadiometer (Seca 214). Height and weight were then used to calculate body mass index (BMI). As part of the baseline survey, participants reported their perceived health status, which was assessed using the Medical Outcomes Study Short-Form; response categories were dichotomized (excellent/very good/good versus fair/poor) [31].

Demographic measures

Examined demographic variables included age, marital/partner status, educational attainment, employment status, income, and number of children in the household. The last two measures were used to determine if participants' household incomes were above or below/borderline the federal poverty line based on the 2010 federal poverty guidelines for income and household size. For example, a family of three with a reported household income falling in the category of $10,000–$19,999 would be classified as being borderline/at the federal poverty level of $18,301 [32], while those with lower incomes were classified as being below the federal poverty level, and those with higher incomes were classified as being above the federal poverty level.

Analysis

The analytic sample included participants who completed the accelerometer protocol at the baseline and 12-month assessments (n = 121, 63.3% of the baseline sample, see Fig. 1.). We calculated descriptive statistics for all key variables at baseline and used t-tests and chi square tests to determine if there were differences between the intervention and usual care groups in sociodemographics, health-related measures, MVPA participation, and in meeting the physical activity recommendation at baseline as assessed by 1-min and 10-min bouts. Likewise, we tested for differences between participants in our analysis sample and those participants excluded due to insufficient accelerometer data.

We employed analyses of covariance (ANCOVA) to assess the relationship between change in MVPA over 12 months, calculated as a change score, and intervention assignment (intervention versus usual care). We used step-wise model selection methods using F-tests (P = .20 entrance criteria and a P = .10 staying criteria) and several criterion-based procedures (best Akaike Information Criterion (AIC), Mallows C_p, SBC or adjusted R^2) to identify the best model from the health-related and demographic variable pool for change in total MVPA minutes per week using 10-min bouts. The pool consisted of available health-related measures (health status, BMI) and demographic characteristics (age, education, employment status, poverty level, marital/partner status and number of children in household) believed to potentially impact physical activity. Although the models identified by each technique were similar, slight variations were present; we selected the model created by our F-test sequence, which also had the best AIC and best Mallow's C_p as the final model. This model included poverty level and BMI as covariates. We used a similar procedure for the 1-min bouts data, but none of these criteria agreed on a single best model. Therefore we selected the model suggested by our significance-based

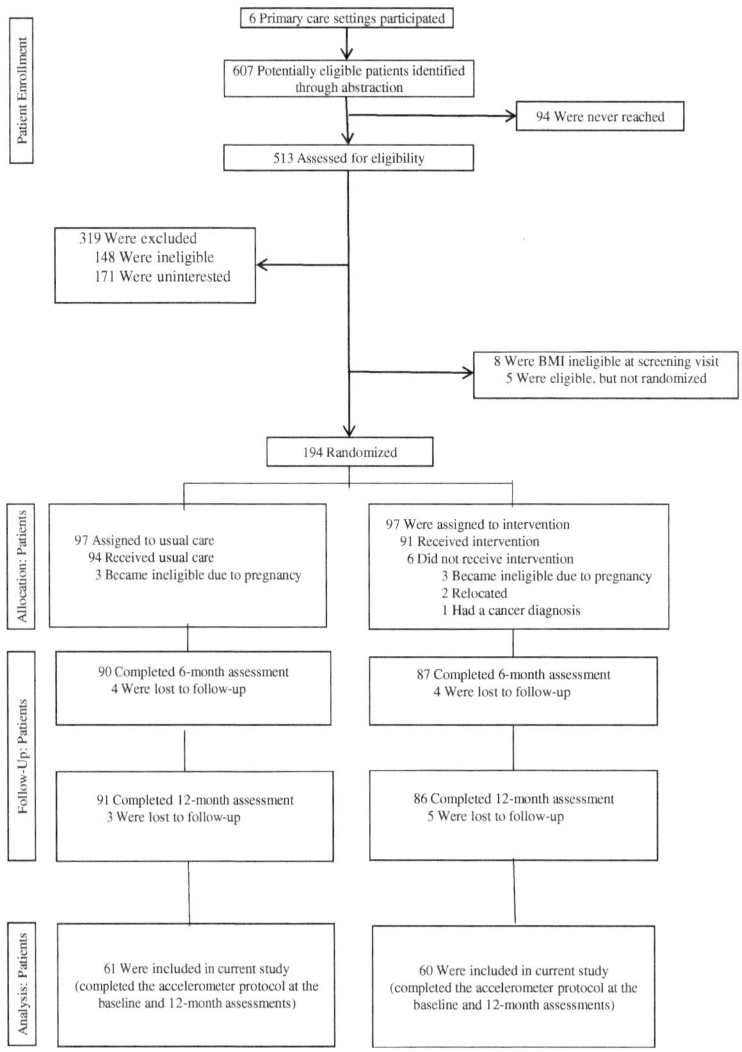

Fig. 1 Consort Diagram

criteria, since it included poverty level and BMI as covariates, which was consistent with the 10-min bout model.

Results

Participants (n = 121) had a mean age of 36.1 (SD = 5.43) years and a mean BMI of 30.24 kg/m^2 (SD = 2.60) (See Table 1.). The majority was employed (78%), not married/partnered (70%), and had a family income that placed them borderline/at or below the federal poverty level (62%). Participants who were excluded due to missing data (n = 64) were younger (mean age ± SD: 34.1 ± 5.4 years versus 36.1 ± 5.4 years, p = .02) and less likely to be employed (59% vs. 78%, p = .01). There were also marginal differences in the likelihood of reporting health as good, very good or excellent (47% versus 62%, p = .054), and of having children (44% versus 29%, p = .051). No significant differences were observed in the remaining demographic or health-related measures between the analytic sample for this study and Shape participants who were excluded due to missing accelerometer data (data not shown). Furthermore, there were no significant differences in the demographic or health-related measures between the intervention group and usual care groups (see Table 1).

About one-third (38%) of participants met the physical activity recommendation at baseline when assessed using 10-min bouts; this percentage increased to 76% when assessed using 1-min bouts (see Table 2). Participants randomly assigned to the usual care group participated in more MVPA during the baseline measurement period (see Table 2). However, there were no significant differences in MVPA participation by either group at 12 months or in the percent of participants meeting the physical activity recommendation at either baseline or 12 months. Furthermore, there was no significant

Table 1 Baseline characteristics of The Shape Program participants with baseline and 12-month accelerometer data (n = 121)

	Total (n = 121)		Usual Care (n = 61)		Intervention (n = 60)		
	%	n	%	n	%	n	P value
Demographics							
Age (mean years)[a]	36.12	5.43	35.62	5.76	36.62	5.07	.32
Education							.997
< high school (HS) diploma	10.08	12	10.00	6	10.17	6	
HS diploma or GED	28.57	34	28.33	17	28.81	17	
Some college or more	61.34	73	61.67	37	61.02	36	
Federal poverty level (FPL)							.90
Above FPL	37.29	44	35.59	21	38.89	23	
Borderline/at FPL	32.20	38	32.20	19	32.20	19	
Below FPL	30.51	36	32.20	19	28.81	17	
Marital/Partner status							.51
Currently married/partnered	29.91	35	32.76	19	27.12	16	
Not married/partnered	70.09	82	67.24	39	72.88	43	
Number of children in household							.20
None	70.54	79	64.81	35	75.86	44	
1 or more	29.46	33	35.19	19	24.14	14	
Employment status							.26
Employed (full or part time)	77.97	92	73.77	45	82.46	47	
Not employed	22.03	26	26.23	16	17.53	10	
Health-related variables							
BMI (kg/m^2)[a]	30.24	2.60	30.27	2.37	30.22	2.76	.92
Perceived health status							.45
Good/Very Good/Excellent	61.67	74	58.55	35	65.00	39	
Fair/Poor	38.33	46	41.67	25	35.00	21	

Note:
[a]Means and standard deviations are presented (vs. % and n).[2] = 150 min of moderate-vigorous PA/week

Table 2 Moderate-vigorous physical activity (MVPA) participation of The Shape Program participants with baseline and 12-month accelerometer data (n = 121)

	Total (n = 121)		Usual Care (n = 61)		Intervention (n = 60)		P value
Met physical activity rec.	%	n	%	n	%	n	
Baseline (1-min bouts)	76.0	92	77.1	47	75.0	45	.83
Baseline (10-min bouts)	38.0	46	41.0	25	35.0	21	.58
12 months (1-min bouts)	69.4	84	75.4	46	63.3	38	.17
12-months (10-min bouts)	31.4	38	34.4	21	28.3	17	.56
Minutes MVPA/week	Mean	SD	Mean	SD	Mean	SD	
Baseline (1-min bouts)	438.69	445.0	546.11	549.90	329.47	266.88	.007
Baseline (10-min bouts)	202.65	308.05	262.33	387.18	141.98	182.00	.03
12-months (1-min bouts)	396.98	471.23	455.00	518.69	337.98	413.54	.17
12-months (10-min bouts)	189.17	327.43	237.54	396.62	140.00	230.65	.10

change in MVPA over the intervention period (see Table 3) or significant difference in changes in MVPA by group assignment over the intervention period (see Table 4).

We conducted a sensitivity analyses that excluded the 9.7% who participated in no moderate to vigorous activity at baseline to determine if the intervention resulted in increased MVPA among participants who were participating in some MVPA at baseline; results remained the same (data not shown).

Discussion

Shape was a multicomponent intervention previously shown to prevent weight gain in a sample of socioeconomically disadvantaged Black women who have overweight or obesity [15], a population with low rates of physical activity [5]. Given the importance of physical activity for weight maintenance [17–20] and overall health benefits independent from weight [33], we wanted to determine whether the Shape intervention increased MVPA. Analyses determined that MVPA did not increase over the 12-month intervention period. This finding, combined with the known efficacy of the Shape intervention, suggests that the weight gain prevention may have been due to dietary changes rather than increases in MVPA. It is possible that participants viewed diet-related changes as being more valuable and/or easier to integrate into their daily lives. It also is conceivable that participants prioritized dietary change goals, since more of the Shape behavioral changes goals focused on dietary changes than on physical activity. Future research in the weight gain prevention intervention arena would be well poised to investigate these beliefs and attitudes. In addition, research is needed to understand how to stress the importance of physical activity for overall health and how to promote both MVPA and dietary changes in weight gain prevention interventions. For example, a recent review of interventions that compared the effects of presenting behaviors either simultaneously or sequentially found that both approaches appeared to be effective on one, but not both outcomes [34]. Thus, additional questions remain for the optimal design of multiple behavior interventions to encourage behavior change across all targeted outcomes.

This study adds to the small body of research examining whether physical activity changes during the course of a weight gain prevention intervention. A recent study of a 2-year weight gain prevention intervention for students attending community college found that the intervention did not increase physical activity or reduce sugar-sweetened beverage intake, but did promote reductions in fast food intake [35]. Another recent randomized controlled trial of a weight gain prevention intervention determined that more than half of the participants [62.0% of sample, 56.3% of completers] maintained their body weight over the 12-month intervention, but energy expenditure did not change [36]. Study participants (n = 87) were premenopausal women between the ages of 18–45 with a BMI >18.5 kg/m^2; 12% were Black.

Interventions that have focused on increasing physical activity among predominantly Black participants have had limited success [37, 38]. The Shape intervention addressed possible structural barriers to physical activity due to lack of access and opportunities [39, 40] by providing intervention participants with a no-cost membership to a local YMCA with available child care vouchers. About three-quarters (70.3%, n = 64) of the women activated their YMCA memberships but use of the memberships was limited, with 42.2% (n = 27) of the women making no subsequent visits to the YMCA over the 12-month intervention period. Women living near/below the federal poverty line and those who met the physical activity guidelines (assessed using 10-min bouts) were more likely to visit the gym at least once after activating their memberships [41]. Although YMCA memberships were provided, the Shape intervention messages primarily emphasized lifestyle-based physical activity changes – such as parking one's car further away – to gain additional steps. It is possible that Shape participants perceived themselves as already being physically active and that this message did not resonate.

Shape health coaches discussed with intervention participants the importance of physical activity and provided strategies such as planning ahead, time management, and seeking social support to promote physical activity. In retrospect, it may have been beneficial to place greater emphasis on accumulating MVPA in 10-min bouts

Table 3 Results from ANCOVA models estimating moderate-vigorous physical activity (MVPA) change over 12 months among participants in the Shape Program (n = 118)

	MVPA at 12 months (1-min bouts) final model				MVPA at 12 months (10-min bouts) final model			
	DF[a]	Type III SS	F value	*P* value	DF	Type III SS	F value	*P* value
Random assignment	1	297,540.98	1.19	.28	1	17,894.45	0.15	.07
BMI (kg/m^2)	1	683,372.27	2.73	.10	1	284,526.03	2.31	.13
Federal poverty level	2	1,457,041.95	2.91	0.06	2	848,682.20	3.44	.04

Note:
[a]*DF* Degrees of freedom

Table 4 Adjusted mean change in weekly moderate-vigorous physical activity (MVPA) among participants in the Shape Program by intervention status estimated by ANCOVA models (*n* = 118)

	Adjusted 12-month mean change in MVPA (95% CI), minutes/week			
	Intervention (*n* = 59)	Control (*n* = 59)	Between group difference	*P* value
1-min bouts	20.50 (−109.09, 150.10)	-80.04 (−209.21, 49.13)	100.54 (−82.20, 283.29)	.29
10-min bouts	7.39 (−83.57, 98.35)	-17.26 (−107.93, 73.40)	24.66 (−103.61, 152.92)	.70

because the classification of bouts had a marked effect on the prevalence estimates of those meeting physical activity recommendations; at baseline, 76% of participants were classified as meeting the recommendation when using 1-min bouts versus 38% when using 10-min bouts. Similarly, a validation study conducted by Wolin et al. [42] found notable differences in mean minutes of moderate physical activity per week among Black women living in public housing when assessed by 1-min or 10-min bouts [660 (SD = 345) versus 91 (SD = 110) minutes/week, respectively]. The increase in the percentage of participants classified as meeting the physical activity recommendation when 1-min bouts were used indicates that study participants did participate in MVPA, but there was a need for bouts of longer duration. Future intervention efforts should focus on helping individuals who participate in short (< 10-min) bouts of MVPA increase the duration of their MVPA.

Study findings should be considered in light of study strengths and limitations. Study strengths include the use of objectively measured MVPA as well as a sample that is often underrepresented in obesity prevention trials [43]. However, as the study was conducted with low-income Black women living in the South, results of the study may have limited generalizability to other overweight and obese populations. In addition, our sample was a subset of the entire study sample, and it is not known whether the inclusion of participants with insufficient accelerometer data may have had an impact on the study findings. It would be informative to conduct qualitative research to determine why participants did not complete the accelerometer protocol, as this research could provide insights into increasing compliance. Furthermore, despite being randomly assigned to study arms, individuals randomized to usual care participated in greater MVPA at baseline when assessed using 1-min and 10-min bouts, although there was no difference in meeting the physical activity recommendation by study arm. Lastly, this study focused on MVPA and did not investigate changes in light intensity physical activity.

Conclusion

In summary, study results determined that Shape was not effective in increasing MVPA among a sample of Black women with overweight or obesity, although prior research determined that the Shape intervention prevented weight gain. Intervention participants may have focused on making dietary changes over increasing physical activity. Results of this study add to the limited extant research examining changes in physical activity occur during the course of a weight gain prevention intervention and can inform future weight gain prevention intervention messages. In addition, the classification of bouts had a marked effect on the prevalence estimates of those meeting physical activity recommendations. More research is needed to understand how to present both physical activity and dietary changes in weight gain prevention interventions and how to stress the importance of physical activity for overall health.

Abbreviations

ANCOVA: Analysis of covariance; BMI: Body mass index; FPL: Federal poverty level; MVPA: Moderate-vigorous physical activity; PA: Physical activity

Acknowledgments

We would like to thank the administration and staff of Piedmont Health for their participation in The Shape Program. We also would like to especially thank the women who participated in Shape.

Funding

The Shape Program was funded by grant R01DK078798 from the National Institute for Diabetes and Digestive and Kidney Diseases.

Authors' contributions

MLG and GGB designed the study. PF oversaw all data collection. SA conducted all analyses. MLG led the drafting of the manuscript. SA, GGB, PF, SFW, LMQ participated in revising the draft versions of the manuscript and provided critical comments during the process. All authors approved the final manuscript.

Competing interests

The authors declare that they have no competing interests.

Author details

[1]Department of Kinesiology and Health Studies, 25 West Independence Way, University of Rhode Island, Kingston, RI 02881, USA. [2]Duke Global Digital Health Science Center, Duke Global Health Institute, Duke University, Durham, NC 27710, USA. [3]Georgetown Lombardi Comprehensive Cancer Center, Georgetown University, Washington, D.C. 20007, USA. [4]Section of General Internal Medicine, Department of Medicine, Boston University, Boston, MA 02118, USA. [5]Department of Psychology and Neuroscience, Duke University, Durham, NC 27708, USA.

References

1. Flegal KM, Carroll MD, Kit BK, Ogden CL. Prevalence of obesity and trends in the distribution of body mass index among US adults, 1999-2010. JAMA. 2012;307:491–7.
2. Ogden CL, Carroll MD, Kit BK, Flegal KM. Prevalence of childhood and adult obesity in the United States, 2011-2012. JAMA. 2014;311:806–14.
3. Flegal KM, Kruszon-Moran D, Carroll MD, Fryar CD, Ogden CL. Trends in obesity among adults in the United States, 2005 to 2014. JAMA. 2016;315:2284–91.
4. Befort CA, Nazir N, Perri MG. Prevalence of obesity among adults from rural and urban areas of the United States: findings from NHANES (2005-2008). J Rural Health. 2012;28:392–7.
5. Roger VL, Go AS, Lloyd-Jones DM, Benjamin EJ, Berry JD, Borden WB, et al. Heart disease and stroke statistics–2012 update: a report from the American Heart Association. Circulation. 2012;125:e2–220.
6. Hooker SP, Hutto B, Zhu W, Blair SN, Colabianchi N, Vena JE, et al. Accelerometer measured sedentary behavior and physical activity in white and black adults: the REGARDS study. J Sci Med Sport. 2016;19:336–41.
7. Lee I-M, Shiroma EJ, Lobelo F, Puska P, Blair SN, Katzmarzyk PT, et al. Effect of physical inactivity on major non-communicable diseases worldwide: an analysis of burden of disease and life expectancy. Lancet. 2012;380:219–29.
8. Ekelund U, Steene-Johannessen J, Brown WJ, Fagerland MW, Owen N, Powell KE, et al. Does physical activity attenuate, or even eliminate, the detrimental association of sitting time with mortality? A harmonised meta-analysis of data from more than 1 million men and women. Lancet. 2016; doi: 10.1016/S0140-6736(16)30370-1
9. Patel AV, Bernstein L, Deka A, Feigelson HS, Campbell PT, Gapstur SM, et al. Leisure time spent sitting in relation to total mortality in a prospective cohort of US adults. Am J Epidemiol. 2010;172:419–29.
10. Matthews CE, George SM, Moore SC, Bowles HR, Blair A, Park Y, et al. Amount of time spent in sedentary behaviors and cause-specific mortality in US adults. Am J Clin Nutr. 2012;95:437–45.
11. Thorp AA, Owen N, Neuhaus M, Dunstan DW. Sedentary behaviors and subsequent health outcomes in adults a systematic review of longitudinal studies, 1996-2011. Am J Prev Med. 2011;41:207–15.
12. Colditz GA, Willett WC, Rotnitzky A, Manson JE. Weight gain as a risk factor for clinical diabetes mellitus in women. Ann Intern Med. 1995;122:481–6.
13. Mozaffarian D, Hao T, Rimm EB, Willett WC, Hu FB. Changes in diet and lifestyle and long-term weight gain in women and men. N Engl J Med. 2011;364:2392–404.
14. Wing RR, Hill JO. Successful weight loss maintenance. Annu Rev Nutr. 2001; 21:323–41.
15. Foley P, Levine E, Askew S, Puleo E, Whiteley J, Batch B, et al. Weight gain prevention among black women in the rural community health center setting: the shape program. BMC Public Health. 2012;12:305.
16. Flynn KJ, Fitzgibbon M. Body images and obesity risk among black females: a review of the literature. Ann Behav Med. 1998;20:13–24.
17. Brown WJ, Kabir E, Clark BK, Gomersall SR. Maintaining a healthy BMI: data from a 16-year study of young Australian women. Am J Prev Med. 2016;51: e165–78.
18. Sternfeld B, Wang H, Quesenberry CP Jr, Abrams B, Everson-Rose SA, Greendale GA, et al. Physical activity and changes in weight and waist circumference in midlife women: findings from the study of Women's health across the nation. Am J Epidemiol. 2004;160:912–22.
19. Pavey TG, Peeters GMEEG, Gomersall SR, Brown WJ. Long-term effects of physical activity level on changes in healthy body mass index over 12 years in young adult women. Mayo Clin Proc. 2016;91:735–44.
20. Pronk NP, Wing RR. Physical activity and long-term maintenance of weight loss. Obes Res. 1994;2:587–99.
21. Hutfless S, Gudzune KA, Maruthur N, Wilson RF, Bleich SN, Lau BD, et al. Strategies to prevent weight gain in adults: a systematic review. Am J Prev Med. 2013;45:e41–51.
22. Bennett GG, Foley P, Levine E, Whiteley J, Askew S, Steinberg DM, et al. Behavioral treatment for weight gain prevention among black women in primary care practice: a randomized clinical trial. JAMA Intern Med. 2013; 173:1770–7.
23. Bandura A. Self-efficacy: toward a unifying theory of behavioral change. Psychol Rev. 1977;84:191–215.
24. Bennett GG, Warner ET, Glasgow RE, Askew S, Goldman J, Ritzwoller DP, et al. Obesity treatment for socioeconomically disadvantaged patients in primary care practice. Arch Intern Med. 2012;172:565–74.
25. Greaney ML, Quintiliani LM, Warner ET, King DK, Emmons KM, Colditz GA, et al. Weight management among patients at community health centers: the "be fit, be well" study, vol. 5. New Rochelle: Obesity and Weight Management. Mary Ann Liebert, Inc.; 2009. p. 222–8.
26. Lanpher MG, Askew S, Bennett GG. Health literacy and weight change in a digital health intervention for women: a randomized controlled trial in primary care practice. J Health Commun. 2016;21(Suppl 1):34–42.
27. Heil DP, Brage S, Rothney MP. Modeling physical activity outcomes from wearable monitors. Med Sci Sports Exerc. 2012;44:S50–60.
28. Heil DP, Bennett GG, Bond KS, Webster MD, Wolin KY. Influence of activity monitor location and bout duration on free-living physical activity. Res Q Exerc Sport. 2009;80:424–33.
29. Heil DP. Predicting activity energy expenditure using the Actical activity monitor. Res Q Exerc Sport. 2006;77:64–80.
30. Haskell WL, Lee I-M, Pate RR, Powell KE, Blair SN, Franklin BA, et al. Physical activity and public health: updated recommendation for adults from the American College of Sports Medicine and the American Heart Association. Med Sci Sports Exerc. 2007;39:1423–34.
31. Stewart AL, Hays RD, Ware JE Jr. The MOS short-form general health survey. Reliability and validity in a patient population. Med. Care. 1988;26:724–35.
32. Office of the Assistant Secretary for Planning and Evaluation. HHS poverty guidelines. Washington, DC: US Department of Health and Human Services; 2010. https://aspe.hhs.gov/2010-hhs-poverty-guidelines. Accessed 28 July 2017
33. Garber CE, Blissmer B, Deschenes MR, Franklin BA, Lamonte MJ, Lee I-M, et al. American College of Sports Medicine position stand. Quantity and quality of exercise for developing and maintaining cardiorespiratory, musculoskeletal, and neuromotor fitness in apparently healthy adults: guidance for prescribing exercise. Med Sci Sports Exerc. 2011;43:1334–59.
34. James E, Freund M, Booth A, Duncan MJ, Johnson N, Short CE, et al. Comparative efficacy of simultaneous versus sequential multiple health behavior change interventions among adults: a systematic review of randomised trials. Prev Med. 2016;89:211–23.
35. Laska MN, Lytle LA, Nanney MS, Moe SG, Linde JA, Hannan PJ. Results of a 2-year randomized, controlled obesity prevention trial: effects on diet, activity and sleep behaviors in an at-risk young adult population. Prev Med. 2016;89:230–6.
36. Metzgar CJ, Nickols-Richardson SM. Effects of nutrition education on weight gain prevention: a randomized controlled trial. Nutr J. 2016;15:31.
37. Banks-Wallace J, Conn V. Interventions to promote physical activity among African American women. Public Health Nurs Blackwell Science Inc. 2002;19: 321–35.
38. Whitt-Glover MC, Keith NR, Ceaser TG, Virgil K, Ledford L, Hasson RE. A systematic review of physical activity interventions among African American adults: evidence from 2009 to 2013. Obes Rev Wiley Online Library. 2014;15:125–45.
39. Richter DL, Wilcox S, Greaney ML, Henderson KA, Ainsworth BE. Environmental, policy, and cultural factors related to physical activity in African American women. Women Health. 2002;36:91–109.
40. Wilcox S, Richter DL, Henderson KA, Greaney ML, Ainsworth BE. Perceptions of physical activity and personal barriers and enablers in African-American women. Ethn Dis. 2002;12:353–62.
41. Greaney ML, Askew S, Foley P, Wallington SF, Bennett GG. Linking patients with community resources: use of a free YMCA membership among low-income black women. Transl Behav Med. 2016; Available from: doi: 10.1007/s13142-016-0431-7
42. Wolin KY, Heil DP, Askew S, Matthews CE, Bennett GG. Validation of the international physical activity questionnaire-short among blacks. J Phys Act Health. 2008;5:746–60.
43. Kumanyika SK, Obarzanek E, Stevens VJ, Hebert PR, Whelton PK, Kumanyaka SK. Weight-loss experience of black and white participants in NHLBI-sponsored clinical trials. Am J Clin Nutr. 1991;53:1631S–8S.

3

Effect and process evaluation of a kindergarten-based, family-involved cluster randomised controlled trial in six European countries on four- to six-year-old children's steps per day: the ToyBox-study

Marieke De Craemer[1*], Maïté Verloigne[1,2], Ilse De Bourdeaudhuij[1], Odysseas Androutsos[3], Violeta Iotova[4], Luis Moreno[5], Berthold Koletzko[6], Piotr Socha[7], Yannis Manios[3], Greet Cardon[1]

Abstract

Background: The ToyBox-intervention is a theory- and evidence-based intervention delivered in kindergartens to improve four- to six-year-old children's energy balance-related behaviours and prevent obesity. The current study aimed to (1) examine the effect of the ToyBox-intervention on increasing European four- to six-year-old children' steps per day, and (2) examine if a higher process evaluation score from teachers and parents was related to a more favourable effect on steps per day.

Methods: A sample of 2438 four- to six-year-old children (51.9% boys, mean age 4.75 ± 0.43 years) from 6 European countries (Belgium, Bulgaria, Germany, Greece, Poland and Spain) wore a motion sensor (pedometer or accelerometer) for a minimum of two weekdays and one weekend day both at baseline and follow-up to objectively measure their steps per day. Kindergarten teachers implemented the physical activity component of the ToyBox-intervention for 6 weeks in total, with a focus on (1) environmental changes in the classroom, (2) the child performing the actual behaviour and (3) classroom activities. Children's parents received newsletters, tip cards and posters. To assess intervention effects, multilevel repeated measures analyses were conducted for the total sample and the six intervention countries separately. In addition, process evaluation questionnaires were used to calculate a total process evaluation score (with implementation and satisfaction as a part of the overall score) for teachers and parents which was then linked with the physical activity outcomes.

Results: No significant intervention effects on four- to six-year-old children' steps per weekday, steps per weekend day and steps per average day were found, both in the total sample and in the country-specific samples (all $p > 0.05$). In general, the intervention effects on steps per day were least favourable in four- to six-year-old children with a low teachers process evaluation score and most favourable in four- to six-year-old children with a high teachers process evaluation score. No differences in intervention effects were found for a low, medium or high parents' process evaluation score.

(Continued on next page)

* Correspondence: marieke.decraemer@ugent.be
[1]Department of Movement and Sport Sciences, Ghent University, Watersportlaan 2, 9000 Ghent, Belgium
Full list of author information is available at the end of the article

(Continued from previous page)

Conclusion: The physical activity component of the ToyBox-intervention had no overall effect on four- to six-year-old children' steps per day. However, the process evaluation scores showed that kindergarten teachers that implemented the physical activity component of the ToyBox-intervention as planned and were satisfied with the physical activity component led to favourable effects on children's steps per day. Strategies to motivate, actively involve and engage the kindergarten teachers and parents/caregivers are needed to induce larger effects.

Keywords: Effect evaluation, Process evaluation, Preschool, Europe, Pedometer, Step counts, ToyBox, RCT

Background

Sufficient levels of physical activity (PA) are associated with numerous positive mental and physical health outcomes, even at preschool age [1]. In addition, PA plays an important role in the prevention of overweight and obesity, and PA tracks from year to year [2–4]. However, many preschool children appear to be insufficiently active [5–9] and do not comply with the PA guidelines of 180 min of total PA per day [10, 11]. For this reason, several interventions targeting an increase in preschoolers' PA have been developed and implemented, with mixed effects as a result [12–18].

The aim of the ToyBox-study was to develop, implement and evaluate a kindergarten-based, family-involved intervention to prevent overweight and obesity in four- to six-year-old preschool children from six European countries (i.e., Belgium, Bulgaria, Germany, Greece, Poland, and Spain). One of the four behaviours on which the intervention focused, was PA (together with sedentary behaviour, water consumption, and snacking behaviour) [19, 20]. The effectiveness of the intervention on objectively measured PA (via accelerometers) has already been evaluated in the Belgian sample, as accelerometers were only used in Belgian preschool children. More specifically, small but positive effects were found in sub-groups such as preschool boys and preschoolers from kindergartens with a high socio-economic status (SES) [21]. However, the effectiveness of the ToyBox-intervention on steps per day in the total sample still has to be investigated. Further, as preliminary results showed that there was a big variance in implementation of the different ToyBox components across kindergartens [22, 23], the effectiveness will be studied as a function of the variability of the implementation of the PA-component of the intervention. Therefore, it is important to examine the relationship between effect evaluation (study outcomes) and process evaluation (intervention implementation and participant satisfaction) in order to better understand the potential effects of a health promotion intervention [24].

A process evaluation should be guided by using a specific framework. The model used in the ToyBox-intervention is the model by Saunders et al. (2005) and is described in detail elsewhere [25, 26]. This model describes and recommends several key elements to conduct a process evaluation, such as *reach* (level of participation in the intervention), *fidelity* (quality of implementation), *dose delivered* (the amount of the intervention that was delivered by the implementers), *dose received – exposure* (the level of active participation and being receptive to or using the materials and resources), *dose received – satisfaction* (the level of satisfaction of the implementer and the target group regarding the intervention) and *context* (within which the ToyBox-intervention was implemented) [25].

Thus, the aim of the current study was (1) to evaluate the effectiveness of the ToyBox-intervention on European preschoolers' objectively measured steps per day in the total sample and in the country-specific samples, and (2) to examine whether a higher level of intervention implementation and satisfaction of the PA-component of the ToyBox-intervention was related to more favourable effects on preschoolers' steps per day in the total sample.

Methods

Study protocol

The kindergarten-based ToyBox-intervention with family involvement, targeting four- to six-year-old preschoolers, has a cluster randomised pre-test post-test design with intervention kindergartens and control kindergartens across six European countries: Belgium, Bulgaria, Germany, Greece, Poland, and Spain. Preschool children and their parents/caregivers were recruited at kindergartens, daycare centers or preschool settings, depending on the country regulations and legislation. In Germany, Bulgaria, Spain and Poland, children/families were recruited from kindergartens, in Greece from kindergartens and daycare centers, and in Belgium from preschool settings. In order to avoid confusion for the reader, all these settings (kindergartens, daycare centers, preschool settings) will be referred to as "kindergartens" in this paper. Additionally, to avoid confusion regarding the term "preschool children" we will use the term "four- to six-year-old children" throughout the manuscript.

Kindergartens were selected in the provinces of West- and Oost-Vlaanderen in Belgium, Varna in Bulgaria, Bavaria in Germany, Attica in Greece, Mazowiecki in Poland, and Zaragoza in Spain. Kindergartens were recruited from different SES backgrounds. Lists of all municipalities that exist within the selected provinces were collected and information on the SES variables was provided (mean years of education for the population aged 25–55 years or annual income). Tertiles were created, based on the selected SES variables, and five municipalities were randomly selected from each tertile (i.e., approximately five municipalities for low SES, five for medium SES, and five for high SES) in each country. Then, 1003 kindergartens within these randomly chosen municipalities across the six countries were randomly selected (with the exclusion of the lowest 20% of the kindergartens with the smallest number of children), and a personal visit was performed to inform the kindergarten staff about the ToyBox-study. In total, 309 kindergartens (30.8%) across the six countries agreed to participate in the study, and all four- to six-year-old children born in 2007 and 2008 (n = 16,798; age at baseline was 3.5–5.5 years old) received an information letter to take home in which the purpose of the study was explained to the parents/caregivers, and the child was invited to wear a pedometer or accelerometer for six consecutive days. Sample size calculations can be found elsewhere [27]. The flow of kindergartens through the study is depicted in Fig. 1, and the flow of participants through the study is depicted in Fig. 2. In total, 7056 parents/caregivers (42.0%) provided consent for their child to participate in the study.

After the recruitment of the kindergartens and the execution of the baseline measurements, kindergartens' municipalities were randomly assigned to the intervention or control condition (ratio 2:1) to avoid contamination between kindergartens in the same municipality. This was done by by the project coordinator (Greece) with the use of a command in Excel, which means that the randomisation occurred automatically and electronically. Kindergartens allocated to the intervention condition received the intervention programme. Kindergartens allocated to the control condition continued with the normal kindergarten curriculum. The ToyBox-intervention was implemented within the school year 2012–2013.

Before the start of the intervention, baseline measurements were performed on weekdays from May to June 2012. On those days, researchers visited intervention and control kindergartens and fitted those preschool children with an accelerometer (Belgium) or a pedometer (other countries) for whom written informed consent from their parents/caregivers had been obtained. One year later, from May to June 2013, follow-up measurements were performed and again, the same children

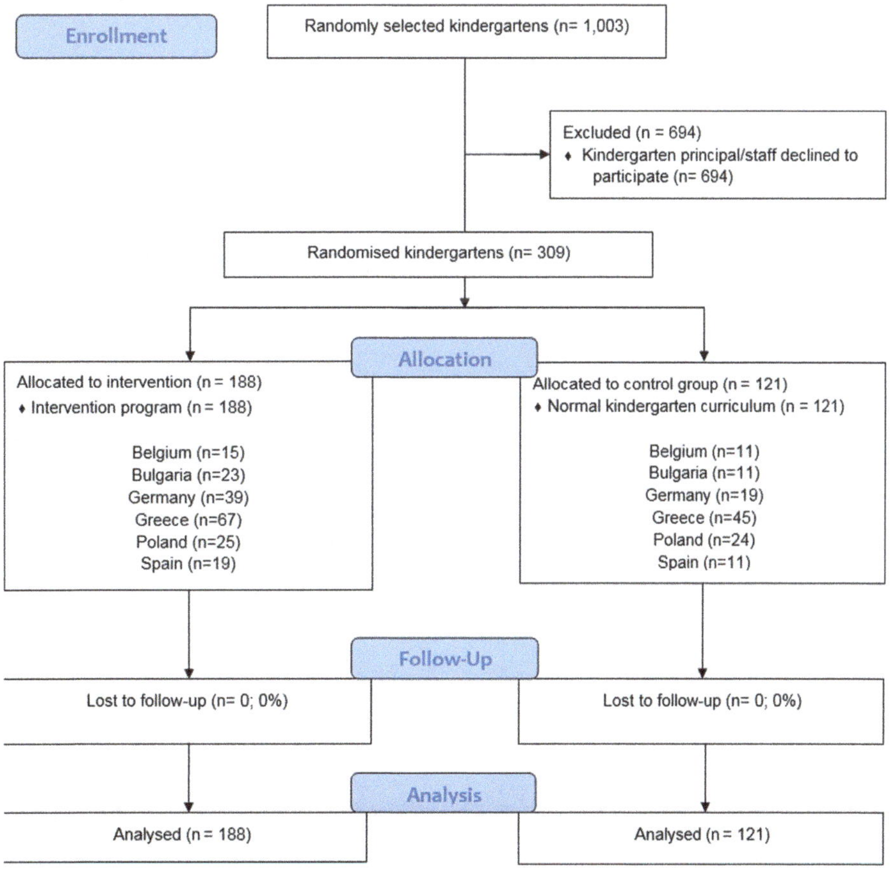

Fig. 1 Flow chart of included kindergartens into the intervention

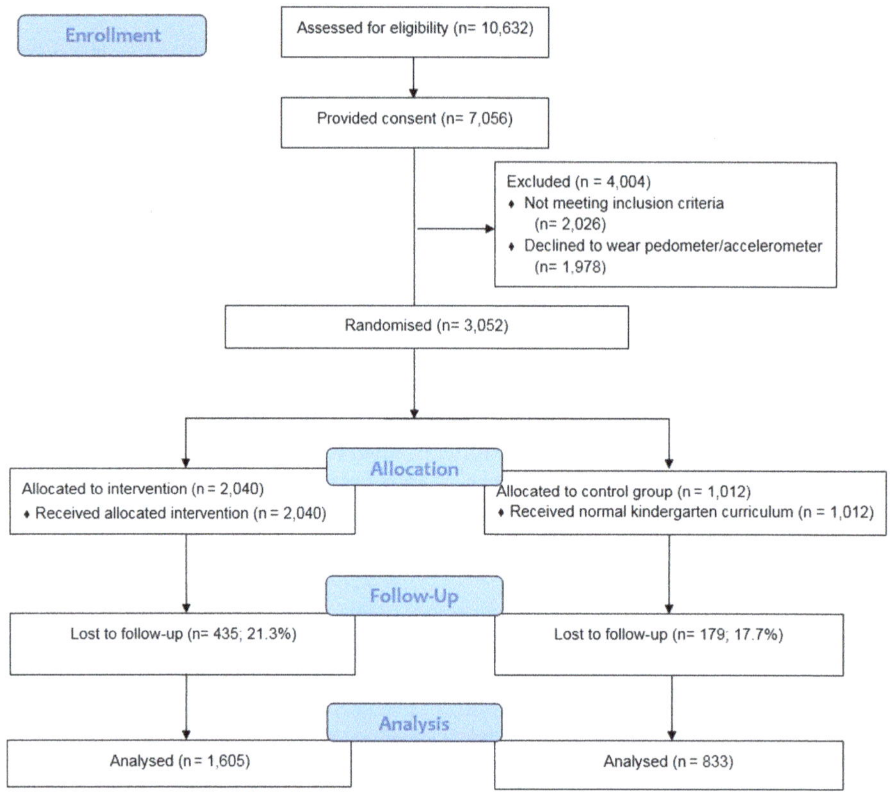

Fig. 2 Flow chart of included four- to six-year-old children with valid pedometer data into the intervention

with written informed consent from both intervention and control kindergartens received a pedometer or accelerometer to objectively measure their step counts.

Ethical statement

The ToyBox-study was approved by the Ethical Committees in all European countries, in line with national regulations (i.e. in Belgium by the Medical Ethics Committee of the Ghent University Hospital; in Bulgaria by the Ethics Committee of the Medical University of Varna; in Germany by the Ethics Committee of the Ludwig Maximilian University of Munich; in Greece by the Bioethics Committee of Harokopio University and the Greek Ministry of Education; in Poland by the Bioethics Committee of the Children's Memorial Health Institute and the Department of Information and Publicity of the Polish Ministry of Education; and in Spain by the Clinical Research Ethics Committee and the Department of Consumers' Health of the Government of Aragón. The ToyBox-study is registered with the clinical trials registry clinicaltrials.gov, ID: NCT02116296.

ToyBox-intervention: PA-component

The kindergarten-based, family-involved ToyBox-intervention was planned and developed following the Intervention Mapping protocol [28, 29]. The intervention included components on water consumption, healthy snacking and sedentary behaviour, as well as a PA-component which will be further discussed below.

The ToyBox-intervention consisted of 24 intervention weeks. The PA-part of the intervention was implemented in weeks 5 until 8 (i.e., 'first focus'), and had a two-week 'repetition period' in weeks 19 and 20. Furthermore, some PA-components were also implemented throughout the whole school year, such as restructuring the classroom (e.g., rearranging the furniture to create space to be physically active, providing equipment (not provided by the researchers) in the classroom that stimulates moving such as balls, big sponge bricks,...) and installing movement landscapes (e.g. large equipment such as wall bars, benches, mats, hoops,...) in the classroom. The ToyBox-intervention was implemented by the kindergarten teachers, who had two 1-h teacher training sessions with the researchers to explain the goals and the material of the ToyBox-study, and to answer kindergarten teachers' questions, prior to the intervention. During the second training session, teachers were provided with the "ToyBox", i.e. a box containing material for the class (including a teachers' guide, four classroom activity guides and a kangaroo hand puppet), and material for the home (including newsletters, tip-cards, and posters for the parents/caregivers). In the classroom activity guide for PA, three different themes were included, namely (1) setting environmental changes in the classroom (i.e., how to rearrange the classroom to make free space for the preschool children to be more active), (2) the preschool child performing the actual behaviour (i.e., being physically active during structured physical education sessions), and (3) classroom activities (i.e., kangaroo stories, and PA excursions). Teachers were asked to allocate a minimum of 1 h per week to use the ToyBox-materials and to implement the ToyBox-intervention in the classroom, while the environmental changes were conducted and retained throughout the project. The 1 h per week recommendation was chosen based on the focus groups that were held before the development of the intervention [30]. Kindergarten teachers clearly mentioned that they already have a busy week schedule and that they only wanted to implement an intervention when it would include ready-to-use materials and when they only had to devote limited time to the implementation. For that reason, we only included 60 min per week as a minimum recommendation, although devoting more time per week or even per day was recommended and encouraged.

To involve the parents/caregivers, four- to six-year-old children received two newsletters, two tip-cards and one poster (with key messages on PA that could be coloured at kindergarten or at home) to take home for their parents/caregivers. The newsletters and tip-cards contained tips and strategies to increase four- to six-year-old children' PA levels. The relevant materials can be found on the ToyBox-website (www.toybox-study.eu).

Instrumentation

PA was assessed by means of steps per day using Omron Walking Style Pro pedometers (HJ-720IT-E2) (Bulgaria, Germany, Greece, Poland, and Spain) and ActiGraph (Pensacola, FL) accelerometers with activated step count function (Belgium). Step counts from the pedometer and accelerometer are comparable and have been validated to measure PA in preschool children [31]. The devices were worn on the right hip, secured by an elastic waist band. Pedometers were only used as a measuring instrument during the baseline and follow-up measurements and not as a monitoring instrument.

Procedure

Four- to six-year-old children wore a motion sensor (pedometer or accelerometer) for six full consecutive days, including two weekend days. Accelerometers were initialised to measure activity counts and step counts in 15-s epochs. Four- to six-year-old children's parents/caregivers received an information letter and were instructed to let their child wear the motion sensor during all waking hours and to remove it only during water-based activities. After data collection, data from pedometers were downloaded using Omron Health Management Software version E1.012, and data from accelerometers were downloaded using ActiLife version 5.5.5-software. Both the first (fitting day) and sixth day (collection day) were omitted, because these days did not have a full day of data and were therefore incomplete. All step counts below 1000 and above 30,000 steps per day were deleted and treated as missing data, which is according to the rules of Rowe et al. (2014) [32]. Four- to six-year-old children's step count data were included in data analyses when they had valid data for a minimum of two weekdays and one weekend day.

Process evaluation: teachers

To investigate the intervention process and satisfaction, teachers had to fill in two logbooks with specific questions regarding the process and satisfaction of the PA component, which were based on the model of Saunders et al. (2005) [25, 26]. The key process evaluation elements that were questioned in the monthly logbooks were "Fidelity", "Dose delivered", and "Dose received – satisfaction" [25, 26]. No information on "Reach", "Dose received – exposure" and "Context" was available.

The specific questions per key element that were used from the monthly logbooks are depicted in Table 1 with an explanation about the score. Teachers filled in a logbook during the "first focus" and during the "repetition period" [33]. This logbook was completed either via phone calls from the researchers to the teachers or via email by the teachers. The questions with answer possibilities on a 5-point-scale were dichotomised based on the mean score. Below the mean was coded into 0, and equal to or higher than the mean was coded into 1. All monthly logbook questions with a score of 0 or 1 were used to calculate the total process evaluation score for each intervention kindergarten by adding up all scores. A higher process evaluation score represents a higher level of intervention implementation and satisfaction. The minimum score was 0 and the maximum score was 26. Based on the teachers' process evaluation score, kindergartens were divided into three groups, based on the tertiles: kindergartens with a low (recoded into 1), a medium (recoded into 2) or a high level (recoded into 3) of implementation and satisfaction. To look for a difference in effect between the intervention group (with three categories of teachers' process evaluation scores: 1, 2, 3) and the control group, the control group (recoded into 0) was added as an extra group (in addition to low, medium and high process evaluation scores).

Process evaluation: parents/caregivers

Also parents/caregivers had to fill in a questionnaire regarding the process of the PA component of the

Table 1 Overview process evaluation questions to calculate the process evaluation score (score on 26) for teachers

	Fidelity = whether the intervention was delivered as intended by the teachers and received by the children	Dose delivered = how much was delivered by the teachers and received by the children	Dose received – satisfaction = how the intervention was received by the teachers
Questionnaire Teachers' physical activity logbook (first focus)	*"When did you deliver the 1st physical activity behaviour newsletter to the parents? Not delivered – in week 5 – in week 6 – in week 7 – in week 8"* 1 = yes (in weeks 5–8) 0 = not delivered *"When did you deliver the 1st physical activity behaviour tip-card to the parents? Not delivered – in week 5 – in week 6 – in week 7 – in week 8"* 1 = yes (in weeks 5–8) 0 = not delivered *"When did you deliver the physical activity behaviour poster to the parents? Not delivered – in week 5 – in week 6 – in week 7 – in week 8"* 1 = yes (in weeks 5–8) 0 = not delivered *"All planned activities were performed. Totally disagree – disagree – neither disagree nor agree – agree – totally agree"* 1 = a score of ≥3.52 0 = a score of <3.52 *"Did you implement the classroom activities as described in the manual for physical activity? Never – rarely – sometimes – often – always"* 1 = score ≥ mean value of 3.60 0 = score < mean value of 3.60 *"Was equipment and space appropriately arranged for physical education lessons? Never – rarely – sometimes – often – always"* 1 = score ≥ mean value of 4.18 0 = score < mean value of 4.18	*"How much time did you devote on physical education lessons on an average weekly basis for this month?"* 1 = score ≥ mean value of 122.4 min/week 0 = score < mean value of 122.4 min/week *"Did you devote on average at least one hour per week in the classroom activities as described in the manual? Never – rarely – sometimes – often – always"* 1 = score ≥ mean value of 4.14 0 = score < mean value of 4.14 Sum score of eight items related to classroom activities for physical activity (implementation of 4 kangaroo stories and 4 excursions) (mean score: 1.90) 1 = a score of ≥1.90 0 = a score of <1.90	*"It was easy to read and understand the text in the Classroom Activity Guide for physical activity"* 1 = score ≥ mean value of 4.07 0 = score < mean value of 4.07 *"The amount of information and activities in the Classroom Activity Guide for physical activity were appropriate"* 1 = score ≥ mean value of 3.85 0 = score < mean value of 3.85 *"It was easy to implement the activities described in the Classroom Activity Guide for physical activity"* 1 = score ≥ mean value of 3.67 0 = score < mean value of 3.67 *"I enjoyed the activities I delivered this month"* 1 = score ≥ mean value of 4.09 0 = score < mean value of 4.09 *"The activities I delivered this month were enjoyed by the children"* 1 = score ≥ mean value of 4.28 0 = score < mean value of 4.28 *"The information presented in the Classroom Activity Guide for physical activity, the content of the material and the way the activities should be delivered are appropriate to achieve the goals"* 1 = score ≥ mean value of 4.00 0 = score < mean value of 4.00
Questionnaire Teachers' physical activity logbook (repetition period)	*"When did you deliver the 2nd physical activity behaviour newsletter to the parents? Not delivered – in week 19 – in week 20"* 1 = yes (in weeks 19–20) 0 = not delivered *"When did you deliver the 2nd physical activity behaviour tip-card to the parents? Not delivered – in week 19 – in week 20"* 1 = yes (in weeks 19–20) 0 = not delivered *"All planned activities were performed. Totally disagree – disagree – neither disagree nor agree – agree – totally agree"* 1 = a score of ≥3.44 0 = a score of <3.44 *"Did you implement the classroom activities as described in the manual for physical activity? Never – rarely – sometimes – often – always"* 1 = score ≥ mean value of 3.58 0 = score < mean value of 3.58 *"Was equipment and space appropriately arranged for physical education lessons? Never – rarely – sometimes – often – always"* 1 = score ≥ mean value of 4.31 0 = score < mean value of 4.31	*"How much time did you devote on physical education lessons on an average weekly basis for this month?"* 1 = score ≥ mean value of 123.3 min/week 0 = score < mean value of 123.3 min/week *"Did you devote on average at least one hour per week in the classroom activities as described in the manual? Never – rarely – sometimes – often – always"* 1 = score ≥ mean value of 3.82 0 = score < mean value of 3.82 Sum score of eight items related to classroom activities for physical activity (implementation of 4 kangaroo stories and 4 excursions) (mean score: 1.55) 1 = a score of ≥1.55 0 = a score of <1.55	*"It was easy to implement the activities described in the Classroom Activity Guide for physical activity"* 1 = score ≥ mean value of 3.68 0 = score < mean value of 3.68 *"I enjoyed the activities I delivered this month"* 1 = score ≥ mean value of 3.92 0 = score < mean value of 3.92 *"The activities I delivered this month were enjoyed by the children"* 1 = score ≥ mean value of 4.12 0 = score < mean value of 4.12
Mean score (± standard deviation)/maximum score	6.23 (±1.13)/11	1.55 (±1.13)/6	5.45 (±2.25)/9

intervention. These questions were also based on the model of Saunders et al. (2005) [25, 26]. The key process evaluation elements that were questioned in the questionnaire for parents were "Dose delivered", "Dose received – exposure" and "Dose received – satisfaction" [25, 26]. No information on "Fidelity", "Reach" and "Context" was available.

The specific questions per key element that were used from the questionnaire are depicted in Table 2 with an explanation about the score. The questions with answer possibilities on a 5-point-scale were dichotomised based on the mean score. All questions with a score of 0 or 1 were used to calculate the total process evaluation score for each parent/caregiver by adding up all scores. Again, a higher process evaluation score represents a higher level of the intervention and satisfaction process. The minimum score was 0 and the maximum score was 17. Based on the parents'/caregivers' process evaluation scores, four- to six-year-old children were divided into three groups, based on tertiles: four- to six-year-old children with a low (recoded into 1), a medium (recoded into 2) or a high level (recoded into 3) of parental process evaluation score. To look for a difference in effect between the intervention group (with three

Table 2 Overview process evaluation questions to calculate the process evaluation score (score on 17) for parents/caregivers

Dose delivered = whether the intervention was delivered as intended by the parents/ caregivers and received by the children	Dose received – exposure = whether the intervention was delivered as intended by the teachers and received by the parents/ caregivers	Dose received – satisfaction = how the intervention was received by the parents/ caregivers
"Did you implement the suggested activities of the ToyBox Newsletters and Tip-cards? Never – rarely – sometimes – often – always" 1 = score ≥ mean value of 3.07 0 = score < mean value of 3.07	*"Did you or your partner receive the materials regarding physical activity?"* (one score for each component: Newsletter 1, Newsletter 2, Tip-card 1, Tip-card 2, Poster) 1 = yes 0 = no & I don't know	*"In general, how easy was it to understand the text in the ToyBox Newsletters and Tip Cards? Very difficult – difficult – easy – very easy"* 1 = score ≥ mean value of 3.45 0 = score < mean value of 3.45
	"Did you or your partner read the materials regarding physical activity?" (one score for each component: Newsletter 1, Newsletter 2, Tip-card 1, Tip-card 2, Poster) 1 = yes 0 = no & I don't know	*"In general, did you find the information provided in the ToyBox Newsletters and Tip Cards trustful? Not at all – to a little degree – neither trustful or not trustful – to some degree – to a large degree"* 1 = score ≥ mean value of 4.39 0 = score < mean value of 4.39
		"In general, how useful did you find the Suggestions and Tips for parents in the ToyBox Newsletters and Tip Cards? Not useful at all – a little useful – somewhat useful – very useful" 1 = score ≥ mean value of 3.25 0 = score < mean value of 3.25
		"Did you/your partner and your child enjoy the ToyBox activities conducted with the family? I did not enjoy it at all – I did not enjoy it so much – I enjoyed it – I enjoyed it a lot" 1 = score ≥ mean value of 2.87 0 = score < mean value of 2.87
		"In general, what did you think about the amount of text in the ToyBox Newsletters and Tip cards? Far too much – too much – about right – too little – far too little" 1 = 3 0 = > 3 & < 3
		"In general, what did you think of the design (colours, lay out, type of letters) of the ToyBox Newsletters and Tip Cards? I did not like it at all – I did not like it so much – I liked it – I liked it a lot" 1 = score ≥ mean value of 3.08 0 = score < mean value of 3.08
Mean score (± standard deviation)/ maximum score 0.33 (±0.47)/1	Mean score (± standard deviation)/ maximum score 4.86 (±4.16)/10	Mean score (± standard deviation)/ maximum score 1.88 (±1.50)/6

categories: 1, 2, 3) and the control group (recoded into 0), the control group was again added as an extra level of implementation and satisfaction.

Statistical analyses

Steps per day were separately calculated for weekdays, weekend days and average days. To take into account that some four- to six-year-old children had more weekend days than others, outcome variables on an average day were calculated using the following formula: ((MEAN(outcome on weekday 1, outcome on weekday 2)*5) + (MEAN(outcome on weekend day 1, outcome on weekend day 2)*2)/7. Prior to all analyses, all outcome measures were first checked for normal distribution (skewness <0.70) and appeared to be normally distributed. Descriptive statistics were computed to describe the characteristics (age, sex) of the sample, and were reported as frequencies (%) or means and standard deviations or percentages.

Multilevel repeated measures analyses were performed using MLwiN 2.31 (Centre for Multilevel Modelling, University of Bristol, UK) to assess the effectiveness of the intervention on steps per weekday, weekend day and average day. Multilevel modeling (five levels: time, child, kindergarten class, kindergarten, country) was used to take clustering of two measurements (baseline and follow-up) of four- to six-year-old children in kindergarten classes in kindergartens in countries into account. For the country-specific analyses, four levels were used (time, child, kindergarten class, kindergarten). All analyses were adjusted for age and sex. Two ß-values will be reported in the results: (1) the ß-value for 'time' is the estimate for the time effect, and can be interpreted as the magnitude of change in the outcome variable going from follow-up to baseline for the reference category (i.e., control group), and (2) the ß-value for 'time*condition' is the estimate for the intervention effect for all outcome variables, which describes the difference between the mean change in the intervention group and the mean change in the control group.

To study if the effect was different regarding the intervention process evaluation score four- to six-year old children's steps per weekday, steps per weekend day and steps per day, multilevel repeated measures analyses ('time*process evaluation score') were performed (five levels: time, child, kindergarten class, kindergarten, country). All analyses were adjusted for children's age and sex. For all analyses, statistical significance level was set at $p < 0.05$.

Results

Descriptive results

In total, 2438 children (51.9% boys, mean age at baseline 4.75 ± 0.43 years) provided valid step count data at baseline and follow-up (drop-out of 71.3%). At baseline, four- to six-year-old children took 10,739 (±3258) steps per weekday, 9690 (±3850) steps per weekend day, and 10,440 (±2898) steps on an average day. At follow-up, they took 10,745 (±3501) steps per weekday, 9028 (±3924) steps per weekend day, and 10,254 (±3059) steps on an average day. Descriptive analyses showed that four- to six-year-old children from the control group significantly took less steps at baseline compared to four- to six-year-old children from the control group, both at weekdays (t = 8.07, p < 0.001) and average days (t = 6.78, p < 0.001). There was no significant difference for steps at weekend days. In addition, 37.4%, 28.9%, and 32.1% of four- to six-year-old children complied with the PA guidelines of 11,500 steps per day [34] on weekdays, weekend days and average days respectively, at baseline. At follow-up, 38.4%, 24.4% and 31.4% of four- to six-year-old children complied with the PA guidelines on weekdays, weekend days and average days, respectively. The CONSORT checklist can be found in Additional file 1.

Intervention effects: total sample

Results obtained from the multilevel repeated measures analyses for the PA outcomes in the total sample are shown in Table 3. No significant intervention effects were found for steps per day, steps per weekday and steps per weekend day.

Country-specific intervention effects

Only one significant intervention effect was found for Bulgarian four- to six-year-old children's steps per day with children from the intervention group having an increase in steps per average day from baseline to follow-up compared to children from the control group who experience a decrease in steps per average day. No other country-specific intervention effects were found, as depicted in Table 4.

Relationship between the teachers' process evaluation score and the effects on four- to six-year-old children's steps per day (total intervention sample)

In total, a teachers' process evaluation score could be calculated for 1605 children (out of 2438), as not all teachers filled in the monthly logbooks. From the 460 teachers who participated in the intervention, 8.1% (n = 41) did not fill in the logbook for PA during the first focus, and 23.3% (n = 107) did not fill in the logbook for PA during the repetition period. The mean teachers' process evaluation score for all intervention kindergartens was 13.49 (±2.56) on a total score of 26 (minimum = 6.50, maximum = 19.00). Kindergartens were divided into three groups, based on the teachers' process evaluation score: (1) kindergartens with the lowest teachers' process evaluation score (score 6.50–

Table 3 Time and interaction effects for steps per average day, steps per weekday and steps per weekend day in the total sample (adjusted for age and sex)

n = 2438 (*I* = 1605; C = 833)		PRE (steps/day)	POST (steps/day)	Time		Time * condition	
				ß	*p*-value	ß	*p*-value
Average day	I	10,898	10,712				
	C	10,280	10,098	−182.23	0.04	−4.27	0.98
Weekday	I	11,205	11,166				
	C	10,412	10,505	92.83	0.70	−131.91	0.44
Weekend day	I	10,118	9563				
	C	9941	9071	−869.88	<0.001	314.84	0.14

I intervention group, *C* control group
Time: the ß-value for 'time' is the estimate for the time effect, and can be interpreted as the magnitude of change in the outcome variable going from follow-up to baseline for the reference group (i.e., control group)
Time*Condition: the ß-value for 'time*condition' is the estimate for the intervention effect for all outcome variables, which describes the difference between the mean change in the intervention group and the mean change in the control group

12.74; $n_{\text{four- to six-year-old children}} = 501$; $n_{\text{kindergartens}} = 36$), (2) kindergartens with a medium teachers' process evaluation score (score 12.75–14.00; $n_{\text{four- to six-year-old children}} = 612$; $n_{\text{kindergartens}} = 32$), and (3) kindergartens with the highest teachers' process evaluation score (score 14.01–19.00; $n_{\text{four- to six-year-old children}} = 492$; $n_{\text{kindergartens}} = 34$). Of all 312 teachers, 37.1% had a low, 29.7% had a medium and 33.2% had a high teachers' process evaluation score. Teachers scored best on dose received (satisfaction; 5.45/9) and fidelity (6.23/11) and had the lowest scores for dose delivered (1.55/6). Detailed information on the scores for each component of the teachers' process evaluation score can be found in Table 1.

Regarding steps per weekday, a significant interaction effect was found between children from the control group and children with a low teachers' process evaluation score, going from baseline to follow-up (β = −553.95 (SE = 235.50); $p = 0.02$). Four- to six-year-old children with a low teachers' process evaluation score significantly decreased their steps per weekday from baseline to follow-up (−461 steps/weekday; $p = 0.01$), while children from the control group did not significantly change their steps per weekday from baseline to follow-up ($p = 0.52$). Furthermore, a significant interaction effect was found between children with a low teachers' process evaluation score and a medium and high teachers' process evaluation score, going from baseline to follow-up (β = 558.57 (SE = 250.95), $p = 0.03$ and β = 682.16 (SE = 264.62), $p = 0.01$). Four- to six-year-old children with a medium teachers' process evaluation score and a high teachers' process evaluation score did not significantly decrease their steps per weekday going from baseline to follow-up ($p = 0.56$ and $p = 0.24$, respectively), while children with a low teachers' process evaluation score significantly decreased their steps per weekday (−461 steps/weekday; $p = 0.01$).

Regarding steps per weekend day, a significant interaction effect was found between children from the control group and children with a high teachers' process evaluation score, going from baseline to follow-up (β = 866.35 (SE = 293.65), $p = 0.003$). Four- to six-year-old children from the control group significantly decreased their steps per weekend day from baseline to follow-up (−870 steps/weekday, $p < 0.001$), while children with a high teachers' process evaluation score did not ($p = 0.99$). Furthermore, a significant interaction effect was found between children with a low and children with a medium teachers' process evaluation score (β = −669.56 (SE = 310.93), $p = 0.03$), and between children with a medium and children with a high teachers' process evaluation score (β = 1095.61 (SE = 312.67), $p < 0.001$). Four- to six-year-old children with a medium teachers' process evaluation score significantly decreased their steps per weekend day from baseline to follow-up (−1099 steps/weekend day, $p < 0.001$), while children with a low teachers' process evaluation score and children with a high teachers' process evaluation score did not show a significant change in their steps between the two time points ($p = 0.06$ and $p = 0.99$, respectively).

Regarding steps per day, a significant interaction effect was found between four- to six-year-old children with a low teachers' process evaluation score and a high teachers' process evaluation score, going from baseline to follow-up (β = 608.98 (SE = 234.10); $p = 0.01$). This means that children with a low teachers' process evaluation score significantly decreased their steps per day from baseline to follow-up (−452 steps/day; $p = 0.01$), while children with a high teachers' process evaluation score did not change their steps per day from baseline to follow-up. No other interaction effects were found for steps per day. All interaction effects between time and teachers' process evaluation score for steps per weekday, steps per weekend day and steps per day can be found in Fig. 3. In addition, Fig. 3 clearly shows that at baseline, four- to six-year-old children from the control group had a lower amount of steps per weekday and steps per average day compared to the intervention group.

Table 4 Time and interaction effects for steps per average day, steps per weekday and steps per weekend day for the six European countries (adjusted for age and sex)

		PRE (steps/day)	POST (steps/day)	Time		Time * condition	
				ß	*p*-value	ß	*p*-value
Belgium (*n* = 540; *I* = 332; C = 208)							
Average day	I	10,453	10,705				
	C	10,475	10,455	−20.15	0.08	271.55	0.23
Weekday	I	11,029	11,149				
	C	10,992	10,969	−23.24	0.32	142.76	0.60
Weekend day	I	9028	9493				
	C	9165	9036	−128.64	0.04	593.53	0.11
Bulgaria (*n* = 78; *I* = 33; C = 45)							
Average day	I	7108	7650				
	C	8708	8074	−633.58	0.20	1175.75	0.03
Weekday	I	6677	7231				
	C	8354	7549	−805.00	0.33	1358.65	0.07
Weekend day	I	8471	8986				
	C	9564	9360	−203.52	0.47	718.51	0.44
Germany (*n* = 212; *I* = 180; C = 32)							
Average day	I	11,808	11,766				
	C	12,048	11,130	−917.75	0.88	875.88	0.21
Weekday	I	12,182	12,131				
	C	12,548	11,739	−809.20	0.87	757.60	0.35
Weekend day	I	10,814	10,797				
	C	10,471	9282	−1189.11	0.96	1171.59	0.24
Greece (*n* = 356; *I* = 260; C = 96)							
Average day	I	9943	10,190				
	C	9003	9301	298.22	0.28	−51.38	0.91
Weekday	I	10,394	10,697				
	C	9143	9718	575.37	0.24	−271.78	0.58
Weekend day	I	8822	8927				
	C	8698	8303	−394.65	0.72	499.64	0.38
Poland (*n* = 837; *I* = 512; C = 325)							
Average day	I	11,475	10,969				
	C	10,686	10,615	−70.67	0.003	−434.55	0.11
Weekday	I	11,589	11,526				
	C	10,662	11,065	403.05	0.75	−465.64	0.13
Weekend day	I	11,186	9574				
	C	10,753	9498	−1255.97	<0.001	−356.81	0.36
Spain (*n* = 415; *I* = 288; C = 127)							
Average day	I	12,954	12,269				
	C	11,554	10,803	−751.10	0.001	65.82	0.87
Weekday	I	13,688	13,089				
	C	11,924	11,518	−406.22	0.02	−193.30	0.67
Weekend day	I	11,096	10,197				
	C	10,649	9036	−1613.30	0.003	713.61	0.19

I intervention group, *C* control group
Time: the ß-value for 'time' is the estimate for the time effect, and can be interpreted as the magnitude of change in the outcome variable going from follow-up to baseline for the reference group (i.e., control group)
Time*Condition: the ß-value for 'time*condition' is the estimate for the intervention effect for all outcome variables, which describes the difference between the mean change in the intervention group and the mean change in the control group

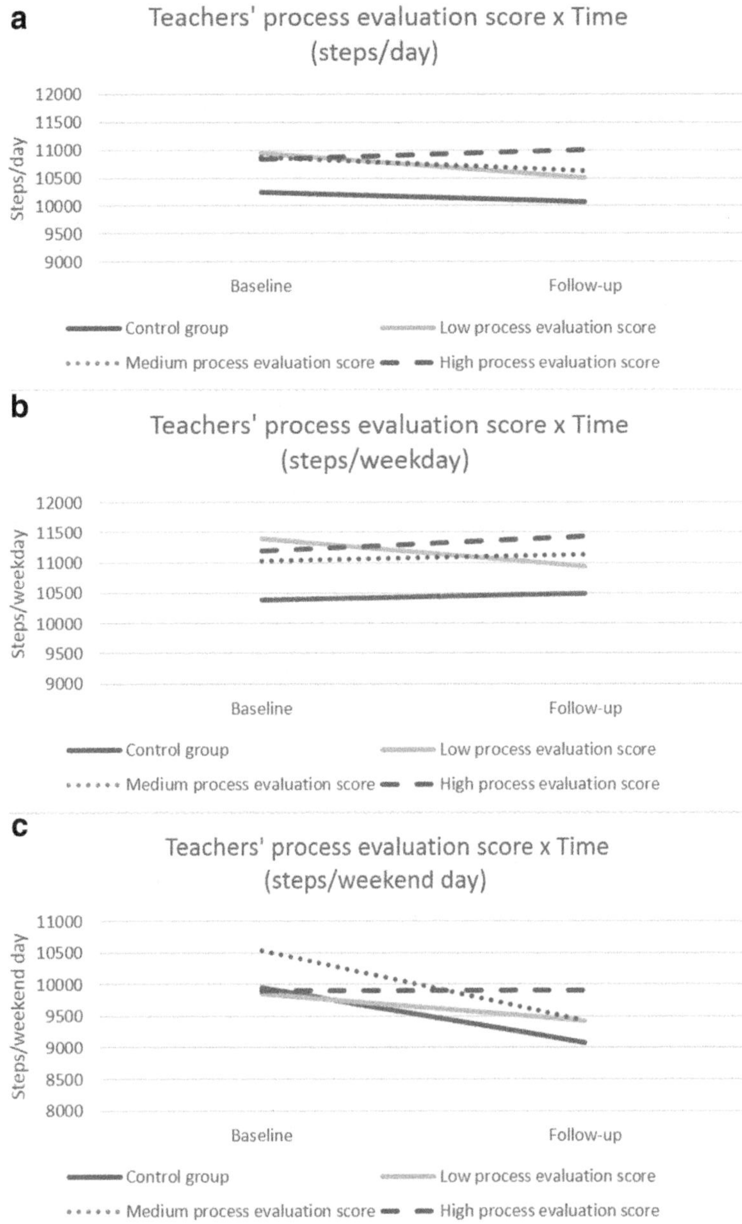

Fig. 3 Teachers' process evaluation score x Time for **a** steps/average day, **b** steps/weekday and **c** steps/weekend day

Relationship between the parents'/caregivers' process evaluation score and the effects on four- to six-year-old children' steps per day (total intervention sample)

In total, a parents'/caregivers' process evaluation score could be calculated for 1420 children (drop-out of 11.5%). The mean parents'/caregivers' process evaluation score for all intervention kindergartens was 6.90 (±3.50) on a total score of 17 (minimum = 0; maximum = 14). Four- to six-year-old children were divided into three groups, based on the parents'/caregivers' process evaluation score: (1) four- to six-year-old children with a low parents'/caregivers' process evaluation score (score 0.00–5.00; $n_{\text{four- to six-year-old children}} = 464$), (2) four- to six-year-old children with a medium parents'/caregivers' process evaluation score (score 6.00–9.00; $n_{\text{four- to six-year-old children}} = 498$), and (3) four- to six-year-old children with a high parents'/caregivers' process evaluation score (score 10.00–14.00; $n_{\text{four- to six-year-old children}} = 458$). Of all parents, 31.8% had a low, 34.7% had a medium, and 33.5% had a high parents'/caregivers' process evaluation score. Parents/caregivers scored best on dose received - exposure (4.86/10) and had the lowest scores for dose received - satisfaction (1.88/6). Detailed information on the scores for each component of the parents'/

caregivers' process evaluation score can be found in Table 2.

For steps per weekday, steps per weekend day and steps per day, no significant interaction effects were found between time and parents'/caregivers' process evaluation score (all $p > 0.05$). This means that there is no difference between baseline and follow-up in steps per weekday, steps per weekend day or steps per day for four- to six-year-old children from the control group and four- to six-year-old children with a low, medium and high parents'/caregivers' process evaluation score.

Discussion

The aim of the present study was twofold. First, we wanted to investigate the effect of the PA-component of the ToyBox-intervention on European four- to six-year-old children's objectively measured steps per day for the total sample, and for the different countries (Belgium, Bulgaria, Germany, Greece, Poland, and Spain). Second, we wanted to examine whether a higher teachers' or parents'/caregivers' process evaluation score was related to more beneficial effects on four- to six-year-old children's steps per day.

For the total sample, no intervention effects were found, which means that the intervention did not cause an effect on four- to six-year-old children's PA in terms of steps per day. Also country-specific analyses revealed no effects on European four- to six-year-old children's steps per day. The lack of effects on children's PA is in line with other published studies targeting four- to six-year-old children's PA levels [16, 17]. One might have expected to find larger effects in four- to six-year-old children from Bulgaria and Greece, as these are the countries with the lowest levels of steps per day at baseline [6], and thus have more room to improve their steps per day. However, after analysing the data, it became clear that even in the countries with low steps per day at baseline, the intervention lacked to show an effect. This lack of effect might be due to the age-related decline of PA in children [35]. Furthermore, the ToyBox-intervention focussed on four different behaviours (i.e., water consumption, healthy snacking, sedentary behaviour and PA) during one school year, which means that only a limited period of time (i.e. 6 weeks) was available to implement the PA-module. However, teachers were encouraged to continue the implementation of different parts of the PA-component of the intervention throughout the school year. A recent systematic review and meta-analysis of randomised control trials showed that implementing interventions for a longer period of time (more than 6 months) enhanced intervention effects [36]. It might be suggested for future interventions to focus on PA for a longer period of time to enhance intervention effects. In addition, parents were only passively involved which might also explain the lack of intervention effects, as four- to six-year-old children spend a considerable amount of time in the presence of their parents [21, 27].

The results from the process evaluation showed a medium teachers' process evaluation score with a mean score of 13.5 on a total of 26. The higher score on fidelity can be explained by the fact that almost all kindergarten teachers handed out the newsletters and tip-cards for the parents/caregivers, based on the set time plan of the ToyBox-intervention. In addition, the higher score for dose received (satisfaction) shows us that kindergarten teachers in general might have enjoyed the intervention components and that they might be convinced about the clarity, appropriateness and the feasibility of the intervention components. The low score for dose delivered can be explained by the fact that the classroom activities were not implemented as intended. Although kindergarten teachers read the Kangaroo stories during the first weeks of intervention implementation, most of them did not implement the proposed excursions. In addition, during the repetition period, less than 25% of kindergarten teachers repeated using the Kangaroo stories and more than 90% of all teachers did not execute the excursions. This shows that excursions might be hard to implement in kindergarten classes, and that the Kangaroo stories can be used for a short period during the intervention, but not for longer implementation periods.

The results in this paper show that there are some differences in effect between the control group and between kindergartens with different process evaluation scores (low to high). For example for steps per weekday, four- to six-year-old children with a medium and high process evaluation score did not decrease their steps from baseline to follow-up, while four- to six-year-old children with a low process evaluation score did. This shows that having teachers that do not implement the intervention as intended (i.e., low teacher process evaluation score) and were not satisfied with the intervention, could have unfavourable effects compared to teachers that implement the intervention in a better way and were satisfied with the intervention or even compared to teachers that did not implement the intervention at all (i.e., control group). This shows that not implementing an intervention (i.e., doing nothing) is better than implementing an intervention with low fidelity to the study protocol. The influence of teachers implementing the intervention as intended (i.e., high teachers' process evaluation score) was still present on weekend days, as children from the control group decreased their steps per weekend day from baseline to follow-up, while children with a high teachers' process evaluation score did not. This shows that teachers implementing the intervention with high fidelity to the study protocol can stop a possible decrease in steps per weekday or weekend day. These age-related declines in PA have been studied before [35] and could thus be ameliorated with the ToyBox-intervention, if implemented with high fidelity and well-liked by the teachers. The results from the current study are very relevant, as our results emphasise the major importance of linking process to effect evaluation. These results are comparable to what has already been found in a recent study by Verloigne et al. (2015) in Belgian children (mean age: 6.0 years old) in which favourable effects were found for primary schools with medium and high process evaluation scores of the IDEFICS-intervention, but these effects were not found in preschool children [37]. Other studies found similar results with favourable effects in the targeted behaviours in adolescents with a higher level of intervention implementation [38–40]. However, in the current study, the variation between the three levels of intervention implementation and satisfaction was very small, and the scores were predominantly medium, which might be the cause of the lack of more and stronger effects. Moreover, the context of the kindergarten setting is different compared to the primary school setting, which might explain the differences observed between the studies. There are some possible reasons why the teachers' process evaluation scores were low in general. In the development of the ToyBox-intervention, focus groups with parents and teachers of four- to six-year-old children were conducted at the beginning of the development-phase, to involve both groups in the development of the intervention [30], which means that they reflected about what could be feasible within an intervention. However, the teachers that were involved in the focus group discussions were not the teachers that eventually had to implement the intervention, which means that focus groups were not used to involve the teachers more in the implementation of the intervention. Furthermore, it might be possible that principals of the intervention kindergartens agreed in participating in the intervention, but that teachers from those kindergartens were not really motivated to implement the intervention (e.g., due to large time investments, busy schedules, etc.). For future interventions, it might be an option to use a participatory health research approach, which means that the target group and the implementers are actively involved in designing and developing an intervention [41, 42]. An option might be to create an interaction with a panel of kindergarten teachers during the development and implementation of the intervention, which enables receiving feedback from the teachers and the development of an intervention that complies with teachers' skills and takes their needs into consideration. This might lead to better process evaluation scores and thus to better effects. In the ToyBox-intervention, only small flexibility and local adaptations were allowed to ensure comparability of results and in an extend that affected the fidelity of the implementation of certain components of the programme. The implementation of future projects in this field should allow more flexibility to meet the local needs, which is what the study of Hawe et al. (2004) suggests. Hawe et al. (2004) recommends to adapt the intervention to the local context. Rather than standardising the components of the intervention, these components could be seen as "mechanisms" in the change process, and can thus take on different forms according to the local context [43].

A low parents'/caregivers' process evaluation score was found with a mean score of 6.90 on a total score of 17. The results suggest that parents/caregivers read and were satisfied with the newsletters, tip-cards and posters for the PA component of the ToyBox-intervention, but that they were not satisfied with for example the usefulness, design and the amount of text of these tools. In addition, results showed that there was no difference in effect between four- to six-year-old children from the control group and four- to six-year-old children with a low, medium or high parents'/caregivers' process evaluation score. This is comparable with the IDEFICS-intervention in which higher levels of parental exposure to the intervention was not related to more favourable effects in children's BMI z-scores, and parental exposure and involvement in the intervention was much less than aimed for [44]. In the ToyBox-intervention, parents/caregivers were only passively involved as they only received newsletters, tip-cards and posters which they had to read. It might thus be possible that passively involving parents/caregivers in increasing four- to six-year-old children's steps per day might not be the way to go forward. Actively involving parents/caregivers might be a more promising strategy in future interventions targeting four- to six-year-old children's steps per day [45–47], and might induce an increase in children's PA.

Based on the information received from both kindergarten teachers and parents/caregivers, the ToyBox-material and/or components could be adapted and revised to meet the comments. For example by providing active toys and/or activity videos for the teachers. In addition, qualitative research could be helpful to investigate kindergarten teachers' and parents'/caregivers' perspectives on what worked and what did not work. The revised material and/or components could then be pilot tested to see whether teachers and parents/caregivers are more satisfied with the intervention components and implement the intervention as intended.

Study strengths are the large sample of four- to six-year-old children that provided valid pedometer data, and the cluster randomised controlled trial with a pre-test post-test design. However, future studies could look into objectively measuring four- to six-year-olds' PA by using hip and wrist accelerometers simultaneously as wrist-worn accelerometers have shown to measure different PA intensities more accurately [48]. Another strength is the use of process evaluation questionnaires for both kindergarten teachers and parents/caregivers. Key elements from the process evaluation model of Saunders et al. (2005) were used to calculate the process evaluation scores for teachers and parents/caregivers, which shows that process evaluation scores were theory-based [25, 26].

Study limitations include the fact that pedometers cannot distinguish between the different PA intensities and are only able to measure in steps per day. Missing data (e.g., during water-based activities) were not imputed, which may have induced bias. Furthermore, there was a large drop-out of four- to six-year-old children due to a lack of valid pedometer data at both baseline and follow-up. Also, there was no objective measurement of intervention implementation as the data for the process evaluation scores were self-reported in both teachers and parents/caregivers. It is possible that both teachers and parents/caregivers overestimated their efforts, which might have introduced bias. In addition, as not all teachers filled in all logbooks and not all parents filled in the process evaluation questionnaire, this also might have induced bias. Future studies could try to incorporate objective methods (e.g., observation) to study process evaluation. Furthermore, teachers' logbooks did not contain specific questions regarding the implementation of the environmental changes in the classroom, which means that valuable information was not recorded. This could however be taken into account by using observations. Another limitation that should be considered is that the differences by countries regarding the process evaluation score and sub-scores of each process evaluation component were not reported. However, this manuscript already gives a general image of the link between effect and process evaluation for all countries combined. Finally, it should be acknowledged that there is no standardised way to calculate process evaluation scores. Although it was based on a method used in previous studies [37, 49, 50], there are still some limitations linked to the method used to calculate the process evaluation scores as not all components of Saunders et al. (2005) were used to calculate the score, and equal weights for each component were used. In addition, there is not yet a consensus on how to operationalise the different process evaluation components [37, 51]. Consequently, the process evaluation scores provide a more general idea of the level of process evaluation of the kindergarten teachers and parents/caregivers. Process evaluation has many components, but implementation and satisfaction were the two that were chosen as the focus for this study. In addition, the current study chose to include satisfaction in the process evaluation score, while other papers in the literature have only included implementation scores to study the relationship between process and effect evaluation.

Conclusion

Overall, the ToyBox-intervention had no effect on European four- to six-year-old children's steps per day. Future European interventions with the aim to increase four- to six-year-old children's steps per day should incorporate country-specific adaptations to increase the effectiveness. The process evaluation scores showed that higher teachers' process evaluation score did not cause a decrease in steps per day, while four- to six-year-old children with a lower score or from the control group did. Therefore, future interventions should search for strategies to motivate the kindergarten teachers to induce larger effects, for instance by using a participatory approach in which kindergarten teachers are involved from the beginning of the study or by providing more active toys and exercise videos. However, this should be combined with actively involving children's parents.

Abbreviations

CONSORT: Consolidated standards of reporting trials; PA: Physical activity; SES: Socio-economic status

Acknowledgements

The ToyBox-study group consists of: **Co-ordinator:** Yannis Manios; **Steering Committee:** Yannis Manios, Berthold Koletzko, Ilse De Bourdeaudhuij, Mai Chin A Paw, Luis Moreno, Carolyn Summerbell, Tim Lobstein, Lieven Annemans, Goof Buijs; **External Advisors:** John Reilly, Boyd Swinburn, Dianne Ward; **Harokopio University (Greece):** Yannis Manios, Odysseas Androutsos, Eva Grammatikaki, Christina Katsarou, Eftychia Apostolidou, Eirini Efstathopoulou; **Ludwig Maximilians Universitaet Muenchen (Germany):** Berthold Koletzko, Kristin Duvinage, Sabine Ibrügger, Angelika Strauß, Birgit Herbert, Julia Birnbaum, Annette Payr, Christine Geyer; **Ghent University (Belgium):** *Department of Movement and Sports Sciences:* Ilse De Bourdeaudhuij, Greet Cardon, Marieke De Craemer, Ellen De Decker and *Department of Public Health:* Lieven Annemans, Stefaan De Henauw, Lea Maes, Carine Vereecken, Jo Van Assche, Lore Pil; **VU University Medical Center EMGO Institute for Health and Care Research (the Netherlands):** EMGO Institute for Health and Care Research: Mai Chin A Paw, Saskia te Velde; **University of Zaragoza (Spain):** Luis Moreno, Theodora Mouratidou, Juan Fernandez, Maribel Mesana, Pilar De Miguel-Etayo, Esther González, Luis Gracia-Marco, Beatriz Oves; **Oslo and Akershus University College of Applied Sciences (Norway):** Agneta Yngve, Susanna Kugelberg, Christel Lynch, Annhild Mosdøl; **University of Durham (UK):** Carolyn Summerbell, Helen Moore, Wayne Douthwaite, Catherine Nixon; **State Institute of Early Childhood Research (Germany):** Susanne Kreichauf, Andreas Wildgruber; **Children's Memorial Health Institute (Poland):** Piotr Socha, Zbigniew Kulaga, Kamila Zych, Magdalena Góźdź, Beata Gurzkowska, Katarzyna Szott; **Medical University of Varna (Bulgaria):** Violeta Iotova, Mina Lateva, Natalya Usheva, Sonya Galcheva, Vanya Marinova, Zhaneta Radkova, Nevyana Feschieva; **International Association for the Study of Obesity (UK):** Tim Lobstein, Andrea Aikenhead; **National Institute for Health Promotion and Disease Prevention (the Netherlands):** Goof Buijs, Annemiek Dorgelo, Aviva Nethe, Jan Jansen; **AOK- Verlag (Germany):** Otto Gmeiner, Jutta Retterath, Julia Wildeis, Axel Günthersberger; **Roehampton University (UK):** Leigh Gibson; **University of Luxembourg (Luxembourg):** Claus Voegele.

Funding
The ToyBox-study is funded by the Seventh Framework Programme (CORDIS FP7) of the European Commission under grant agreement n° 245,200. The content of this article reflects only the authors' views and the European Community is not liable for any use that may be made of the information contained therein.

Authors' contributions
All authors read, critically reviewed and approved the final manuscript, and participated in the ToyBox-project. MDC was responsible for the data collection, performed the analysis and wrote the manuscript. MV helped with data analysis.

Competing interests
The authors declare that they have no competing interests.

Author details
[1]Department of Movement and Sport Sciences, Ghent University, Watersportlaan 2, 9000 Ghent, Belgium. [2]Research Foundation Flanders, Brussels, Belgium. [3]Department of Nutrition and Dietetics, Harokopio University, School of Health Science & Education, E. Venizelou 70, 17671 Athens, Greece. [4]Medical University Varna, Clinic of Paediatric Endocrinology, UMHAT "St. Marina", "Hr. Smirnenski" Blvd, Varna, Bulgaria. [5]University of Zaragoza, GENUD (Growth, Exercise, Drinking behaviour and Development), C/Corona de Aragón 42, 50009 Zaragoza, Spain. [6]University of Munich Medical Centre, Dr. von Hauner Children's Hospital, Lindwurmstr.4, 80337 Munich, Germany. [7]Children's Memorial Institute, Al. Dzieci Polskich 20, 04-730 Warsaw, Poland.

References
1. Timmons BW, Leblanc AG, Carson V, Connor Gorber S, Dillman C, Janssen I, Kho ME, Spence JC, Stearns JA, Tremblay MS. Systematic review of physical activity and health in the early years (aged 0–4 years). Appl Physiol Nutr Metab. 2012;37:773–92.
2. Janz KF, Dawson JD, Mahoney LT. Tracking physical fitness and physical activity from childhood to adolescence: the muscatine study. Med Sci Sports Exerc. 2000;32:1250–7.
3. Kelder SH, Perry CL, Klepp KI, Lytle LL. Longitudinal tracking of adolescent smoking, physical activity, and food choice behaviors. Am J Public Health. 1994;84:1121–6.
4. Jones RA, Hinkley T, Okely AD, Salmon J. Tracking physical activity and sedentary behavior in childhood: a systematic review. Am J Prev Med. 2013;44:651–8.
5. Hinkley T, Salmon J, Okely AD, Crawford D, Hesketh K. Preschoolers' physical activity, screen time, and compliance with recommendations. Med Sci Sports Exerc. 2012;44:458–65.
6. De Craemer M, Lateva M, Iotova V, De Decker E, Verloigne M, De Bourdeaudhuij I, Androutsos O, Socha P, Kulaga Z, Moreno L, et al. Differences in Energy Balance-Related Behaviours in European Preschool Children: The ToyBox-Study. PLoS One. 2015;10:e0118303.
7. Timmons BW, Naylor PJ, Pfeiffer KA. Physical activity for preschool children–how much and how? Can J Public Health. 2007;98(Suppl 2):S122–34.
8. Oliver M, Schofield GM, Kolt GS. Physical activity in preschoolers: understanding prevalence and measurement issues. Sports Med. 2007;37:1045–70.
9. Bornstein DB, Beets MW, Byun W, McIver K. Accelerometer-derived physical activity levels of preschoolers: a meta-analysis. J Sci Med Sport. 2011;14:504–11.
10. Institute of Medicine of the National Academies. Early Childhood Obesity Prevention Policies. Washington (DC), US: The National Academies Press; 2011.
11. National physical activity recommendations for children 0–5 years. [http://www.health.gov.au/internet/main/publishing.nsf/Content/F01F92328EDADA5BCA257BF0001E720D/$File/Move%20and%20play%20every%20day%205yrs.PDF].
12. Van Cauwenberghe E, De Bourdeaudhuij I, Maes L, Cardon G. Efficacy and feasibility of lowering playground density to promote physical activity and to discourage sedentary time during recess at preschool: a pilot study. Prev Med. 2012;55:319–21.
13. Van Cauwenberghe E, De Craemer M, De Decker E, De Bourdeaudhuij I, Cardon G. The impact of a teacher-led structured physical activity session on preschoolers' sedentary and physical activity levels. J Sci Med Sport. 2013;16:422–6.
14. Cardon G, Labarque V, Smits D, De Bourdeaudhuij I. Promoting physical activity at the pre-school playground: the effects of providing markings and play equipment. Prev Med. 2009;48:335–40.
15. Hannon JC, Brown BB. Increasing preschoolers' physical activity intensities: an activity-friendly preschool playground intervention. Prev Med. 2008;46:532–6.
16. Bellows LL, Davies PL, Anderson J, Kennedy C. Effectiveness of a physical activity intervention for Head Start preschoolers: a randomized intervention study. Am J Occup Ther. 2013;67:28–36.
17. Reilly JJ, Kelly L, Montgomery C, Williamson A, Fisher A, McColl JH, Lo Conte R, Paton JY, Grant S. Physical activity to prevent obesity in young children: cluster randomised controlled trial. BMJ. 2006;333:1041.
18. Bayer O, von Kries R, Strauss A, Mitschek C, Toschke AM, Hose A, Koletzko BV. Short- and mid-term effects of a setting based prevention program to reduce obesity risk factors in children: a cluster-randomized trial. Clin Nutr. 2009;28:122–8.
19. Manios Y, Grammatikaki E, Androutsos O, Chinapaw MJ, Gibson EL, Buijs G, Iotova V, Socha P, Annemans L, Wildgruber A, et al. A systematic approach for the development of a kindergarten-based intervention for the prevention of obesity in preschool age children: the ToyBox-study. Obes Rev. 2012;13(Suppl 1):3–12.
20. Manios Y, Androutsos O, Katsarou C, Iotova V, Socha P, Geyer C, Moreno L, Koletzko B, De Bourdeaudhuij I. Designing and implementing a kindergarten-based, family-involved intervention to prevent obesity in early childhood: the ToyBox-study. Obes Rev. 2014;15(Suppl 3):5–13.
21. De Craemer M, De Decker E, Verloigne M, De Bourdeaudhuij I, Manios Y, Cardon G. The effect of a kindergarten-based, family-involved intervention on objectively measured physical activity in Belgian preschool boys and girls of high and low SES: the ToyBox-study. Int J Behav Nutr Phys Act. 2014;11:38.
22. Flynn MA, McNeil DA, Maloff B, Mutasingwa D, Wu M, Ford C, Tough SC. Reducing obesity and related chronic disease risk in children and youth: a synthesis of evidence with 'best practice' recommendations. Obes Rev. 2006;7(Suppl 1):7–66.
23. De Bourdeaudhuij I, Van Cauwenberghe E, Spittaels H, Oppert JM, Rostami C, Brug J, Van Lenthe F, Lobstein T, Maes L. School-based interventions promoting both physical activity and healthy eating in Europe: a systematic review within the HOPE project. Obes Rev. 2011;12:205–16.
24. Wilcox S, Laken M, Parrott AW, Condrasky M, Saunders R, Addy CL, Evans R, Baruth M, Samuel M. The faith, activity, and nutrition (FAN) program: design of a participatory research intervention to increase physical activity and improve dietary habits in African American churches. Contemp Clin Trials. 2010;31:323–35.
25. Saunders RP, Evans MH, Joshi P. Developing a process-evaluation plan for assessing health promotion program implementation: a how-to guide. Health Promot Pract. 2005;6:134–47.
26. Androutsos O, Apostolidou E, Iotova V, Socha P, Birnbaum J, Moreno L, De Bourdeaudhuij I, Koletzko B, Manios Y. Process evaluation design and tools used in a kindergarten-based, family-involved intervention to prevent obesity in early childhood. The ToyBox-study. Obes Rev. 2014;15(Suppl 3):74–80.
27. De Craemer M, De Decker E, Verloigne M, De Bourdeaudhuij I, Manios Y, Cardon G. The effect of a cluster randomised control trial on objectively measured sedentary time and parental reports of time spent in sedentary activities in Belgian preschoolers: the ToyBox-study. Int J Behav Nutr Phys Act. 2016;13:1.
28. De Craemer M, De Decker E, De Bourdeaudhuij I, Verloigne M, Duvinage K, Koletzko B, Ibrugger S, Kreichauf S, Grammatikaki E, Moreno L, et al. Applying the Intervention Mapping protocol to develop a kindergarten-based, family-involved intervention to increase European preschool children's physical activity levels: the ToyBox-study. Obes Rev. 2014;15(Suppl 3):14–26.
29. Bartholomew LK, Parcel GS, Kok G, Gottlieb NH, Fernandez ME. Planning Health Promotion Programs: An Intervention Mapping Approach. 3rd ed. San-Francisco: Jossey-Bass; 2011.
30. De Craemer M, De Decker E, De Bourdeaudhuij I, Deforche B, Vereecken C, Duvinage K, Grammatikaki E, Iotova V, Fernandez-Alvira JM, Zych K, et al. Physical activity and beverage consumption in preschoolers: focus groups

with parents and teachers. BMC Public Health. 2013;13:278.
31. De Craemer M, De Decker E, Santos-Lozano A, Verloigne M, De Bourdeaudhuij I, Deforche B, Cardon G: Validity of the Omron pedometer and the actigraph step count function in preschoolers. J Sci Med Sport. 2015;18(3):289–93.
32. Rowe DA, Mahar MI, Raedeke TD, Lore J. Measuring physical activity in children with pedometers: Reliability, reactivity, and replacement of missing data. Pediatr Exerc Sci. 2004;16:343–54.
33. Duvinage K, Ibrugger S, Kreichauf S, Wildgruber A, De Craemer M, De Decker E, Androutsos O, Lateva M, Iotova V, Socha P, et al. Developing the intervention material to increase physical activity levels of European preschool children: the ToyBox-study. Obes Rev. 2014;15(Suppl 3):27–39.
34. De Craemer M, De Decker E, De Bourdeaudhuij I, Verloigne M, Manios Y, Cardon G. The translation of preschoolers' physical activity guidelines into a daily step count target. J Sports Sci. 2015;33:1051–7.
35. Wong SH, Huang WY, He G. Longitudinal changes in objectively measured physical activity differ for weekdays and weekends among Chinese children in Hong Kong. BMC Public Health. 2015;15:1310.
36. Kamath C, Vickers K, Ehrlich A, McGovern L, Johnson J, Singhal V, Paulo R, Hettinger A, Erwin P, Montori V. Clinical review: behavioral interventions to prevent childhood obesity: a systematic review and metaanalyses of randomized trials. J Clin Endocrinol Metab. 2008;93:4606–15.
37. Verloigne M, Ahrens W, De Henauw S, Verbestel V, Marild S, Pigeot I, De Bourdeaudhuij I. Process evaluation of the IDEFICS school intervention: putting the evaluation of the effect on children's objectively measured physical activity and sedentary time in context. Obes Rev. 2015;16(Suppl 2):89–102.
38. Saunders RP, Ward D, Felton GM, Dowda M, Pate RR. Examining the link between program implementation and behavior outcomes in the lifestyle education for activity program (LEAP). Eval Program Plann. 2006;29:352–64.
39. Story M, Mays RW, Bishop DB, Perry CL, Taylor G, Smyth M, Gray C. 5-a-day Power Plus: process evaluation of a multicomponent elementary school program to increase fruit and vegetable consumption. Health Educ Behav. 2000;27:187–200.
40. Gray HL, Contento IR, Koch PA. Linking implementation process to intervention outcomes in a middle school obesity prevention curriculum, 'Choice, Control and Change'. Health Educ Res. 2015;30:248–61.
41. International Collaboration for Participatory Health Research: Position Paper 1: What is Participatory Health Research?. 2013.
42. Wright MT, Gardner B, Roche B, von Unger H, Ainlay C. Building an international collaboration on participatory health research. Prog Community Health Partnersh. 2010;4:31–6.
43. Hawe P, Shiell A, Riley T. Complex interventions: how "out of control" can a randomised controlled trial be? BMJ. 2004;328:1561–3.
44. De Bourdeaudhuij I, Verbestel V, De Henauw S, Maes L, Marild S, Moreno LA, Barba G, Siani A, Kovacs E, Konstabel K, et al. Implementation of the IDEFICS intervention across European countries: perceptions of parents and relationship with BMI. Obes Rev. 2015;16(Suppl 2):78–88.
45. Campbell KJ, Hesketh KD. Strategies which aim to positively impact on weight, physical activity, diet and sedentary behaviours in children from zero to five years. A systematic review of the literature. Obes Rev. 2007;8:327–38.
46. Hesketh KD, Campbell KJ. Interventions to prevent obesity in 0–5 year olds: an updated systematic review of the literature. Obesity (Silver Spring). 2010;18(Suppl 1):S27–35.
47. Golan M. Parents as agents of change in childhood obesity–from research to practice. Int J Pediatr Obes. 2006;1:66–76.
48. Johansson E, Larisch LM, Marcus C, Hagstromer M. Calibration and Validation of a Wrist- and Hip-Worn Actigraph Accelerometer in 4-Year-Old Children. PLoS ONE [Electronic Resource]. 2016;11:e0162436.
49. Latomme J, Cardon G, De Bourdeaudhuij I, Iotova V, Koletzko B, Socha P, Moreno L, Androutsos O, Manios Y, De Craemer M. Effect and process evaluation of a kindergarten-based, family-involved intervention with a randomized cluster design on sedentary behaviour in 4- to 6- year old European preschool children: The ToyBox-study. PLoS ONE [Electronic Resource]. 2017;12:e0172730.
50. Pinket AS, Van Lippevelde W, De Bourdeaudhuij I, Deforche B, Cardon G, Androutsos O, Koletzko B, Moreno LA, Socha P, Iotova V, et al. Effect and Process Evaluation of a Cluster Randomized Control Trial on Water Intake and Beverage Consumption in Preschoolers from Six European Countries: The ToyBox-Study. PLoS ONE [Electronic Resource]. 2016;11:e0152928.
51. Griffin TL, Pallan MJ, Clarke JL, Lancashire ER, Lyon A, Parry JM, Adab P, Investigators WST: Process evaluation design in a cluster randomised controlled childhood obesity prevention trial: the WAVES study. Int J Behav Nutr Phys Act. 2014;11:112.

4

The role of self-regulatory skills and automaticity on the effectiveness of a brief weight loss habit-based intervention: secondary analysis of the 10 top tips randomised trial

Nathalie Kliemann[1], Victoria Vickerstaff[2], Helen Croker[1], Fiona Johnson[1], Irwin Nazareth[2] and Rebecca J. Beeken[1,3*]

Abstract

Background: Habit-interventions are designed to promote the automaticity of healthy behaviours and may also enhance self-regulatory skills during the habit-formation process. A recent trial of habit-based advice for weight loss (10 Top Tips; 10TT), found that patients allocated to 10TT lost significantly more weight over 3 months than those allocated to usual care, and reported greater increases in automaticity for the target behaviours. The current study aimed to test the hypothesis that i) 10TT increased self-regulatory skills more than usual care, and ii) that self-regulatory skills and automaticity changes mediated the effect of 10TT on weight loss.

Methods: 537 obese patients from 14 primary care practices in the UK were randomized to receive 10TT or usual care. Patients in the 10TT group received a leaflet containing tips for weight loss and healthy habits formation, a self-monitoring log book and a wallet-sized shopping guide on how to read food labels. Patients were weighed and completed validated questionnaires for self-regulation and automaticity at baseline and 3-month follow-up. Within-group and Between-group effects were explored using Paired T-test and ANCOVA, respectively. Mediation was assessed using bootstrapping to estimate indirect effects and the sobel test.

Results: Over 3 months patients who were given 10TT reported greater increases in self-regulatory skills (Mean difference: .08; 95% CI .01; .15) than those who received usual care. Changes in self-regulatory skills and automaticity over 3 months mediated the effect of the intervention on weight loss (β = .52, 95% Bias Corrected CI .17; .91).

Conclusions: As hypothesised, 10TT enhanced self-regulatory skills and changes in self-regulatory skills and automaticity mediated the effect of the intervention on weight loss. This supports the proposition that self-regulatory training and habit formation are important features of weight loss interventions.

Trial registration: This study was prospectively registered with the International Standard Randomised Controlled Trials (ISRCTN16347068) on 26 September 2011.

Keywords: Self-regulation, Habit formation, Automaticity, Weight loss, Intervention

* Correspondence: r.beeken@leeds.ac.uk
[1]Department of Behavioural Science & Health, University College London, London, England
[3]Leeds Institute of Health Sciences, University of Leeds, Level 10, Worsley Building, Clarendon Way, Leeds LS2 9NL, England
Full list of author information is available at the end of the article

Background

Obesity is a growing public health concern that affects more than 600 million adults worldwide [1, 2] and increases risk for chronic diseases [2, 3]. There is therefore a need to find effective interventions to help individuals with obesity to lose weight and to prevent weight gain at the population level. While commercial programmes are promising, they require a certain level of motivation on the part of the individual, such as attendance at group sessions over a prolonged period of time.

Evidence from recent studies suggests that brief habit-based interventions [4, 5], may be an innovative approach for promoting weight loss, even when conscious motivation is low [5]. Habit-based interventions promote the repetition of target behaviours in a consistent context in order to make them become more automatic and habitual [6, 7]. Habits are formed through learned associations between a cue or stimulus with a response, so that when a cue is encountered it automatically generates an impulse toward action [8]. Although interest is growing in habit-formation approaches [5, 7, 9], weight loss interventions applying this approach are still scarce [10, 11] and their mechanisms of action are not completely understood. Improving the theoretical understanding of how habit-based interventions bring about weight loss is pressing, as it may provide guidance on the development of more effective interventions [12] to tackle the obesity epidemic.

A recent habit-based weight loss intervention, called 10 Top Tips (10TT), was developed as a leaflet to promote a set of everyday healthy eating and activity behaviours [10] in obese patients (n = 537) from primary care in the UK [4]. The advice for turning these target behaviours into habits involved the recommendation of making specific plans and repeating the behaviours in a consistent context, as well as monitoring performance daily using a log book. The active treatment was defined as the first three months [6], which is the period usually required to form habits [9, 13]. The results of this trial demonstrated that over three months patients allocated to 10TT lost 0.87 kg (95% CI -1.47; –.027, adjusted mean) more than those allocated to usual care. Furthermore, patients who received 10TT reported a greater increase in automaticity of the target behaviours (adjusted sum difference = 8.45, 95% CI =2.59, 14.32) over three months, which suggests that 10TT was more effective at establishing new habits by the end of the intervention period. However, whether this increase in automaticity was the mechanism behind the observed weight loss remains to be explored.

The process of habit formation may also require self-regulatory skills to translate the intended behaviour into action and override unwanted automated responses [9, 14]. Self-regulation refers broadly to the multiple processes involved in goal-directed behaviour [15] and encompasses the ability to alter behaviour, thoughts, feelings, attention and environment in the pursuit of personal goals [16–19]. The capacity to self-regulate behaviour is considered to be a relatively stable construct [20], but one that can be improved through practice [21, 22]. Since, the habit acquisition phase within 10TT involves actions such as setting goals, planning, self-monitoring and reviewing progress [23], it is possible that it may also enhance self-regulatory skills. Recent studies have suggested that self-regulatory skills may be an important individual factor that helps individuals to achieve, as well as maintain a healthy weight and diet [21, 24, 25]. Examining the impact of the 10TT intervention on self-regulatory skills may deepen our understanding of the mechanisms underlying the effectiveness of habit-based weight loss interventions.

Therefore, the current study aimed to explore the mechanisms behind the weight loss observed in the 10TT trial. Specifically, this study aimed to investigate the effect of 10TT on self-regulatory skills and whether changes in self-regulatory skills and automaticity mediated the effect of the intervention on weight loss over three months. Data from returned 10TT log books were also explored to provide an indication of engagement with the intervention, and how this related to changes in self-regulatory skills, automaticity and weight loss. We hypothesised that i) 10TT increased self-regulatory skills more than usual care, ii) that self-regulatory skills and automaticity changes mediated the effect of 10TT on weight loss and iii) that patients with the greatest improvement in self-regulatory skills, automaticity and weight would be more engaged in terms of their use of the log books.

Methods

Study design

This study is a secondary analysis from a two-arm, individually-randomised (1:1 ratio), controlled trial in obese adults in primary care, comparing the 10TT intervention with 'usual care'. The active treatment was defined as the first three months. The protocol of the trial has been published elsewhere [6]. Ethical approval was granted by South East London Research Ethics Committee 2 via IRAS (Ref No. 10/H0802/59, Approval granted 9th July 2010). The trial was conducted in accordance with the CONSORT 2010 guidelines (see Additional file 1).

Participants and recruitment

Participants were patients from General Practices in England, who were classified as obese (BMI ≥ 30) and were 18 years or older. Patients were excluded if they were pregnant; terminally ill; or unable to provide informed consent due to mental incapacity or active psychotic illness. A total of 14 General Practices across England were selected through the General Practice Research Framework, to represent socio-economically deprived and ethnic diverse populations; and both urban and rural areas. Detailed information about the 14 practices included in this study has been published elsewhere [4, 6]. All obese patients registered in these practices were invited to take part in the study from August 2010 to October 2011. However, when the number of patients with obesity registered in the practice exceeded 500, a random sample of 500 was selected and invited. The practices sent a letter to eligible participants including the information sheet and an 'expression of interest' form. Potential participants met with a health professional, who checked their eligibility, explained the study and took informed consent.

Randomisation

Randomisation took place after eligibility was confirmed and after completion of baseline measures. It was done by telephoning a central randomisation service (Health Service Research Unit at Aberdeen) to ensure allocation concealment. A computer-based list generated random permuted blocks of size 2 to 4. The randomisation was stratified by practice in order to have a socio-economic balance between the groups.

10TT

Participants randomised to 10TT received the 10TT leaflet, a self-monitoring log book and a wallet sized shopping guide on how to read food labels. These were provided to patients at their baseline appointment by a trained health professional (nurses or health care assistants), who spent about 30 min talking through the leaflet with the patients, following a standardized script. After providing the patients with the materials and information about the intervention, there was no further clinical contact. Participants could request more log books when necessary and were instructed to return the completed ones by post in a provided free-post envelope. Further information about the intervention content has been previously published [6].

Usual care

Patients randomised to usual care received the practice's usual care, which consisted of referring patients to community programmes (12 weekly sessions) or to a health professional not involved in the trial for a discussion on healthy eating (usually at least 2 appointments). Detailed information about the usual care received by participants has been previously published [4].

Blinding

Participants were not blinded to their group condition. However, the assessment at 3 months was done by health professionals blinded to participant condition allocation.

Measures

Demographic characteristics

Socio-demographic characteristics, including gender, age, ethnic origin and education, were obtained from health records.

Anthropometric measures

Body weight (in kg) was measured using TANITA scales supplied to the practices for use only in this study and height (in cm) was taken using the Practice equipment. Weight changes from baseline to 3-month follow-up were calculated.

Behavioural measures

Self-regulatory skills were assessed using the validated 31-item Self-Regulation Questionnaire- SRQ [26], adapted for eating and weight self-regulatory skills. The adaptation consisted of changing the wording to make the items apply specifically to weight and dietary self-regulation. For example, 'I'm able to accomplish goals I set for myself' was changed to 'I'm able to accomplish weight loss goals I set for myself'. The Likert response scale was changed from 5 to 4 options by removing the 'uncertain or unsure' option. The scores ranged from 1 (strongly disagree) to 4 (strongly agree). As the original scale has only one factor [26], the outcome for self-regulatory skills was the mean score for the 31 items. Baseline data for the adapted questionnaire showed it had good internal reliability (Cronbach's alpha of .88). The mean score for the 31 items and the mean change from baseline to 3 month follow-up were calculated.

The automaticity of the 10 targeted eating and activity behaviours plus self-weighing behaviour was assessed using a single item taken from the 12-item Self-Report Habit Index [27], asking how much each of the behaviours were done automatically on a 7-point Likert scale from 'none of the time' to 'all of the time'. The scores ranged from 1 to 7. For some of the target behaviours more than one question was generated to better assess the automaticity of the behaviour. For example, for 'Focus on your food' behaviour, two questions on how automatically people eat in front of the TV and at a table were generated (see Additional file 2: Table S2). The mean score for the automaticity of all 16 behaviours was calculated as well as the mean change from baseline to 3-month follow-up for each behaviour (see Additional file 3: Table S3).

10TT log books

The log books had tick sheets, where participants could record whether they managed each tip and record their weight every day. They also contained notes and planning sheets, where participants could write down how they aimed to achieve each tip every week. Data from the 10TT log books returned at 3 months were: the number of weeks the self-monitoring, weight recording and planning sections were used, the number of times the target behaviours were managed at least 5 times per week and the average number of tips managed per week. The use of the 10TT log books in relation to the level of change in self-regulatory skills, automaticity and weight over 3 months were explored using ranked percentiles: percentile <75 represented medium to small changes and percentile ≥75 represented large changes.

Sample size

The trial was powered to detect a significant weight difference between the intervention and control group as published previously [6]. Therefore, the analyses presented in this study should be considered exploratory.

Statistical analyses

Data were analysed using SPSS version 22.0 (SPSS Inc). All analyses were according to intention-to-treat. Initially a completer analysis was performed using complete data at baseline and follow-up for each outcome. Participants with more than 20% of missing data for the self-regulation and automaticity questionnaires were excluded from the completer analysis. When there were up to 20% missing data for these questionnaires the individual median score was imputed. Baseline descriptive analyses were applied. To explore baseline differences between the completers and non-completers at 3 months, chi-square tests for categorical variables and t-tests for continuous variables were applied.

Following the trial's analysis plan [6], we checked for clustering by GP practice by running unconstrained models in the mixed effect models and calculating the intracluster correlation coefficients (ICC). All ICCs were less than 0.05, demonstrating that there were low levels of clustering.

Changes in self-regulatory skills were assessed using paired t-tests for the within-group analysis and ANCOVA, controlling for baseline levels of self-regulation, age, gender and baseline weight, for the between-group analysis. Regression models were used to explore whether baseline data for self-regulation predicted the effect of the intervention on self-regulatory skills changes at 3 month follow-up. The model was adjusted for age, gender and baseline weight and included an interaction term (group condition by predictor).

In the present study we also explored the mediation effects of self-regulatory and automaticity mean changes on the relationship between group condition and weight change at three month follow-up using bootstrapping to estimate indirect effects, and the sobel test. The method used for the mediation analysis was the Baron and Kenny [28], in which the paths of the mediation model are estimated through a series of regression analyses. The sobel test, also called the *product-of-coefficient*, has been widely used in the literature for estimating the indirect effect, but is also considered a conservative method. Since this study tested multiple mediators, Preacher and Hayes [29] recommend also using bootstrapping for testing indirect effects. Bootstrapping is a method that does not impose normality of the sampling distribution and involves multiple resampling of the data set, estimation of the indirect effects and the construct of the confidence interval for the indirect effect [29]. Mean changes in automaticity and in self-regulatory skills over 3 months were tested as mediators, since increases in these constructs were hypothesised to be the underlying mechanisms leading to weight loss. Mediation analyses were adjusted for gender, age, baseline weight, baseline self-regulation mean score and baseline automaticity mean score. Indirect effects were calculated for the total effect, for each mediator and for the contrast of the indirect effects against each other. A 95% Bias Corrected Bootstrapped Confidence Interval was calculated for each indirect effect. Correlations between changes in self-regulation and automaticity in each group condition were also examined.

We performed sensitivity analysis to investigate the potential effect of missing responses for the outcomes using multiple imputations at baseline and follow-up. Multiple imputation models were stratified by study arm and included socio-demographics and self-regulation, automaticity and weight data. A set of 100 imputations were performed.

Finally, descriptive analyses were performed for the data collected from the log books and presented per level of changes in self-regulatory skills, automaticity and weight over three months. Baseline differences were checked between those who sent back the log book and those who did not, using chi-square tests for categorical data and t-tests for continuous data.

Results

Participants flow and characteristics

Figure 1 displays the flow diagram of the study participation during the first 3-month of the trial. A total of 537 obese patients were eligible to take part in the study; 267 were randomised to the intervention group and 270 to the control group. As shown in Table 1, most of the participants were female (~65%), white (~95%), and approximately half of the participants did not have a degree (~47%). Age, weight, BMI, self-regulation score, and automaticity score at baseline were similar between the two arms. A total of 380 and 381 participants provided data on self-regulation and automaticity at baseline and 3 months (post-intervention), respectively. The non-completers were not significantly different at baseline in socio-demographic characteristics, weight, self-regulation and automaticity outcomes from those who provided data at both time

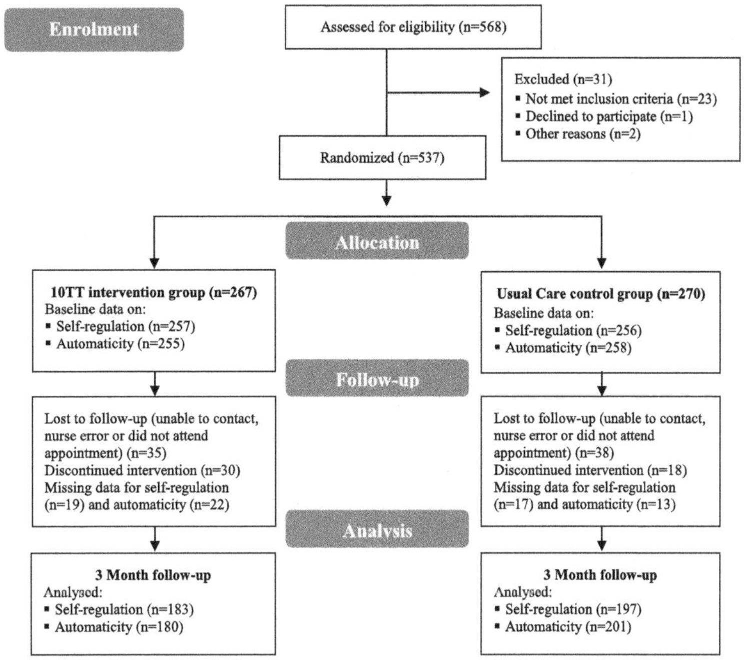

Fig. 1 Flow diagram of participation during the study period

points. The only exception was age, which was significantly greater among completers for self-regulation and automaticity than non-completers.

Post-intervention effect on self-regulatory skills changes

Self-regulatory skills increased significantly over 3 months in both groups ($p < .001$ for all analyses). The between-group analyses showed that at three month follow-up, participants who were given the 10TT intervention had a mean change in self-regulatory skills .08 (95% CI .01; .15, $p = .019$) greater than those who received usual care (Table 2). Sensitivity analysis using multiple imputations gave similar results.

Regression models adjusted for age, gender and baseline weight indicated that lower baseline self-regulatory skills predicted greater changes in self-regulation (B = –.22 SE = .06, $p < .001$) at 3 month follow-up. This result did not differ by arm, as no interaction between baseline data and group condition was found. Analyses using multiple imputations mirrored the results found for completers.

Mediation analysis

As shown in the preliminary results for this trial, over three months the intervention group lost 1.68 kg (SD 3.20) and the control group 0.84 kg (SD 2.83) and the difference of 0.87 (95% CI -1.47; –.27) was statistically significant [4]. Also, the automaticity of the target behaviours increased significantly more in the 10TT group compared to usual care group condition (adjusted sum difference = 8.45, 95% CI =2.59; 14.32 or adjusted mean changes = .21, 95% CI .07; .35). The present study assessed whether self-regulatory and automaticity mean changes mediated the effect of the intervention on weight changes at three months, when controlling for gender, age, baseline weight, baseline self-regulation and baseline automaticity. The results show the intervention condition significantly predicted self-regulation and automaticity changes, which in turn significantly predicted weight changes at 3 months (Fig. 2). The total effect was significant, while the direct effect was non-significant. Using bootstrapping, the results also indicated that the indirect effects of each mediator, as well as the total effect, were significant. The indirect effect of the contrast of the indirect effects was non-significant. This means that there was no difference in the strength of the indirect effect between the mediators. The sobel test was also assessed and was significant for both mediators: self-regulation changes ($z = 2.35$, $p = .010$) and automaticity changes ($Z = 1.99$, $p = .046$). Therefore, changes in both self-regulatory skills and automaticity mediated the effect of the intervention on weight change at 3 month. The sensitivity analysis using multiple imputations showed similar results for both mediators: self-regulation changes ($z = 2.54$, $p = .01$) and automaticity changes ($z = 1.97$, $p = .004$).

Regarding the correlation between changes in self-regulatory skills and automaticity, it represented a medium effect in the intervention group ($r = 0.32$ at 3 months) and in the control group ($r = 0.39$ at 3 months). Analyses using multiple imputations provided similar results.

Table 1 Baseline characteristics by randomised group and by completers and non-completers at 3 months for self-regulation and automaticity outcomes

	All participants		Self-regulation outcome		Automaticity outcome	
Characteristics	Intervention group (*N* = 267)	Control group (*N* = 270)	Completers[i] (N-380)	Non-completers (*N* = 157)	Completers[i] (*N* = 381)	Non-completers (*N* = 156)
Age (in years)						
Mean (SD)	57.0 (12.8)	57.6 (12.5)	58.5 (11.7)	54.3 (14.4)**	58.7 (11.7)	53.9 (14.3)**
Gender						
Female, % (n)	66.7 (178)	64.8 (175)	64.5 (245)	68.8 (108)$^{\Delta}$	65.1 (248)	67.3 (105)$^{\Delta}$
Ethnic group						
White[a], % (n)	94.7 (252)	95.2 (255)	95.3 (362)	92.9 (145)$^{\Delta}$	94.8 (361)	94.2 (146)$^{\Delta}$
Other[b], % (n)	5.3 (15)	4.9 (13)	4.7 (18)	7.1 (11)$^{\Delta}$	5.2 (20)	5.8 (9)$^{\Delta}$
Qualification						
Non-degree[c], % (n)	49.6 (129)	44.4 (116)	46.2 (172)	49.0 (73)$^{\Delta}$	45.4 (169)	51.0 (76)$^{\Delta}$
Degree[d], % (n)	28.8 (75)	34.9 (91)	33.9 (126)	26.8 (40)$^{\Delta}$	33.1 (123)	28.9 (43)$^{\Delta}$
Other[e], % (n)	21.5 (56)	20.7 (54)	19.9 (74)	24.2 (36)$^{\Delta}$	21.5 (80)	20.1 (30)$^{\Delta}$
Weight[f] (in kg)						
Mean (SD)	100.4 (17.0)	101.2 (17.5)	100.7 (16.7)	101.3(18.9)$^{\Delta}$	100.4 (17.07)	102.06 (18.3)$^{\Delta}$
BMI[f] (in kg/m^2)						
Mean (SD)	36.1 (4.7)	36.5 (5.4)	36.2 (4.9)	36.5 (5.4)$^{\Delta}$	36.2 (5.04)	36.6 (5.2)$^{\Delta}$
Self-regulation[g]						
Mean (SD)	2.4(.3)	2.4 (.3)	2.4 (.3)	2.4 (.3)$^{\Delta}$	2.4 (.36)	2.4 (.37)$^{\Delta}$
Automaticity[h]						
Mean (SD)	4.4 (1.0)	4.5 (.9)	2.4 (.3)	2.4 (.3)$^{\Delta}$	4.5 (.9)	4.4 (1.0)$^{\Delta}$

**$p < .001$ $^{\Delta}p > .05$
[a]White British, White Irish or other White background
[b]African, other black background, Indian, Pakistani, Bangladeshi, Chinese, other Asian background, White and Black Caribbean, White and Asian, other mixed background or other ethnic origin
[c]GCSE/School certificate/O-level/CSE, Vocational qualifications or A-level or equivalent
[d]Degree or Post-graduate degree
[e]Still studying, other or do not wish to answer
[f]Data at baseline was available for 536 participants
[g]Self-regulatory skills score ranged from 1 (strongly disagree) to 4 (strongly agree) and data at baseline was available for 513 participants
[h]Automaticity score ranged from 1 (disagree) to 7 (agree) and data at baseline was available for 513 participants
[i]Data at baseline and 3 months

Descriptive analysis of the 10TT log books

Table 3 presents the descriptive data from the returned 10TT log books. Around 40% of those who received 10TT returned the log books at 3 months. The baseline differences between those who sent back the log book and those who did not were similar to the differences found for completers and non-completers at 3 months. The only exception was for automaticity, which was slightly greater among participants who sent the log book back (M = 4.9 vs M = 4.6, $p = .041$). The majority of participants used the self-monitoring sheets correctly and for a median time of 13 weeks. However, those who showed the greatest changes in self-regulatory skills, automaticity and weight used the self-monitoring sheet for around 14, 14 and 15 weeks, respectively. Most participants recorded their weight for around 13 weeks, but those with the greatest changes in weight recorded it for 15 weeks. In terms of planning, the majority of participants made plans to achieve their behavioural goals for around 10 weeks. However, those with the greatest changes in automaticity did it for 11 weeks. People were expected to manage all 10 target behaviours, however most managed 5 tips per week. People who showed the highest improvement in self-regulatory skills and weight loss managed around 6 tips per week and those with the greatest improvement in automaticity managed 7 tips per week.

Discussion

This study is the first to explicitly assess the potential mechanisms of a brief habit-based intervention for weight loss in a population-based sample of obese adults. The study showed that 10TT promoted changes in self-regulatory skills and that these changes, alongside changes in automaticity, mediated the effect of 10TT on weight loss. Furthermore, participants who engaged

Table 2 Effect of the intervention on self-regulation at 3-month follow-up

	Intervention group					Control Group					Mean diff[c] (95% CI)	P
Characteristics	N	Baseline M (SE)	3 M M (SE)	Diff (95% CI)	P	N	Baseline M (SE)	3 M M (SE)	Diff (95% CI)	P		
Completer analysis												
Self-regulatory skills[a]	183	2.46 (.02)	2.68 (.03)	.22 (.16;.27)	<.001	197	2.49 (.02)	2.62 (.03)	.12 (.08;.17)	<.001	.08 (.01;.15)	.019
Sensitivity analyses[b]												
Self-regulatory skills[a]	267	2.46 (.02)	2.68(.03)	.21 (.16;.26)	<.001	270	2.49 (.02)	2.61 (.03)	.12 (.07;.17)	<.001	.08 (.01;.14)	.012

[a]Self-regulatory skills score ranged from 1 (strongly disagree) to 4 (strongly agree)
[b]Sensitivity analysis using multiple imputation to deal with missing data
[c]Adjusted for gender, age, baseline weight and baseline data for self-regulation

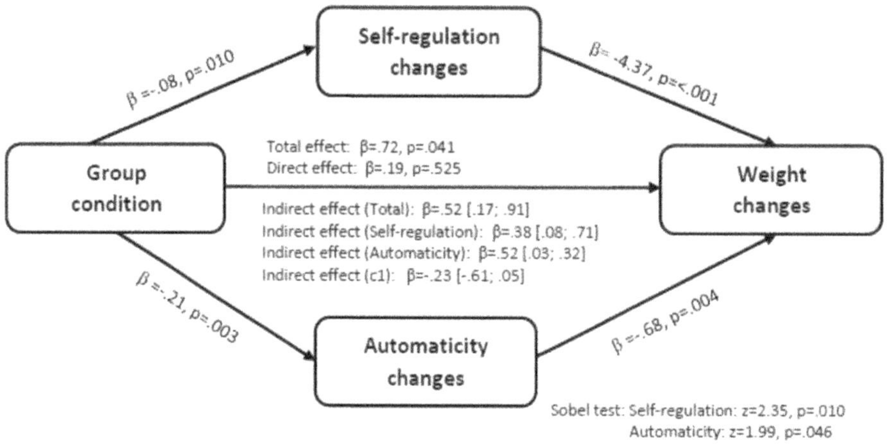

Fig. 2 Mediation of self-regulation and automaticity changes on the effect of group condition on weight loss at 3 month

more with the intervention in terms of number of weeks monitoring the target behaviours, recording weight, and making plans, experienced the greatest changes in self-regulatory skills, automaticity and weight.

The results of this study are in line with the suggestion that habit-based interventions help people to improve their self-regulatory capacity, since they require people to make goals, plan and monitor their behaviour [9, 14]. This is comparable to other intervention studies that have applied planning techniques, in which changes in self-regulatory skills were found over a short [30, 31] and long period of time [32]. However, this is the first study to show that a planning technique within a habit intervention improves self-regulatory skills. Importantly, the 10TT intervention was particularly effective at promoting self-regulatory skills among those patients who had poor self-regulation skills at baseline, although ceiling effects may have affected this result. However, due to the nature of 10TT (a brief, self-help intervention), the specificity and relevance of the goals and plans formed by the participants is not known. The quality of plans is relevant for habit formation, as they need to be context specific in order to make the target behaviour become more automatic. Future studies should assess the quality of plans made by participants and explore how this relates to habit formation.

According to the previous results of this trial, patients who received the 10TT also experienced greater increases in automaticity than those who received usual care at 3 months [4]. The present study demonstrated that changes in both self-regulatory skills and automaticity mediated the effect of 10TT on weight loss at 3 months. Given that the majority of studies do not assess the mechanism for an intervention's success [32], this is an important finding which suggests the intervention works as it is intended to. This is also in line with recent evidence suggesting that nutrition and weight loss interventions that include self-regulation components tend to be more effective [33, 34]. The observed correlation between changes in automaticity and self-regulatory skills also adds to our understanding of the habit-formation process, as it suggests that self-regulatory skills may be required for the development of automaticity [35, 36]. Self-regulatory skills are thought to help individuals to act according to an intended behaviour [9, 14] and may also help to both suppress impulse tendencies toward temptations [15] and prevent the loss of healthy habits when environmental cues change [10].

The log book data showed that participants who monitored their weight and target behaviours more frequently, and who made more plans, showed the greatest improvement in self-regulatory skills and automaticity, and also experienced the greatest weight loss. This is an indication that the intervention worked best when engaged with and adhered to. Although the difference in self-monitoring between those who showed the greatest and lowest engagement was only around 1 to 2 weeks, this fits with habit theory. According to Lally and Gardner [9] habit formation may vary widely and habits can be formed over as little as 18 days as many as 254 days, depending on the complexity of the behaviour, and as other aspects. Furthermore, a study conducted by Lange, Richert, Koring, Knoll, Schwarzer and Lippke [31] showed that significant improvements in self-regulation can be observed over just a week. Future studies should explore ways to improve engagement and adherence, for example the use of novel technologies to facilitate self-monitoring. In addition, the 10TT intervention only addresses forming habits and does not include a self-regulatory training component to help participants break existing habits. This could be important because breaking habits require more effortful self-regulatory skills in order to disrupt cue-response associations [9]. Future studies should explore the effect of adding self-regulatory training specifically focused on

Table 3 Descriptive data from the log books per level of changes in self-regulatory skills, automaticity and weight over 3 months (Only 10TT participants)

Changes over 3 months	All 10TT participants[a]		10TT participants that returned the Log books[b]		Used self-monitoring sheets		Recorded weight		Made plans		N° times tips were managed ≥5 d/w	Tips managed per week
	N	M (SD)	% (N)	M (SD)	Total % (N)	N° weeks MED	Total % (N)	N° weeks MED	Total % (N)	N° weeks MED	MED	MED
Self-regulation												
Per percentile[c]												
< 75	130	.03 (.22)	38.4 (50)	−.01 (.21)	100 (50)	13	90.0 (45)	13	92.0 (46)	10	76.5	5.5
≥ 75	53	.68 (.27)	35.3 (24)	.67 (.24)	100 (24)	14	91.6 (22)	13	95.8 (23)	10	92.0	6.5
Automaticity												
Per percentile[c]												
< 75	122	.24 (.59)	38.5 (47)	.26 (.47)	95.7 (45)	13	91.5 (43)	13	93.6 (44)	10	70.0	5.5
≥ 75	58	1.54 (.59)	44.8 (26)	1.69 (.74)	100 (26)	14	88.5 (23)	13	92.3 (24)	11	97.5	7.5
Weight												
Per percentile[c]												
< 75	144	−.12 (1.7)	35.4 (51)	−.42 (1.5)	96.1 (49)	13	86.3 (44)	12	92.2 (47)	9	67.0	5.5
≥ 75	56	−5.7 (2.7)	44.6 (25)	−5.7 (3.5)	100 (25)	15	96.0 (24)	15	96.0 (24)	10	90.0	6.5

3 months was equivalent to 15 weeks
M mean, *SD* Standard deviation, *MED* Median
[a]All 10TT participants with data for the outcome
[b]All 10TT participants who sent the log books back and had data for the outcomes
[c]Changes to the outcome over 3 months categorised according to the percentile, that is - <75 = medium to low changes and ≥75 = greater changes

breaking habits to the current advice on forming habits. This could potentially enhance the effects of the 10TT intervention.

A strength of this study was that the intervention was delivered by health professionals from primary care across England, which provides direct evidence for its effectiveness in clinical practice. However, there are limitations concerning the generalisability of the results, which were presented with the previous findings from this trial [4]. Briefly, participants were not blinded to their condition, although the 3-month follow-up assessment was done by a health professional blinded to condition allocation. Ethnic minorities and men were under-represented and the sample was slightly older compared with the population of adults with obesity described in the Health Survey of England.

There are also limitations related specifically to the current analyses. The results for changes in self-regulation and automaticity should be interpreted as exploratory, as the trial was only powered to detect differences in weight change between the group conditions. Self-regulation was measured using an adapted version of the SRQ, which excluded the middle response option from the original version to encourage people to commit one way or the other, but as a consequence may have increased the risk of ceiling effects. Future studies should aim to replicate these analyses using a valid and reliable measure of eating self-regulatory skills, such as the recently developed Self-Regulation Questionnaire of Eating Behaviour (SREBQ) [37]. The automaticity of the target behaviours was assessed using only one item from the 12-item Self-report Habit Index [27], and may not be comprehensive enough to assess habit formation. Future studies should consider using the shortened 4-item version of this questionnaire, which has been recently validated [38]. In this study, automaticity also represented the overall score for the automaticity of the target behaviours. As a consequence, it was not possible to draw conclusions about which behaviours had become habitual and it may have overestimated the effect of the intervention. Future studies should explore changes in each of the eating, activity and self-weighing behaviours and their automaticity separately using valid and reliable measures, as opposed to single items.

Furthermore, given the measures used in this study were all self-report, changes in self-regulatory skills and automaticity may represent the individuals perception of change, rather than actual change. Objective and technologic-based methods to assess nutrition, physical activity and healthy behaviours could promote more accurate data on these behaviours [39]. Other aspects may have also played a role on the effect of the intervention on weight loss that were not included in these analyses. For example, social support has also been identified as an important aspect of behaviour change [40], and this should be further explored. In addition, the analysis of the pathways was missing data for the variables of interest (compromising internal validity) and of course nullifying randomisation so that the results are more in keeping with that of a cohort study analysis rather than a RCT. Finally, qualitative analysis on the specificity of plans made by the participants and their relationship with habit formation could also further the understanding of the effect of this intervention.

Conclusions

In conclusion, our findings suggest that a habit-based intervention can enhance self-regulatory skills, especially among people with lower levels of self-regulatory skills at baseline. Furthermore, changes in self-regulation and automaticity are the underlying mechanisms by which 10TT promoted weight loss in adults with obesity, supporting the theoretical basis of the intervention. This study also provided evidence that greater engagement with the intervention was associated with greater improvements in self-regulatory skills, automaticity and weight loss. Future studies should explore whether the effect of the 10TT intervention on self-regulation and automaticity can be enhanced through facilitating engagement with the log books (e.g. through digital self-monitoring) and the effect of adding self-regulatory training for breaking existing habits on weight loss.

Additional files

Additional file 1: CONSORT 2010 checklist of information to include when reporting a randomised trial*

Additional file 2: Table S1. 10 Target eating and activity behaviours plus self-weighing and the 16 automaticity questions

Additional file 3: Table S2. Descriptive data of the automaticity of each target behaviour

Abbreviations

10TT: 10 Top Tips intervention; BMI: Body Mass Index; SREBQ: Self-Regulation of Eating Behaviour Questionnaire; SRQ: Self-Regulation Questionnaire

Acknowledgements

Researchers involved in this study were supported by YCR, CRUK, CAPES, UCL, Marie Curie and NIHR. The views expressed in this publication are those of the authors and not necessarily those of YCR, CRUK, CAPES, UCL, Marie Curie and NIHR.

Funding

The trial was funded by the Medical Research Council – National Prevention Research Initiative. RJB is supported by Yorkshire Cancer Research Academic Fellowship funding, FJ and HC are funded by Cancer Research UK, NK by CAPES/BRASIL, VV by Marie Curie and National Institute for Health Research and IN is a core funded member of staff at University College London.

Authors' contributions
RB, IN, and HC designed the research; NK and VV analysed the data; NK wrote the first draft of the paper; All authors read, edited, and approved the final manuscript.

Competing interests
The authors declare that they have no competing interests.

Author details
[1]Department of Behavioural Science & Health, University College London, London, England. [2]Department of Primary Care & Population Health, University College London, London, England. [3]Leeds Institute of Health Sciences, University of Leeds, Level 10, Worsley Building, Clarendon Way, Leeds LS2 9NL, England.

References
1. Finucane MM, Stevens GA, Cowan MJ, et al. National, regional, and global trends in body-mass index since 1980: systematic analysis of health examination surveys and epidemiological studies with 960 country-years and 9.1 million participants. Lancet. 2011;377:557–67.
2. Afshin A, Forouzanfar MH, Reitsma MB, et al. Health effects of overweight and obesity in 195 countries over 25 years. N Engl J Med. 2017;377:13–27.
3. WHO. Global status report on noncommunicable diseases 2014 no. 978 92 4 156485, vol. 4. Geneva: World Health Organization; 2014.
4. Beeken RJ, Leurent B, Vickerstaff V, et al. A brief intervention for weight control based on habit-formation theory delivered through primary care: results from a randomised controlled trial. Int J Obes. 2017;41:246–54.
5. Rothman AJ, Sheeran P, Wood W. Reflective and automatic processes in the initiation and maintenance of dietary change. Ann Behav Med. 2009;38:S4–S17.
6. Beeken RJ, Croker H, Morris S, et al. Study protocol for the 10 top tips (10TT) trial: randomised controlled trial of habit-based advice for weight control in general practice. BMC Public Health. 2012;12:667.
7. Verplanken B, Wood W. Interventions to break and create consumer habits. J Public Policy & Mark. 2006;25:90–103.
8. Gardner B. A review and analysis of the use of 'habit' in Understanding, predicting and influencing health-related behaviour. Health psych rev. 2014; 9:1–19.
9. Lally P, Gardner B. Promoting habit formation. Health Psych Rev. 2013;7:S137–58.
10. Lally P, Chipperfield A, Wardle J. Healthy habits: efficacy of simple advice on weight control based on a habit-formation model. Int J Obes. 2008;32:700–7.
11. Gardner B. A review and analysis of the use of 'habit' in understanding, predicting and influencing health-related behaviour. Health Psych Rev. 2015;9:277–95.
12. Craig P, Dieppe P, Macintyre S, et al. Developing and evaluating complex interventions: the new Medical Research Council guidance. Int J Nurs Stud. 2013;50:587–92.
13. Lally P, Van Jaarsveld CHM, Potts HWW, Wardle J. How are habits formed: modelling habit formation in the real world. Eur J Soc Psychol. 2010;40:998–1009.
14. Nederkoorn C, Houben K, Hofmann W, Roefs A, Jansen A. Control yourself or just eat what you like? Weight gain over a year is predicted by an interactive effect of response inhibition and implicit preference for snack foods. Health Psychol. 2010;29:389–93.
15. Baumeister RF, Gailliot M, DeWall CN, Oaten M. Self-regulation and personality: how interventions increase regulatory success, and how depletion moderates the effects of traits on behavior. J Pers. 2006;74:1773–801.
16. Boekaerts M, Maes S, Karoly P. Self-regulation across domains of applied psychology: is there an emerging consensus? Appl Psychol: an international review. 2005;54:149–54.
17. Carver CS, Scheier MF. On the self-regulation of behavior. New York: Cambridge University Press; 2001.
18. De Vet E, De Ridder D, Stok M, et al. Assessing self-regulation strategies: development and validation of the tempest self-regulation questionnaire for eating (TESQ-E) in adolescents. Int J Behav Nutr Phys Act. 2014;11:106.
19. Moilanen KL. The adolescent self-regulatory inventory: the development and validation of a questionnaire of short-term and long-term self-regulation. J Youth Adolesc. 2007;36:835–48.
20. Hagger MS. The multiple pathways by which trait self-control predicts health behavior. Ann Behav Med. 2014;48:282–3.
21. Johnson F, Pratt M, Wardle J. Dietary restraint and self-regulation in eating behavior. Int J Obes. 2012;36:665–74.
22. Hofmann W, Schmeichel BJ, Baddeley AD. Executive functions and self-regulation. Trends Cogn Sci. 2012;16:174–80.
23. Muraven M, Baumeister RF. Self-regulation and depletion of limited resources: does self-control resemble a muscle? Psychol Bull. 2000;126:247–59.
24. Kroese FM, Evers C, De Ridder DTD. How chocolate keeps you slim. The effect of food temptations on weight watching goal importance, intentions, and eating behavior. Appetite. 2009;53:430–3.
25. de Wit JB, Stok FM, Smolenski DJ, et al. Food culture in the home environment: family meal practices and values can support healthy eating and self-regulation in young people in four European countries. Appl Psychol Health Well Being. 2015;7:22–40.
26. Carey KB, Neal DJ, Collins SE. A psychometric analysis of the self-regulation questionnaire. Addic Behav. 2004;29:253–60.
27. Verplanken B, Orbell S. Reflections on past behavior: a self-report index of habit strength. J Appl Soc Psychol. 2003;33:1313–30.
28. Baron RM, Kenny DA. The moderator mediator variable distinction in social psychological-research - conceptual, strategic, and statistical considerations. J Pers Soc Psychol. 1986;51:1173–82.
29. Preacher KJ, Hayes AF. Asymptotic and resampling strategies for assessing and comparing indirect effects in multiple mediator models. Behav Res Methods. 2008;40:879–91.
30. Kreausukon P, Gellert P, Lippke S, Schwarzer R. Planning and self-efficacy can increase fruit and vegetable consumption: a randomized controlled trial. J Behav Med. 2012;35:443–51.
31. Lange D, Richert J, Koring M, et al. Self-regulation prompts can increase fruit consumption: a one-hour randomised controlled online trial. Psychol Health. 2013;28:533–45.
32. Luszczynska A, Tryburcy M, Schwarzer R. Improving fruit and vegetable consumption: a self-efficacy intervention compared with a combined self-efficacy and planning intervention. Health Educ Res. 2007;22:630–8.
33. Michie S, Abraham C, Whittington C, et al. Effective techniques in healthy eating and physical activity interventions: a meta-regression. Health Psychol. 2009;28:690–701.
34. Dombrowski SU, Knittle K, Avenell A, Araujo-Soares V, Sniehotta FF. Long term maintenance of weight loss with non-surgical interventions in obese adults: systematic review and meta-analyses of randomised controlled trials. Br Med J. 2014;348:g2646.
35. Bargh JA, Williams EL. The automaticity of social life. Curr Dir Psychol Sci. 2006;15:1–4.
36. Neal DT, Wood W, Drolet A. How do people adhere to goals when willpower is low? The profits (and pitfalls) of strong habits. J Pers Soc Psychol. 2013;104:959–75.
37. Kliemann N, Beeken RJ, Wardle J, Johnson F. Development and validation of the self-regulation of eating behaviour questionnaire for adults. Int J Behav Nutr Phys Act. 2016;13:87.
38. Gardner B, Abraham C, Lally P, de Bruijn GJ. Towards parsimony in habit measurement: testing the convergent and predictive validity of an automaticity subscale of the self-report habit index. Int J Behav Nutr Phys Act. 2012;9:102.
39. Bruening M, van Woerden I, Todd M, et al. A mobile ecological momentary assessment tool (devilSPARC) for nutrition and physical activity behaviors in college students: a validation study. J Med Internet Res. 2016;18:e209.
40. Christakis NA, Fowler JH. The spread of obesity in a large social network over 32 years. N Engl J Med. 2007;357:370–9.

5

Self-reported eating rate is associated with weight status in a Dutch population

Janet H.W. van den Boer, Jentina Kranendonk, Anne van de Wiel, Edith J.M. Feskens, Anouk Geelen and Monica Mars*

Abstract

Background: Observational studies performed in Asian populations suggest that eating rate is related to BMI. This paper investigates the association between self-reported eating rate (SRER) and body mass index (BMI) in a Dutch population, after having validated SRER against actual eating rate.

Methods: Two studies were performed; a validation and a cross-sectional study. In the validation study SRER (i.e., 'slow', 'average', or 'fast') was obtained from 57 participants (men/women = 16/41, age: mean ± SD = 22.6 ± 2. 8 yrs., BMI: mean ± SD = 22.1 ± 2.8 kg/m^2) and in these participants actual eating rate was measured for three food products. Using analysis of variance the association between SRER and actual eating rate was studied. The association between SRER and BMI was investigated in cross-sectional data from the NQplus cohort (i.e., 1473 Dutch adults; men/women*n* = 741/732, age: mean ± SD = 54.6 ± 11.7 yrs., BMI: mean ± SD = 25.9 ± 4.0 kg/m^2) using (multiple) linear regression analysis.

Results: In the validation study actual eating rate increased proportionally with SRER (for all three food products $P < 0.01$). In the cross-sectional study SRER was positively associated with BMI in both men and women ($P = 0.03$ and $P < 0.001$, respectively). Self-reported fast-eating women had a 1.13 kg/m^2 (95% CI 0.43, 1.84) higher BMI compared to average-speed-eating women, after adjusting for confounders. This was not the case in men; self-reported fast-eating men had a 0.29 kg/m^2 (95% CI -0.22, 0.80) higher BMI compared to average-speed-eating men, after adjusting for confounders.

Conclusions: These studies show that self-reported eating rate reflects actual eating rate on a group-level, and that a high self-reported eating rate is associated with a higher BMI in this Dutch population.

Keywords: Eating behavior, Eating style, Microstructure of eating, Eating fast, Speed of eating, Overweight

Background

Eating rate, the amount of food consumed per unit of time, has attracted attention for its potential role in preventing and treating obesity [1]. Slower eating is expected to reduce food intake and consequently body weight. Calories that pass quickly through the oral cavity go largely undetected and do not bring about an adequate satiety response, resulting in an increased intake [2]. Moreover, eating rate is a personal characteristic – some people tend to eat faster than others, or vice versa [3–5] – and eating rate could therefore affect long-term energy intake and consequently body weight. A recent meta-analysis has shown that the amount of food eaten can be altered by (experimentally) manipulating eating rate [6]. Furthermore, research indicates that eating rate might affect long-term energy intake and weight status [1, 7–9].

The relation between (self-reported) eating rate, energy intake and BMI has been studied in a number of cross-sectional studies, predominantly Asian. The results in general indicate that a higher self-reported eating rate (SRER) is associated with a higher long-term energy intake, though the results are not conclusive [10, 11].

* Correspondence: monica.mars@wur.nl
Division of Human Nutrition, Wageningen University, P.O. Box 17, 6700 AA Wageningen, The Netherlands

Furthermore, a recent study by Fogel et al. [12] showed that the actual eating rate of Singaporean children was positively associated with BMI. Regarding adults, a recent review and meta-analysis by Ohkuma et al. [7] showed that self-reported fast eaters were more likely to be overweight (BMI $\geq$ 25 kg/m^2) compared to self-reported slow eaters; All studies reported a positive association between eating rate and weight status, although there was a large variation in magnitude of the association. In addition, positive associations have been found between SRER and weight gain in longitudinal studies [13, 14]. For example, Tanihara et al. [13] found that male office workers who reported to be fast eaters on average gained 1.9 kg over a period of 8 years while the other male office workers only gained 0.7 kg on average.

This research consistently showed that SRER is associated with energy intake and BMI, but the generalizability of these findings is questionable. The studies in this field of research are limited to Asian populations, predominantly Japanese. To date only Leong et al. [15] investigated the association between SRER and BMI in a non-Asian population (i.e., New Zealand). This study, however, only included women, relied on self-reported data for height and weight, and did not collect data on energy intake. More research is needed to see if similar (positive) associations between SRER, energy intake and BMI exist in non-Asian populations, despite differences in diet, habits and ethnicity [7].

Furthermore, data on the validity of self-reported eating rate is limited [10, 16–18]. To our knowledge only Petty et al. [18] validated SRER against actual eating rate (g/min). They showed that, on a group-level, actual eating rate increased with increasing SRER-categories (i.e., slow, medium and fast). They, however, only validated SRER for one food product (i.e., pasta), and they did not address how well SRER reflects the actual eating rate of individuals.

Hence we aimed to validate self-reported eating rate and investigate its relation with energy intake and objectively assessed weight status in Dutch men and women. First we conducted a laboratory study validating self-reported eating rate in three foods varying in structure, after which we analyzed self-reported eating rate and different measures of weight status (i.e., BMI, waist circumference and body fat percentage) in a large, Dutch cohort study (i.e., NQplus [19]).

Methods

Study 1: Validation SRER

Study population and design

Students were recruited through posters at university buildings and student housing in Wageningen. Students who did not like the food products offered were excluded from participation. In total 64 students participated. Seven of them were excluded from the analyses; six because of a technical error and one because of mobile phone usage during the test session.

SRER and actual eating rate were obtained from participants during a single visit to the university in October–November 2013. This allowed for comparison between SRER and actual eating rate within persons. Participants were told that the aim of the study was to pilot test lunch products for another study.

Procedure

Participants were instructed not to eat anything in the 2 h prior to their lunch at the university. First they filled out a questionnaire on their eating behavior which included a question on eating rate: "How would you describe your eating rate compared with others? 'Very slow', 'slow', 'average', 'fast' or 'very fast'?". This question was based on previous research [10, 15]. Subsequently the participants received three lunch products: first a soft bun with cheese, then apple, and finally vanilla custard. Serving sizes differed between participants. The total lunch offered represented a normal lunch in terms of energy content; i.e., 20% of the daily energy requirement of the individual participants, which was estimated using the Schofield equation while assuming a moderate physical activity level [20, 21]. Participants pressed the spacebar of the laptop in front of them with the first bite of a product and again when they swallowed the last bite. The time between pressing the spacebars was recorded, which represents the time spent eating. Intake was measured by weighing the products prior to and after consumption. Actual eating rate was determined by dividing the intake in grams by the time spent eating in minutes for each product separately.

Furthermore, before the consumption of each product and at the end participants rated their level of satiety using visual analogue scales (0-100 mm); Feelings of hunger (Not at all-Extremely), fullness (Not at all-Extremely), satiety (Not at all-Extremely), desire to eat (Very weak-Very strong) and prospective consumption (Nothing at all-A very large amount) were rated [22]. Overall satiety scores were calculated by extracting the average of the scores for hunger, desire to eat and prospective consumption from the average of the scores for fullness and satiation [22]. Moreover, after the consumption of each product participants indicated how much they liked the product (1, Dislike very much – 5 Like very much).

Study 2: Association between SRER and weight status

Study population and design

This study investigates data from NQplus, an ongoing cohort study designed to: validate a newly developed FFQ, start a reference database for nutrition research and study associations between diet and intermediate health outcomes [19, 23]. The cohort consists of adults (20–70 years old) randomly selected from households in Wageningen, Renkum, Ede, Arnhem and Veenendaal. Participants were recruited via letters and emails between May 2011 and March 2013. In total 2048 people were included. SRER was available of 1642 participants; The other participants either did not answer the eating rate question, or dropped out before receiving the question. Finally, 1473 participants were included in the analyses, as other data (i.e., data on age, smoking, education level, emotional eating, restraint eating, and/or external eating) was missing for 169 out of the 1642 participants with SRER.

Since registration the participants received a number of questionnaires (which twice included the eating rate question). Additionally, anthropometric measurements were taken. The collected data was used for the cross-sectional analysis of the association between SRER and weight status.

Online questionnaires

General characteristics At baseline participants reported their highest completed education, which was categorized into three groups; low (i.e., no education, primary education, lower or preparatory vocational education, or lower general secondary education), medium (i.e., intermediate vocational education or apprenticeship, or higher general secondary education or pre-university secondary education) and high (i.e., higher vocational education or university). Additionally, the participants completed a semi-quantitative food frequency questionnaire (FFQ) on last month's intake which was used to calculate average daily energy intake. This FFQ has been found to be valid to assess mean energy intake in large samples and for ranking individuals [24].

Furthermore, the participants received the 'Dutch Eating Behavior Questionnaire' (DEBQ) [25]. The DEBQ contains 33 items; 13 items reflect emotional eating, ten items reflect external eating and ten items reflect restrained eating. Average scores were calculated to obtain sub scores for emotional, external and restrained eating. Usual physical activity was assessed using two questionnaires: i.e., the 'Activity Questionnaire for Adults and Adolescents' (AQUAA) for sedentary activity [26], and the 'Short questionnaire to assess health-enhancing physical activity' (SQUASH) for moderate-to-vigorous activity [27]. Both sedentary and moderate-to-vigorous activity were determined in minutes per week, and were converted to hours per week for the analyses.

Self-reported eating rate Participants twice received a questionnaire that included the eating rate question (see validation study). The median time in between was 12.1 months. In the analyses we used the SRER off the first time the participants answered the eating rate-question. SRER-data from the second time the participants answered the eating rate-question was only used to test repeatability.

Anthropometrics

Anthropometric measurements were performed twice. The median time in between was 12.9 months. Height was measured, without footwear, to the nearest 0.1 cm using a stadiometer (SECA, Hamburg, Germany). Weight was measured to the nearest 0.1 kg using a digital scale (SECA, Hamburg, Germany), after taking of footwear and heavy clothes and removing heavy items from the pockets. Waist circumference was measured between the lowest rib and the iliac crest to the nearest 0.5 cm using a non-elastic flexible tape (SECA, Hamburg, Germany), after removing thick clothes from that area. This measurement was performed twice and the average of those measurements was used for analyses. Finally, body fat percentage was measured using a DEXA-scan (Lunar Prodigy Advance; GE Healthcare, Madison, Wisconsin, United States).

For the current analyses we used the anthropometric data of the visit closest to the first time the eating rate-question was answered. On average there were 165 (±91) days between answering the eating rate-question for the first time and the anthropometric measurements.

Statistical analyses

SPSS (IBM SPSS Statistics, Version 20, IBM Corporation, Armonk, NY, USA) was used for the statistical analyses. Means and standard deviations are given, unless stated otherwise. *P*-values of <0.05 were considered statistically significant. Normality was judged by visual inspection using QQplots; all data were normally distributed.

SRER was split into three categories for the analyses, as in both studies only few participants reported to be a very slow or very fast eater; The 'very slow' category was combined with the 'slow'-category and the 'fast' category with the 'very fast'-category.

Study 1: Validation SRER

By means of analysis of variance it was investigated whether there was a linear trend between SRER and actual eating rate. Post-hoc analyses (Gabriel's procedure) were performed to identify differences in actual eating rate between SRER-categories. To investigate how well SRER reflects the actual eating rate of individuals, the level of agreement between SRER and tertiles of actual eating rate was determined by calculating kappa (κ) (i.e., chance-corrected proportional agreement) [28].

Furthermore, correlation analyses were performed to investigate the association between the eating rate of the lunch products, between eating rate and liking, and between eating rate and satiety. Independent t-tests were performed to investigate whether eating rate differed between men and women.

Study 2: Association between SRER and weight status

Data were analyzed for the total population and for men and women separately, as both eating rate and BMI are sex-dependent [29, 30]. Kappa (κ) was calculated to assess the level of agreement between answers of participants that answered the eating rate-question on two separate occasions [28]. One-way analyses of variance, independent samples T-tests and chi-square tests were performed to check whether the participant characteristics (e.g., weight status and intake) differed between males and females and between the SRER-categories. Linear regression analysis was performed to investigate whether there was a linear trend between the SRER-categories and participant characteristics.

Furthermore, multiple linear regression analyses were performed to investigate the association between SRER and BMI with adjustment for potential confounders. First a crude model was tested with two dummy variables of SRER; one for comparing fast with average eating rate, one for comparing slow with average eating rate. In a second model age, smoking and education level were added. In the third and main model DEBQ-scores (i.e., emotional, restrained and external eating) were added. In an additional model, 'Model X,' energy intake, moderate-to-vigorous activity and sedentary activity were added to the main model. Suspected under reporters of energy intake (i.e., reported energy intake/calculated basal metabolic rate < 1.35 [31]) were excluded. Due to the exclusion of suspected under reporters and missing data 'Model X' is based on a small subset of the total sample, and is therefore not considered to be the main model. Furthermore, it was investigated whether there was a linear trend between the SRER-categories and BMI in the different models by replacing the dummy variables with the categorical variable for SRER.

Finally, odds ratios for overweight (i.e., BMI ≥ 25 kg/m^2) were determined for self-reported fast eaters (compared to self-reported slow plus average-speed eaters) by means of logistic regression analyses, taking into account potential confounders (i.e., age, smoking, education level, emotional eating, restrained eating and external eating).

Results

Study 1: Validation SRER

In total 57 (men/women n = 16/41) participants (22.6 ± 2.8 years old, self-reported BMI of 22.1 ± 2.8 kg/m^2) were included. Eleven participants reported to be a slow eater (i.e., very slow (n = 1) or slow (n = 10)), 27 participants reported to be an average speed eater, and 19 participants reported to be a fast eater (i.e., fast (n = 18) or very fast (n = 1)). Eating rate (g/min) increased proportionally with SRER for all three lunch products (bread with cheese F (1, 51) = 10.45, P < 0.01; apple F (1, 43) = 12.79, P < 0.01; vanilla custard F (1, 49) = 13.12, P < 0.01) (Fig. 1). Post-hoc analyses showed that eating rate was significantly higher in self-reported fast eaters compared to self-reported slow and average-speed eaters, but did not differ between self-reported slow and average-speed eaters.

The level of agreement between SRER and actual eating rate-tertiles was fair; for all three lunch products a κ-value of 0.25 was found [28]. Within all lunch products actual eating rate-tertiles corresponded with SRER in 50% of the cases, while in about 10% of the cases the actual eating rate-quartiles and SRER showed the

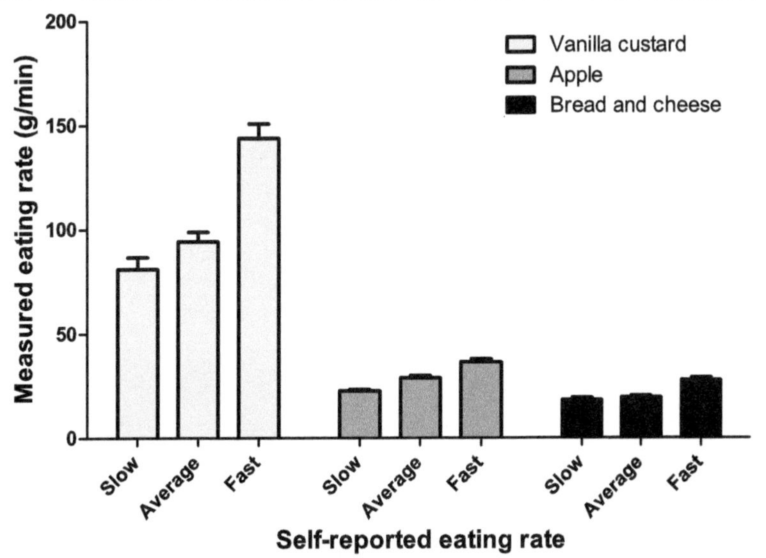

Fig. 1 Actual eating rate within self-reported eating rate-categories (n = 57)

opposite; e.g., indicated to be a slow eater, while actual eating rate was in the highest tertile.

Furthermore, how fast participants consumed one lunch product was correlated with how fast they ate the other lunch products (bread with cheese x apple, $r = .54$ $P < 0.001$; bread with cheese x vanilla custard, $r = .50$ $P < 0.001$; apple x vanilla custard, $r = .69$ $P < 0.001$). Liking was correlated with eating rate in vanilla custard ($r = .37$, $P < 0.01$), but not in bread with cheese ($r = -.02$, $P = 0.90$) and apple ($r = .16$, $P = .28$). Moreover, eating rate was not associated with the satiety score at the start of consumption for all three lunch products (bread with cheese, $r = -.13$ $P = 0.37$; apple, $r = .07$ $P = 0.66$; vanilla custard, $r = -.12$ $P = 0.41$). Finally, men ate all three lunch products faster than women (bread with cheese t (52) = −4.84, $P < 0.001$; apple t (44) = −6.22, $P < 0.001$, vanilla custard t (50) = −4.65, $P < 0.001$).

Table 1 Characteristics of the men and women participating in NQplus

	Men			Women			*P*
	n	Mean	SD	n	Mean	SD	
Age (yrs.)	741	57.5	10.6	732	51.8	12.0	<0.001[a]
Height (cm)	741	180.4	6.8	732	168.6	6.3	<0.001[a]
Weight (kg)	741	86.0	12.8	732	71.8	13.2	<0.001[a]
BMI (kg/m^2)	741	26.4	3.5	732	25.3	4.4	<0.001[a]
Waist circumference (cm)	737	96.9	10.7	731	85.8	11.6	<0.001[a]
Body fat percentage (%)	683	24.7	6.6	613	34.9	7.7	<0.001[a]
Energy intake (MJ/day)	691	9.5	2.6	654	7.8	2.1	<0.001[a]
Energy intake (MJ/day)[c]	288	11.7	2.1	296	9.4	1.6	<0.001[a]
Emotional eating score	741	1.94	0.65	732	2.28	0.74	<0.001[a]
Restrained eating score	741	2.87	0.73	732	3.13	0.68	<0.001[a]
External eating score	741	2.70	0.43	732	2.71	0.45	0.48[a]
Moderate-to-vigorous activity (hours/week)	696	33.9	18.5	666	35.3	16.9	0.13[a]
Sedentary activity (hours/week)	696	36.6	21.0	666	36.4	34.0	0.90[a]
		n	%		n	%	
Prevalence of overweight[d]		460	62.1		322	44.0	<0.001[b]
Prevalence of obesity[e]		118	15.9		91	12.4	0.06[b]
Self-reported eating rate							
Very slow		5	0.7		13	1.8	<0.001[b]
Slow		54	7.3		104	14.2	
Average		315	42.5		408	55.7	
Fast		316	42.6		183	25.0	
Very fast		51	6.9		24	3.3	
Education level [f]							
Low		111	15.0		122	16.7	0.58[b]
Medium		217	29.3		219	29.9	
High		413	55.7		391	53.4	
Smoking status							
Non-smoker		664	89.6		676	92.3	0.07[b]
Smoker		77	10.4		56	7.7	

[a]Independent samples T-test
[b]Chi-square test
[c]Suspected under reporters (i.e., reported energy intake/calculated basal metabolic rate < 1.35) excluded
[d]BMI ≥25 kg/m^2
[e]BMI ≥30 kg/m^2
[f]Education level: low (i.e., no education, primary education, lower or preparatory vocational education, or lower general secondary education), medium (i.e., intermediate vocational education or apprenticeship, or higher general secondary education or pre-university secondary education) and high (i.e., higher vocational education or university)

Study 2: Association between SRER and weight status

Data from 741 men and 732 women is included in the main analyses (Table 1). On average, men were 57.5 ± 10.6 years old and had a BMI of 26.4 ± 3.5 kg/m^2 whereas women were 51.8 ± 12.0 years old and had a BMI of 25.3 ± 4.4 kg/m^2. Collectively, ages ranged from 21.7–77.0 yrs. old and BMI from 16.8–57.6 kg/m^2 for the two groups.th=tlb=

Table 1 shows the prevalence of all five SRER-categories in men and women. The SRER-categories were distributed differently for men and women (chi-square, $P < 0.001$); compared to women, men more often reported to be fast eaters. Furthermore, 931 participants (men/women = 458/ 473) answered the eating rate question twice (Table 2). A κ-value of 0.64 was found for the level of agreement between the answers to both questions.

Tables 3 and 4 show the characteristics of the participants by SRER-category (i.e., slow, average, fast). A positive linear association was found between BMI and SRER-category in both men ($r = .08$, $P = 0.03$) and women ($r = .16$, $P < 0.001$). Also waist circumference and body fat percentage showed a positive association with SRER in women (waist circumference $r = .10$, $P < 0.01$; body fat percentage $r = .14$, $P < 0.001$), but not in men (waist circumference $r = .01$, $P = 0.74$; body fat percentage $r = .01$, $P = 0.71$). In addition SRER was positively associated with moderate-to-vigorous activity, restrained eating and external eating in men, and positively associated with emotional, restrained and external eating in women.

In both men and women SRER was not associated with energy intake before excluding participants suspected of under reporting energy intake (Table 3). In total, 754 participants (men/women = 399/355) were identified as underreporting their energy intake. After excluding these participants SRER was positively associated with energy intake in men ($r = .13$, $P = 0.03$ ($n = 296$)) and women ($r = .17$, $P < 0.01$ ($n = 288$)). In turn, energy intake was positively associated with BMI in men and women after excluding suspected under reporters and adjusting for sedentary and moderate-to-vigorous activity; regression coefficients were 0.28 kg/m^2 /MJ (95% CI: 0.12, 0.44) for men and 0.55 kg/m^2/MJ (95% CI: 0.30, 0.79) for women (men/wome*n* = 273/281).

Model 3 in Table 5 shows the associations between SRER-categories and BMI after adjusting for age, smoking, education level, emotional eating, restrained eating, and external eating. BMI was 1.13 kg/m^2 higher in self-reported fast-eating women compared to self-reported average-speed-eating women. The BMI of self-reported slow-eating women was not significantly different from that of self-reported average-speed-eating women. In men the BMI of both self-reported slow- and fast-eaters was not significantly different from that of self-reported average-speed-eaters. The relation between SRER and BMI was not significantly different between men and women (interaction effect in multiple linear regression: $P = 0.06$). Furthermore, when energy intake, moderate-to-vigorous activity and sedentary activity were added to the main model, the results remained similar (men/ women = 273/281) (Table 5, Model X).

Finally, self-reported fast eaters were at higher risk to be overweight (i.e., BMI ≥ 25 kg/m^2) compared to the other participants (i.e., self-reported average- plus slow-speed eaters) with an adjusted odds ratio of 1.73 (95% CI: 1.38, 2.17). Within women this adjusted odds ratio was 2.05 (95% CI: 1.44, 2.91), while within men this was 1.13 (95% CI: 0.82, 1.56). These odds ratios were not significantly different for men and women (interaction effect in logistic regression: $P = 0.09$).

Table 2 Frequency of self-reported eating rate-categories (SRER) in participants that answered the eating rate question twice[a]

		SRER second time				
		Very slow	Slow	Average	Fast	Very fast
SRER first time	Very slow	13	3	0	0	0
	Slow	5	87	23	2	0
	Average	0	36	367	58	0
	Fast	1	0	49	226	18
	Very fast	0	0	2	18	23

[a]κ-value = 0.64

Discussion

In these studies self-reported eating rate was validated against actual eating rate, and the association between self-reported eating rate (SRER) and weight status was investigated in a Dutch population. The validation study confirmed that self-reported eating rate was positively associated with actual eating rate. The cross-sectional data from the NQplus cohort showed that self-reported eating rate was positively associated with BMI among both men and women. After adjusting for confounders self-reported eating rate remained significantly associated with BMI in women; fast eaters had on average a 1.13 kg/m^2 higher BMI compared to average-speed eaters. In men this relation was no longer significant after adjusting for confounders; nonetheless, the direction of the association was still in the expected direction. Overall, self-reported fast eaters were more likely to be overweight compared to self-reported non-fast eaters.

These findings are in line with previous studies investigating the association between SRER and weight status. In the current study the adjusted odds ratio for being overweight, comparing self-reported fast eaters to non-fast eaters, was 1.73 (95% CI: 1.38, 2.17); where Ohkuma et al. [7] found a pooled odds ratio of 2.15 (95% CI, 1.84–2.51) in their meta-analysis. This shows that previous findings

Table 3 Characteristics (mean ± SD) of the participants by self-reported eating rate-category, within the total population and in men and women separately

	Self-reported eating rate									P ANOVA	P linear trend
	Slow			Average			Fast				
	n	mean	SD	n	mean	SD	n	mean	SD		
Total											
Age (yrs.)	176	53.0	13.1	723	55.1	11.0	574	54.6	12.1	0.11	.42
BMI (kg/m^2)	176	24.8	4.1	723	25.5	4.0	574	26.6	3.9	<0.001	<0.001
Waist circumference (cm)	175	88.2	13.1	721	90.4	12.3	572	93.6	12.2	<0.001	<0.001
Body fat percentage (%)	145	29.9	9.0	647	30.2	8.6	504	28.6	8.8	0.01	0.01
Energy intake (MJ/day)	158	8.4	2.3	662	8.5	2.4	525	8.9	2.7	<0.01	<0.01
Energy intake (MJ/day) [a]	75	9.9	1.8	300	10.2	2.0	209	11.3	2.4	<0.001	<0.001
Emotional eating	176	2.13	0.69	723	2.06	0.71	574	2.17	0.73	0.02	0.09
Restrained eating	176	2.86	0.79	723	3.01	0.72	574	3.03	0.69	0.03	0.03
External eating	176	2.61	0.48	723	2.67	0.42	574	2.78	0.43	<0.001	<0.001
Moderate-to-vigorous activity (h/day)	164	35.4	19.5	663	33.8	17.0	535	35.4	18.0	0.24	0.53
Sedentary activity (h/day)	164	37.6	35.0	663	35.5	29.0	534	37.4	24.4	0.45	0.68
Men											
Age (yrs.)	59	57.9	10.7	315	58.2	10.0	367	56.7	11.1	0.16	0.10
BMI (kg/m^2)	59	25.7	3.9	315	26.3	3.4	367	26.7	3.5	0.09	0.03
Waist circumference (cm)	58	96.1	10.9	314	97.0	10.7	365	96.9	10.7	0.82	0.74
Body fat percentage (%)	52	23.8	6.9	294	24.9	6.8	337	24.7	6.4	0.56	0.71
Energy intake (MJ/day)	54	10.0	2.4	295	9.3	2.5	342	9.5	2.8	0.25	0.89
Energy intake (MJ/day) [a]	27	11.5	1.6	125	11.4	2.0	136	12.0	2.2	0.04	0.03
Emotional eating	59	2.01	0.68	315	1.85	0.61	367	2.01	0.67	<0.01	0.053
Restrained eating	59	2.65	0.79	315	2.84	0.75	367	2.92	0.69	0.02	<0.01
External eating	59	2.62	0.48	315	2.64	0.42	367	2.76	0.43	0.001	<0.001
Moderate-to-vigorous activity (h/day)	57	31.5	19.0	298	32.6	17.8	341	35.4	18.9	0.10	0.04
Sedentary activity (h/day)	57	37.6	19.4	298	35.0	18.8	341	37.8	22.9	0.23	0.30
Women											
Age (yrs.)	117	50.6	13.5	408	52.7	11.1	207	50.8	12.9	0.09	0.75
BMI (kg/m^2)	117	24.4	4.2	408	25.0	4.3	207	26.4	4.6	<0.001	<0.001
Waist circumference (cm)	117	84.2	12.4	407	85.3	10.9	207	87.6	12.3	0.02	<0.01
Body fat percentage (%)	93	33.2	8.3	353	34.6	7.4	167	36.5	7.7	<0.01	<0.001
Energy intake (MJ/day)	104	7.6	1.8	367	7.8	2.0	183	7.8	2.3	0.58	0.39
Energy intake (MJ/day) [a]	48	9.0	1.1	175	9.4	1.5	73	9.8	1.9	0.02	<0.01
Emotional eating	117	2.19	0.69	408	2.22	0.73	207	2.45	0.74	0.001	<0.001
Restrained eating	117	2.97	0.77	408	3.4	0.66	207	3.21	0.65	<0.01	<0.001
External eating	117	2.60	0.48	408	2.69	0.43	207	2.82	0.44	<0.001	<0.001
Moderate-to-vigorous activity (h/day)	107	37.5	19.5	365	34.7	16.4	194	35.3	16.4	0.31	0.41
Sedentary activity (h/day)	107	37.7	41.1	365	35.9	35.2	193	36.6	27.0	0.90	0.87

[a]Suspected under reporters (i.e., reported energy intake/calculated basal metabolic rate < 1.35) excluded

from Asian populations may translate to non-Asian populations. The current study was the first to investigate this association in a non-Asian population that included men and objectively measured height, weight, waist circumference and body fat percentage.

Eating rate is expected to affect weight status via energy intake. If people eat fast, calories pass through the oral cavity quickly, are not sensed and do not bring about an adequate satiety response, resulting in an increased intake [32–36]. The current findings are in line

Table 4 Frequency of participant characteristics by self-reported eating rate-category, within the total population and in men and women separately

	Self-reported eating rate						*P* chi-square test
	Slow		Average		Fast		
	n	%	n	%	n	%	
Total[a]							
Prevalence of overweight[d]	75	42.6	354	49.0	353	61.5	<0.01
Prevalence of obesity[e]	18	10.2	89	12.3	102	17.8	<0.01
Prevalence of smoking	19	10.8	56	7.7	58	10.1	0.23
Education level[f]							
Low	29	16.5	126	17.4	78	13.6	0.19
Medium	44	25.0	220	30.4	172	30.0	
High	103	58.5	377	52.1	324	56.4	
Men[b]							
Prevalence of overweight[d]	29	49.2	196	62.2	235	64.0	0.09
Prevalence of obesity[e]	6	10.2	48	15.2	64	17.4	0.33
Prevalence of smoking	6	10.2	31	9.8	40	10.9	0.71
Education level[f]							
Low	12	20.3	52	16.5	47	12.8	0.37
Medium	13	22.0	92	29.2	112	30.5	
High	34	57.6	171	54.3	208	56.7	
Women[c]							
Prevalence of overweight[d]	46	39.3	158	38.7	118	57.0	<0.001
Prevalence of obesity[e]	12	10.3	41	10.0	38	18.4	0.01
Prevalence of smoking	13	11.1	25	6.1	18	8.7	0.16
Education level[f]							
Low	17	14.5	74	18.1	31	15.0	0.46
Medium	31	26.5	128	31.4	60	29.0	
High	69	59.0	206	50.5	116	56.0	

[a]Slow, *n* = 176; Average, *n* = 723; Fast, *n* = 574
[b]Slow, *n* = 59; Average, *n* = 315; Fast, *n* = 367
[c]Slow, *n* = 117; Average, *n* = 408; Fast, *n* = 207
[d]BMI ≥25 kg/m^2
[e]BMI ≥30 kg/m^2
[f]Education level: low (i.e., no education, primary education, lower or preparatory vocational education, or lower general secondary education), medium (i.e., intermediate vocational education or apprenticeship, or higher general secondary education or pre-university secondary education) and high (i.e., higher vocational education or university)

with this. After excluding suspected under reporters, energy intake was positively associated with BMI. More importantly, energy intake was positively associated with SRER. Previous studies also found positive relations between energy intake and SRER, although not always statistically significant. More accurate measurements of energy intake might reveal stronger relations between energy intake, SRER and BMI. The problem with dietary assessment methods is that the measurement error depends on BMI; overweight people are more likely to underreport energy intake [24]. Excluding under-reporters does not completely resolve this issue.

Furthermore, the validation study confirms that on a group level self-reported eating rate reflects actual eating rate in young adults. Actual eating rate increased proportionally with SRER-categories, and like Petty et al. [18], we found that actual eating rate was significantly higher in self-reported fast eaters compared to self-reported slow and average-speed eaters. We assumed that these findings will also translate to older adults, as eating rate appears to be a stable personal characteristic [3–5]. Moreover, we did not find an association between SRER and age in the cross-sectional study.

However, when examining the results of the validation study at the individual level, only half of the participants correctly classified themselves according to their actual eating rate. The kappa-values showed that after correcting for chance the remaining agreement between SRER

Table 5 Association between self-reported eating rate (SRER) and BMI within the total population and in men and women separately according to multiple linear regression analysis and linear trend analyses

Independent variables	Model 1[a]		Model 2[b]		Model 3[c]		Model X[d]	
	Partial regression coefficient	95% CI or *P*	Partial regression coefficient	95% CI or *P*	Partial regression coefficient	95% CI or *P*	Partial regression coefficient	95% CI or *P*
Total		(*n* = 1473)		(n = 1473)		(n = 1473)		(*n* = 554)
SRER-categories								
Slow	−0.69	(−1.35, −0.03)	−0.57	(−1.22, 0.08)	−0.48	(−1.11, 0.15)	−0.47	(−1.20, 0.27)
Average	0.00	(reference)	0.00	(reference)	0.00	(reference)	0.00	(reference)
Fast	1.03	(0.59, 1.47)	1.09	(0.66, 1.52)	0.90	(0.48, 1.32)	0.58	(0.05, 1.10)
Linear trend		<0.001		<0.001		<0.001		<0.01
Men		(n = 741)		(n = 741)		(n = 741)		(n = 273)
SRER-categories								
Slow	−0.57	(−1.55, 0.41)	−0.56	(−1.51, 0.40)	−0.47	(−1.40, 0.47)	−0.42	(−1.49, 0.65)
Average	0.00	(reference)	0.00	(reference)	0.00	(reference)	0.00	(reference)
Fast	0.40	(−0.14, 0.93)	0.51	(−0.001, 1.03)	0.29	(−0.22, 0.80)	0.28	(−0.38, 0.94)
Linear trend		0.03		<0.01		0.08		0.18
Women		(*n* = 732)		(n = 732)		(n = 732)		(*n* = 281)
SRER-categories								
Slow	−0.56	(−1.46, 0.34)	−0.44	(−1.34, 0.45)	−0.24	(−1.11, 0.63)	−0.34	(−1.36, 0.67)
Average	0.00	(reference)	0.00	(reference)	0.00	(reference)	0.00	(reference)
Fast	1.40	(0.67, 2.14)	1.51	(0.78, 2.23)	1.13	(0.43, 1.84)	0.71	(−0.15, 1.56)
Linear trend		<0.001		<0.001		<0.01		0.06

[a]Crude model
[b]Crude model with age, smoking and level of education
[c]Crude model with age, smoking, level of education, emotional eating, restrained eating and external eating
[d] Crude model with age, smoking, level of education, emotional eating, restrained eating, external eating, energy intake, moderate-to-vigorous activity and sedentary activity (excl. Suspected under reporters of energy intake; i.e., reported energy intake/calculated basal metabolic rate < 1.35)

and tertiles of actual eating rate was only 25%, which is considered 'fair' [28]. As such, SRER might not be a good measure for actual eating rate at the individual level. In the cross-sectional study, however, SRER was used as a measure of eating rate on a group-level. Furthermore, this imperfect agreement between SRER and actual eating rate might mean that the results of the cross-sectional analysis underestimate the true association between eating rate and BMI.

Different explanations exist for the agreement between SRER and actual eating rate being only fair. First, people might not be aware of their eating rate, although this does not seem to be the case. There is good agreement between the answers of people that answered the eating rate question twice, which shows that they have a fixed image of their eating rate. Second, people might interpret eating rate differently than scientists. Third, people are limited to their own observations to evaluate their eating rate and that of others. People do not monitor their eating rate like scientists would: i.e., using a stopwatch and kitchen scale. So how do they answer the eating rate-question? They, for example, could base their answer on how long it takes them to finish one portion or the length of their meals. Finally, they could use different people as a reference.

More intervention studies are needed to investigate if there is a causal relation between (self-reported) eating rate and BMI, and whether this is mediated by long-term energy intake. Based on evidence from experimental studies, these intervention studies should focus on increasing oral sensory exposure time. Some interventions targeting eating rate have already been examined. Spiegel et al. [1] included advice on reducing eating rate in a weight loss program. Participants successfully reduced eating rate, which resulted in weight loss. However, the slower eating rate was not maintained over time. McGee et al. [8] performed a four-month intervention with an 'oral volume restriction device'. This device was worn in the upper palate during a meal, which reduced bite size and thereby eating rate. Participants that used the device most lost more weight. Further advancements could be made by using new technologies, which offer useful tools for both monitoring and altering eating rate. The SPLENDID-system and 10SFork constitute examples of such new technologies [37, 38]. Both provide real-time feedback on eating rate. Usage of such technologies seems to be the logical next step for future research.

Conclusions

The two current studies showed that 1) self-reported eating rate reflects actual eating rate on a group-level, but not at the individual level, and 2) that self-reported fast eating is associated with a higher BMI in a Dutch, adult population, although this association was more pronounced in women. Lowering eating rate might be a promising strategy in tackling obesity. However, first more empirical evidence is needed to confirm the causal relationship between (self-reported) eating rate and BMI, and to show the effectiveness of interventions targeting eating rate.

Abbreviations

AQUAA: Activity questionnaire for adults and adolescents; BMI: Body mass index; CI: Confidence interval; DEBQ: Dutch eating behavior questionnaire; SQUASH: Short questionnaire to assess health-enhancing physical activity; SRER: Self-reported eating rate

Acknowledgements

Not applicable.

Funding

None.

Authors' contributions

AW, EF, AG and MM were involved in the conception and design of the studies. EF, AG, AW, JK and JB were involved in the data collection. JB analyzed the data and wrote the manuscript. EF, AG and MM provided guidance on the analysis and write-up. JK, AW, EF, AG and MM commented on drafts of the manuscript. All authors read and approved the final manuscript.

Competing interests

The authors declare that they have no competing interests.

References

1. Spiegel TA, Wadden TA, Foster GD. Objective measurement of eating rate during Behavioral treatment of obesity. Behav Ther. 1991;22:61–7.
2. de Graaf C, Kok FJ. Slow food, fast food and the control of food intake. Nat Rev Endocrinol. 2010;6:290–3.
3. Zijlstra N, Mars M, Stafleu A, de Graaf C. The effect of texture differences on satiation in 3 pairs of solid foods. Appetite. 2010;55:490–7.
4. Brown WE, Langley KR, Martin A, Macfie HJH. Characterization of patterns of chewing behavior in human-subjects and their influence on texture-perception. J Texture Stud. 1994;25:455–68.
5. Devezeaux de Lavergne M, Derks JAM, Ketel EC, de Wijk RA, Stieger M. Eating behaviour explains differences between individuals in dynamic texture perception of sausages. Food Qual Prefer. 2015;41:189–200.
6. Robinson E, Almiron-Roig E, Rutters F, de Graaf C, Forde CG, Tudur Smith C, Nolan SJ, Jebb SA. A systematic review and meta-analysis examining the effect of eating rate on energy intake and hunger. Am J Clin Nutr. 2014;100:123–51.
7. Ohkuma T, Hirakawa Y, Nakamura U, Kiyohara Y, Kitazono T, Ninomiya T. Association between eating rate and obesity: a systematic review and meta-analysis. Int J Obes. 2015;39:1589–96.
8. McGee TL, Grima MT, Hewson ID, Jones KM, Duke EB, Dixon JB. First Australian experiences with an oral volume restriction device to change eating Behaviors and assist with weight loss. Obesity. 2012;20:126–33.
9. Ford AL, Bergh C, Sodersten P, Sabin MA, Hollinghurst S, Hunt LP, Shield JP. Treatment of childhood obesity by retraining eating behaviour: randomised controlled trial. BMJ. 2010;340:b5388.
10. Sasaki S, Katagiri A, Tsuji T, Shimoda T, Amano K. Self-reported rate of eating correlates with body mass index in 18-y-old Japanese women. Int J Obes Relat Metab Disord. 2003;27:1405–10.
11. Sakurai M, Nakamura K, Miura K, Takamura T, Yoshita K, Nagasawa SY, Morikawa Y, Ishizaki M, Kido T, Naruse Y, et al. Self-reported speed of eating and 7-year risk of type 2 diabetes mellitus in middle-aged Japanese men. Metabolism. 2012;61:1566–71.
12. Fogel A, Goh AT, Fries LR, Sadananthan SA, Velan SS, Michael N, Tint M-T, Fortier MV, Chan MJ, Toh JY, et al. Faster eating rates are associated with higher energy intakes during an ad libitum meal, higher BMI and greater adiposity among 4·5-year-old children: results from the growing up in Singapore towards healthy outcomes (GUSTO) cohort. Br J Nutr. 2017;117:1042–51.
13. Tanihara S, Imatoh T, Miyazaki M, Babazono A, Momose Y, Baba M, Uryu Y, Une H. Retrospective longitudinal study on the relationship between 8-year weight change and current eating speed. Appetite. 2011;57:179–83.
14. Otsuka R, Tamakoshi K, Yatsuya H, Murata C, Sekiya A, Wada K, Zhang HM, Matsushita K, Sugiura K, Takefuji S, et al. Eating fast leads to obesity: findings based on self-administered questionnaires among middle-aged Japanese men and women. J Epidemiol. 2006;16:117–24.
15. Leong SL, Madden C, Gray A, Waters D, Horwath C. Faster self-reported speed of eating is related to higher body mass index in a nationwide survey of middle-aged women. J Am Diet Assoc. 2011;111:1192–7.
16. Ekuni D, Furuta M, Takeuchi N, Tomofuji T, Morita M. Self-reports of eating quickly are related to a decreased number of chews until first swallow, total number of chews, and total duration of chewing in young people. Arch Oral Biol. 2012;57:981–6.
17. Ohkuma T, Fujii H, Iwase M, Kikuchi Y, Ogata S, Idewaki Y, Ide H, Doi Y, Hirakawa Y, Mukai N, et al. Impact of eating rate on obesity and cardiovascular risk factors according to glucose tolerance status: the Fukuoka diabetes registry and the Hisayama study. Diabetologia. 2013;56:70–7.
18. Petty AJ, Melanson KJ, Greene GW. Self-reported eating rate aligns with laboratory measured eating rate but not with free-living meals. Appetite. 2013;63:36–41.
19. van Lee L, Feskens EJ, Meijboom S, Hooft van Huysduynen EJ, Van't Veer P, de Vries JH, Geelen A. Evaluation of a screener to assess diet quality in the Netherlands. Br J Nutr. 2016;115:517–26.
20. Jongvolwassenen, inneming macronutriënten per eetmoment [http://www.rivm.nl/Documenten_en_publicaties/Wetenschappelijk/Tabellen_grafieken/Leefstijl_Voeding/VCP/Jongvolwassenen_2003/Jongvolwassenen_inneming_macronutri_nten_per_eetmome].
21. WHO: Joint FAO/WHO/UNU Expert Consultation on Energy and Protein Requirements (1981: Rome, Italy). In Technical Report Series no 724. Geneva; 1985.
22. Blundell J, De Graaf C, Hulshof T, Jebb S, Livingstone B, Lluch A, Mela D, Salah S, Schuring E, Van Der Knaap H, Westerterp M. Appetite control: methodological aspects of the evaluation of foods. Obes Rev. 2010;11:251–70.
23. Sluik D, Brouwer-Brolsma EM, de Vries JHM, et al. Associations of alcoholic beverage preference with cardiometabolic and lifestyle factors: the NQplus study BMJ Open. 2016;6:e010437. doi:10.1136/bmjopen-2015-010437.
24. Siebelink E, Geelen A, de Vries JH. Self-reported energy intake by FFQ compared with actual energy intake to maintain body weight in 516 adults. Br J Nutr. 2011;106:274–81.
25. Van Strien T, Frijters JER, Bergers GPA, Defares PB: The Dutch eating behavior questionnaire (DEBQ) for assessment of restrained, emotional, and external eating behavior. Int J Eating Disorders. 1986;5:295–15.
26. Chinapaw MJM, Slootmaker SM, Schuit AJ, van Zuidam M, van Mechelen W. Reliability and validity of the activity questionnaire for adults and adolescents (AQuAA). BMC Med Res Methodol. 2009;9:58.
27. Wendel-Vos GC, Schuit AJ, Saris WH, Kromhout D. Reproducibility and relative validity of the short questionnaire to assess health-enhancing physical activity. J Clin Epidemiol. 2003;56:1163–9.
28. Altman DG. Practical statistics for medical research. 1st ed. London; New York: Chapman and Hall; 1991.

29. Deurenberg P, Weststrate JA, Seidell JC. Body mass index as a measure of body fatness: age- and sex-specific prediction formulas. Br J Nutr. 1991;65:105–14.
30. van den Boer JH, Mars M. Modeling of eating style and its effect on intake. Appetite. 2015;86:25–30.
31. Johansson L, Solvoll K, Bjorneboe GE, Drevon CA. Under- and overreporting of energy intake related to weight status and lifestyle in a nationwide sample. Am J Clin Nutr. 1998;68:266–74.
32. de Graaf C. Texture and satiation: the role of oro-sensory exposure time. Physiol Behav. 2012;107:496–501.
33. Wijlens AG, Erkner A, Alexander E, Mars M, Smeets PA, de Graaf C. Effects of oral and gastric stimulation on appetite and energy intake. Obesity (Silver Spring). 2012;20:2226–32.
34. Bolhuis DP, Lakemond CMM, de Wijk RA, Luning PA, de Graaf C. Both a higher number of sips and a longer oral transit time reduce ad libitum intake. Food Qual Prefer. 2014;32:234–40.
35. Spetter MS, Mars M, Viergever MA, de Graaf C, Smeets PA. Taste matters - effects of bypassing oral stimulation on hormone and appetite responses. Physiol Behav. 2014;137:9–17.
36. Zijlstra N, de Wijk RA, Mars M, Stafleu A, de Graaf C. Effect of bite size and oral processing time of a semisolid food on satiation. Am J Clin Nutr. 2009;90:269–75.
37. Maramis C, Diou C, Ioakeimidis I, Lekka I, Dudnik G, Mars M, Maglaveras N, Bergh C, Delopoulos A: Preventing obesity and eating disorders through behavioural modifications: The SPLENDID vision. Transforming Healthcare Through Innovations in Mobile and Wireless Technologies (MOBIHEALTH), Athens, 2014 4th International Conference on Wireless Mobile Communication and Healthcare.
38. Hermsen S, Frost JH, Robinson E, Higgs S, Mars M, Hermans RCJ: Evaluation of a Smart Fork to Decelerate Eating Rate. Journal of the Academy of Nutrition and Dietetics. 2016;116:1066-68.

6

Investigating the importance of the local food environment for fruit and vegetable intake in older men and women in 20 UK towns: a cross-sectional analysis of two national cohorts using novel methods

S. Hawkesworth[1], R.J. Silverwood[2], B. Armstrong[1], T. Pliakas[1], K. Nanchahal[1], C. Sartini[3], A. Amuzu[4], G. Wannamethee[3], J. Atkins[4], S.E. Ramsay[5], J.P. Casas[6], R.W. Morris[7], P.H. Whincup[8] and Karen Lock[1,9*]

Abstract

Background: Local neighbourhood environments can influence dietary behavior. There is limited evidence focused on older people who are likely to have greater dependence on local areas and may suffer functional limitations that amplify any neighbourhood impact.

Methods: Using multi-level ordinal regression analysis we investigated the association between multiple dimensions of neighbourhood food environments (captured by fine-detail, foot-based environmental audits and secondary data) and self-reported frequency of fruit and vegetable intake. The study was a cross-sectional analysis nested within two nationally representative cohorts in the UK: the British Regional Heart Study and the British Women's Heart and Health Study. Main exposures of interest were density of food retail outlets selling fruits and vegetables, the density of fast food outlets and a novel measure of diversity of the food retail environment.

Results: A total of 1124 men and 883 women, aged 69 – 92 years, living in 20 British towns were included in the analysis. There was strong evidence of an association between area income deprivation and fruit and vegetable consumption, with study members in the most deprived areas estimated to have 27% (95% CI: 7, 42) lower odds of being in a higher fruit and vegetable consumption category relative to those in the least deprived areas. We found no consistent evidence for an association between fruit and vegetable consumption and a range of other food environment domains, including density of shops selling fruits and vegetables, density of premises selling fast food, the area food retail diversity, area walkability, transport accessibility, or the local food marketing environment. For example, individuals living in areas with greatest fruit and vegetable outlet density had 2% (95% CI: -22, 21) lower odds of being in a higher fruit and vegetable consumption category relative to those in areas with no shops.

Conclusions: Although small effect sizes in environment-diet relationships cannot be discounted, this study suggests that older people are less influenced by physical characteristics of neighbourhood food environments than is suggested in the literature. The association between area income deprivation and diet may be capturing an important social aspect of neighbourhoods that influence food intake in older adults and warrants further research.

Keywords: Diet, Older people, Food environment, Fruit and vegetables

* Correspondence: Karen.Lock@lshtm.ac.uk
[1]Faculty of Public Health and Policy, London School of Hygiene and Tropical Medicine, London WC1E 7HT, UK
[9]London School of Hygiene & Tropical Medicine, 15-17 Tavistock Place, London, UK
Full list of author information is available at the end of the article

Background

Consumption of a healthy diet is fundamental to promoting health and preventing disease throughout the life-course, particularly in older adulthood [1–3]. It is estimated that by 2050 more than 2 billion people will be aged over 60 [4] and diet quality will be important for healthy aging [5]. Consumption of higher amounts of fruit and vegetables is protective for cardiovascular disease and various cancers [6–8], while inadequate fruit and vegetable intake in older age can increase incidence and severity of these diseases [9, 10]. However, older individuals tend to consume poor quality diets, lacking fruits and vegetables, and lower than recommended intakes of a range of nutrients [11]. National UK survey data suggests that older individuals are not eating recommended levels of fruits and vegetables, with fewer than half of people over 65 years achieving the 5-a-day guidelines [12].

There are many factors influencing dietary intake in older people, from individual health status, medication and personal preferences, to social and environmental factors including cultural norms and place of residence [13]. Policies and interventions to support healthy eating in this age group have tended to focus on individual behavior change for particular diseases or improving food in care settings [14, 15]. However, taking an ecological public health perspective considers how food purchase and diet patterns may be independently influenced by factors such as the neighbourhood food environment [16]. Exposure to poor quality food environments in deprived areas amplifies individual-level risk factors for a poor diet [17] and policies that promote enabling environments may act to make individual diet-change easier [18].

The food environment has been defined as encompassing the collective physical, economic, policy and sociocultural surroundings, opportunities and conditions that influence people's food and beverage choices and nutritional status [19]. Different components of the food environment can influence food purchasing decisions and serve as barriers or facilitators to a healthy diet including the variety, quality and price of available foods and also structural aspects such as the spatial accessibility of retail outlets [20]. Studies of these contextual determinants of diet have predominantly considered associations with food availability that is measured in terms of proximity to, or density of, food retail outlets (the 'community nutrition environment'), or the in-store environment, including the cost and store location of healthy and unhealthy foods (the 'consumer nutrition environments') [21].

There is some evidence, mainly from the USA, that the local food retail environment may be associated with dietary patterns in adults [22, 23]. When looking at specific aspects of the diet, increased fruit and vegetable consumption has been shown to be associated with better access to supermarkets [24] or other food stores [25, 26]. However, these findings are not universal, are often not repeated in other country settings and rarely consider the influences on older age groups [27]. The dietary intake of older people may be particularly influenced by the local neighbourhood environment as barriers and facilitating factors for accessing healthy diets are likely to be magnified by deteriorating physical and cognitive functioning as people age [28].

The built environment comprises a broad range of physical features that could have an impact on food purchase and diet including urban design, land use and transportation provision. Studies of the community nutrition environment have predominantly focused on access to, or density of, food provisioning facilities such as supermarkets [26, 29, 30] without considering the potential influence of other built environment features [31] and few studies consider multiple dimensions of the urban environment or their potential interactions [32]. Most food environment and diet research investigates either the perception of food access or use secondary data sources that record locations or density of food retail premises often used as a simple proxy for food availability [33]. Primary environmental data collection audits are rarely employed on a large scale in food studies but have important advantages in terms of capturing more accurate and fine-detail environmental exposures.

The current study aimed to investigate the association between the neighbourhood food environment, captured through foot-based audits, and self reported fruit and vegetable consumption amongst older individuals from two national cohorts in the UK. The objective was to explore more complex attributes of the neighbourhood food environment that hypothetically influence access to, and availability of, healthy food for older people beyond simple measures of food retail density. These included a novel approach to measure area food retail diversity, measures of transport provision, locally visible marketing of unhealthy food, and physical factors of the built environment that affect walkability which are of relevance to older people.

Methods

This cross-sectional study of the food environment was nested within two nationally representative cohort studies that defined the environmental areas that were assessed. The British Regional Heart Study (BRHS) was established in 1978-80, recruiting 7735 men from primary care centres in 24 British towns into an on-going prospective population-based cohort study [34]. In 1999-2000, a parallel women's cohort study (the British Womens' Heart and Health Study, BWHHS) was established recruiting a total of 4286 women in 23 towns [35]. In 2010-12, survivors from both cohorts were sent a follow-up questionnaire containing lifestyle questions including some relevant to their usual diet. No specific dietary, physiological or nutritional characteristics were considered when selecting the current study population. Ethical approval was provided by the National Research Ethics Service (NRES) Committee for London.

Dietary questions were based on the frequency of consumption of various foods in a typical week. The current analysis focuses on the primary outcome of self-reported frequency of the consumption of fresh fruit and green vegetables/salads derived from questionnaire data. In the BRHS, the number of days each week study participants reported eating "green vegetables, salads", "fresh vegetables" (average of reported summer and winter consumption) and "fresh fruit" (average of reported summer and winter consumption) were combined by averaging then splitting the observed distribution by tertiles to give a three-level categorical variable: "low", "medium" and "high" fruit and vegetable consumption. In the BWHHS, the number of times each week study participants reported eating "green vegetables", "salads" (average of reported summer and winter consumption) and "fresh fruit" (average of reported summer and winter consumption) were similarly combined and split into a three-level categorical variable. The study-specific fruit and vegetable consumption variables were then combined across the studies.

Potential confounding factors and effect modifiers were available from previous survey rounds: socio-economic status was defined at cohort baseline as the longest held occupation (men) or the highest occupational class of the study member and their husband (women); age was defined by date-of-birth and long-standing illness, disability or infirmity and car ownership were self-reported from the current survey round.

Environmental data

A neighbourhood environment audit tool (OPECR - Older People's Environments and CVD Risk tool) was developed to capture neighbourhood features relevant to CVD risk factor behaviours in older adults. The tool is described in detail elsewhere [36] and features many fine-detail indicators relevant to the community food environment including the presence of different types of food retail outlets such as supermarkets, convenience stores and fast food restaurants, and in addition quantified the presence of unhealthy food advertising. We applied the tool through foot-based audits in 20 BWHS and 19 BRHS study towns across the UK: 17 from England and 3 from Scotland. Lower Layer Super Output Areas (LSOA) (geographic areas containing between 1000 and 3000 individuals) were chosen as the unit of data collection in England [37], whilst the broadly equivalent datazones (DZ) were used in Scotland (areas containing 500 – 1000 individuals) [38].

The audit tool was developed in 2009 and piloted in 2 study towns, with the remaining towns audited between 2012 and 2014 [36]. Trained fieldworkers worked across multiple study towns to maximise data collection consistency. Fieldworkers worked in pairs systematically recording all relevant aspects of the OPECR tool for both sides of a road or 'segment'. Inter-observer reliability was found to be high with agreement ranging from 'substantial' for more subjective variables to 'excellent' for objective estimates such as the presence of shops and services [36]. All roads within an LSOA/DZ were audited and considered one data collection 'segment'. Any urban LSOA/DZ where at least one cohort member lived was eligible for inclusion in the audit but large semi-rural areas were excluded if they were not contiguous with the study town or if they included ≤3 cohort members. Environmental data were collected on paper pro-formas and entered into an Access database before being exported into Stata 14.0 (Stata Corporation, College Station, TX) and cleaned prior to analysis.

The audit tool captured various features of the local food environment that influence food access and availability such as the presence of all types of food retail outlets (supermarkets, convenience stores, fast food outlets, cafes, pubs and restaurants) and aspects of the neighbourhood built environment that could affect physical activity and access for older people. Our main exposures of interest were the density of shops selling fruit and vegetables, the density of fast food restaurants and the diversity of the food retail environment. From the audit data, the recorded number of shops selling fruit and vegetables ("Independent convenience/general stores", "Small supermarkets" and "Large supermarkets with parking") per segment were summed across each LSOA/DZ and standardised by area to give the density of shops selling fruit and vegetables. This was then analysed as a three-level categorical variable: "No shops" (0 shops per km^2), "Fewer shops" ($0 <$ shops per $km^2 < 3.5$), "More shops" ($3.5 \geq$ shops per km^2). Similarly, the recorded number of fast food outlets per segment was summed across each LSOA/DZ and standardised by LSOA/DZ area to give the density of fast food outlets, which was analysed as a three-level categorical variable: "No fast food outlets" (0 fast food outlets per km^2), "Fewer fast food outlets" ($0 <$ fast food outlets per $km^2 < 4.5$), "More fast food outlets" ($4.5 \geq$ fast food outlets per km^2).

We also measured the diversity of the neighbourhood food retail environment using a spatial entropy score, a measure of evenness or diversity of a set of attributes in a given area which has been widely used in the built environment and health literature to reflect land use mix [39]. It ranges from 0 to 1, with 0 representing a homogeneous area, covered by a single attribute, and a value of 1 representing heterogeneity, where all attributes are equally distributed. We calculated a spatial entropy score from audit data using four types of food premises: all food shops ("Independent convenience/general stores", "Small supermarkets", "Large supermarkets with parking" and "Other food shops"), restaurants and cafes, pubs and fast food outlets to reflect the diversity of the food retail environment at the LSOA/DZ level. This was analysed as a three-level categorical variable: "no food retail outlets present" (0 outlets per km^2), "low diversity" (0 < outlets per km^2 < 3.5) and "high diversity" (3.5 ≥ outlets per km^2).

In addition, we investigated the potential impact of other dimensions of the neighbourhood built environment on fruit and vegetable intake. This included factors affecting access to shops such as public transport provision, defined as the density of bus stops/km^2, summed across, and standardised by, LSOA/DZ. Bus transport was selected as older people in England are entitled to free bus travel and is likely to be the main form of public transport use at a local level. The neighbourhood food marketing environment was characterised by recording, during the foot based audits, the number of adverts (present in shop windows, billboards and other external locations) promoting sugary drinks, unhealthy snacks/junk foods and alcoholic drinks. The total count of unhealthy food and drink adverts was standardised by LSOA/DZ area to describe the unhealthy food marketing environment categorized into: "no adverts present" (0 adverts per km^2), "Fewer adverts" (0 < adverts per km^2 < 7.9), "More adverts" (7.9 ≥ adverts per km^2).

The influence of the physical built environment on walkability and features affecting access to food shops was captured by a number of variables on the audit tool including many relating to features of road and path quality. To reduce the dimensionality of these data a latent class analysis (LCA) was conducted, described in detail elsewhere [40]. Ten variables related to road and path quality, known to be associated with older peoples' mobility and collected by the foot-based audit, were included in the LCA: 'quality of pavement', 'lowered curbs', 'barriers on pavement', 'pavement width', 'pedestrian traffic', 'road use', 'road connectivity', 'traffic calming measures', 'lamp posts' and 'road crossings'. A 3-class model was considered most appropriate with the classes characterised as "poor quality walking environment" (9.9% of segments), "medium quality walking environment" (57.0%) and "good quality walking environment" (33.1%). The three classes were assigned a score (0, 1 and 2), the mean of which across the LSOA/DZ is referred to as the "road quality score".

Finally, several routine data sources were also used in the analysis. Street connectivity was used as a standard proxy for walkability index: data on the number of road nodes/interconnections within an LSOA/DZ were obtained from the 2015 Ordinance Survey (Digimap Meridian 2 National) and used to generate street connectivity defined as number of intersections per km^2. Population density was also included in the analysis and was defined based on mid-year population estimates for 2010 obtained from the Office of National Statistics [41] and the Scottish Neighbourhood Statistics [42]. Estimates were used to generate area level population density per km^2 smoothed using a 5 km radius buffer. Area social deprivation was defined from the income deprivation domain of the 2010 Index of Multiple Deprivation (IMD) [43] and the 2009 Scottish Index of Multiple Deprivation (SIMD) [44]. For both these indices, LSOA/DZ rank was used to define the relative deprivation.

Statistical methods

Study members were eligible to be included in the analysis if their LSOA/DZ of residence was covered by the foot-based environmental audit and they did not self-report having 'severe' or worse difficulties getting about outdoors. Multilevel ordinal logistic regression models were used with fruit and vegetable consumption ("low", "medium" and "high") as the outcome. The 3-level structure underlying the data (study members nested within LSOA/DZ nested within towns) was accounted for, with random intercepts at the LSOA/DZ and town levels.

For each area-level exposure of interest (density of shops selling fruit and vegetables, density of fast food outlets, diversity of food retail environment, food marketing environment, road and path quality score, transport provision, area income, street connectivity and population density) sequentially adjusted models were fitted as follows: i) Unadjusted; ii) Adjusted for potential confounding variables (sex, age, adult social class, long-standing illness, disability or infirmity, country); iii) Additionally adjusted for all other area-level exposures of interest. Study members were included in a given analysis if they had data available for each exposure of interest and each potentially confounding variable, in addition to the outcome. For each model we assessed the proportional odds assumption using several statistical tests.

Interactions between each exposure of interest and sex, age, adult social class, long-standing illness, disability or infirmity and country were examined using Wald tests in the minimally adjusted model. To aid interpretation of the analyses we examined cross-tabulations and calculated polychoric correlations between each pair of area-level explanatory variables. All analyses were conducted using Stata 14.0 (Stata Corporation, College Station, TX).

Results

A total of 2901 men and 2871 women lived in the 20 towns targeted for the environmental audit. Of these, 2007 study members (1124 men, 883 women) living in 740 areas (LSOAs/DZs) had complete data on diet outcomes, exposures of interest and confounders and were included in the analysis. There was a median of 2 (range 1-20) study members per LSOA/DZ and a median of 105 (range 31-158) study members per town.

The distribution of fruit and vegetable consumption responses from the two cohorts are shown in Table 1. From both cohorts a high proportion of individuals reported eating fruit at least once a day (39.0%-64.9%) with a lower proportion reporting to eat vegetables and salads. There was generally a positive correlation between the area-level explanatory variables that were considered in the analysis, ranging from 0.12 to 0.83 (Table 2). However, there was no evidence of correlation between diversity of the food retail environment and population density. There was evidence that all the individual-level confounders, with the exception of sex, were associated with fruit and vegetable consumption (Table 3). Older age, lower adult social class, long-standing illness, disability or infirmity, and living in Scotland were all associated with lower fruit and vegetable consumption. For example, those aged 85 and over had 22% (95% confidence interval (CI): −4, 42%) lower odds of being in a higher fruit and vegetable consumption category relative to those aged less than 75 (Table 3).

We found no evidence for an association with fruit and vegetable consumption and our main exposures of interest: density of shops selling fruit and vegetables, density of fast food outlets or the diversity of the food retail environment (Table 3). In contrast, there was strong evidence that area income deprivation was associated with fruit and vegetable consumption with study members in the most income-deprived areas estimated to have 27% (95% CI: 7, 42%) lower odds of being in a higher fruit and vegetable consumption category relative to those in the least deprived areas (Table 4). The evidence of the association remained after adjustment for other exposures of interest (Table 4).

There was weak evidence of an association between population density and fruit and vegetable consumption (Table 4). People living in areas with the highest population density were estimated as having 19% (95% CI: -1, 34) lower odds of being in a higher fruit and vegetable consumption category relative to areas with lowest population density, (Table 4). There was no evidence of associations between the remaining area-level exposures of interest and fruit and vegetable consumption, including the marketing or physical environments (Table 4).

There was no convincing evidence of effect modification by any of the variables examined (data not shown), though there was a suggestion of effect modification by car ownership (p = 0.03). In those who did not own a car there was evidence that diversity of the food retail environment was associated with fruit and vegetable consumption (OR 1.85 (95% CI 1.25, 2.73) and OR 1.45 (95% CI 0.97, 2.16) for low and high diversity respectively (relative to no food retail outlets present)). For those who did own a car there was no evidence that diversity of the food retail environment was associated with fruit and vegetable consumption (OR 0.96 (95% CI 0.77, 1.29) and OR 1.05 (95% CI 0.80, 1.40) for low and high diversity respectively).

Discussion

This large, nationally representative study investigated the association between multiple dimensions of the community food environment and fruit and vegetable consumption in older men and women living in the UK. It is one of the largest studies worldwide to explore how the built environment may influence diet in older age, and

Table 1 Distribution of diet question responses among the 2007 participants (n = 1124 men, 883 women) contributing to the analysis

BRHS[a]	Number of days consumed each week							Monthly	Rarely/never
	7	6	5	4	3	2	1		
Fresh fruit (summer)	445 (41.5)	82 (7.7)	107 (10.0)	106 (9.9)	113 (10.6)	81 (7.6)	34 (3.2)	43 (4.0)	60 (5.6)
Fresh fruit (winter)	404 (39.0)	70 (6.8)	102 (9.8)	98 (9.5)	119 (11.5)	85 (8.2)	50 (4.8)	43 (4.2)	65 (6.3)
Fresh vegetables (summer)	260 (23.7)	152 (13.9)	186 (17.0)	164 (15.0)	156 (14.2)	94 (8.6)	32 (2.9)	29 (2.6)	23 (2.1)
Fresh vegetables (winter)	239 (22.3)	140 (13.1)	160 (15.0)	175 (16.4)	149 (13.9)	114 (10.7)	39 (3.6)	32 (3.0)	22 (2.1)
Green vegetables, salads	185 (17.1)	144 (13.3)	150 (13.9)	166 (15.4)	189 (17.5)	113 (10.5)	64 (5.9)	43 (4.0)	26 (2.4)
BWHHS[b]	More than once a day	Once a day	Most days	One or two days a week	Less than once a week	Never			
Fresh fruit (summer)	382 (43.4)	189 (21.5)	191 (21.7)	81 (9.2)	31 (3.5)	6 (0.7)			
Fresh fruit (winter)	282 (32.2)	243 (27.7)	186 (21.2)	111 (12.7)	42 (4.8)	12 (1.4)			
Salads (summer)	94 (10.7)	165 (18.9)	215 (24.6)	320 (36.6)	60 (6.9)	21 (2.4)			
Salads (winter)	43 (5.0)	91 (10.6)	96 (11.2)	313 (36.5)	245 (28.6)	69 (8.1)			
Green vegetables	78 (8.9)	237 (27.1)	344 (39.4)	169 (19.3)	37 (4.2)	9 (1.0)			

[a]British Regional Heart Study
[b]British Womens Heart and Health Study

Table 2 Polychoric correlations between each pair of area-level explanatory variables. Restricted to LSOAs contributing to the analysis ($N = 740$)

	Density of fast food outlets	Diversity of food retail environment	Unhealthy food marketing environment	Road quality score	Transport	Area-level income	Walkability	Population density[f]
Density of shops selling fruit and vegetables	0.64	0.75	0.66	0.19	0.34	0.38	0.36	0.25
Density of fast food outlets		0.81	0.55	0.25	0.31	0.42	0.42	0.23
Diversity of food retail environment[a]			0.58	0.15	0.13	0.26	0.13	−0.05
Unhealthy food marketing environment[b]				0.12	0.24	0.24	0.24	0.21
Road quality score[c]					0.32	0.29	0.30	0.24
Transport						0.29	0.59	0.59
Area-level income[d]							0.40	0.36
Walkability[e]								0.83

[a]Diversity of food retail environment calculated using a spatial entropy score taking into account four types of food premises: all food shops, restaurants and cafes, pubs and fast food restaurants

[b]Unhealthy marketing environment defined from a count of unhealthy food and drink adverts within an area including those promoting sugary drinks, unhealthy snacks/junk food and alcohol

[c]Road quality score calculated from latent class analysis including 10 variables: 'quality of pavement'; 'lowered curbs'; 'barriers on pavement'; 'pavement width'; 'pedestrian traffic'; 'road use'; 'road connectivity'; 'traffic calming measures'; 'lamp posts' and 'road crossings' (full details in Additional file 1)

[d]Income deprivation score and crime score generated from the 2010 Index of Multiple Deprivation LSOA rank (IMD: www.gov.co.uk/government/statistics/english-indices-of-deprivation-2010) or the 2009 Scottish Index of Multiple Deprivation datazone rank (SIMD: http://www.gov.scot/Topics/Statistics/SIMD) to define relative deprivation of an area for England and Scotland respectively

[e]Area walkability generated from street connectivity defined as the number of road nodes/interconnections per km^2 within an LSOA/datazone obtained from 2015 Ordinance Survey (Digimap Meridian 2 National)

[f]Population densitiy obtained from mid-year population estimates from 2010 from the Office of National Statistics (www.ons.gov.uk) and the Scottish Neighbourhood Statistics (www.sns.gov.uk). Estimates used to generate population density per km^2 at the area level smoothed using a 5 km radius buffer

considers a more diverse and comprehensive range of potential neighbourhood environmental influences than any previous study. These include a novel measure of the diversity of food provision in an area, local transport provision and local food marketing. Overall, we found no evidence that the density or diversity of the food retail environment were associated with fruit and vegetable consumption. In contrast, area-level income deprivation was associated with diet; individuals living in the most deprived areas had the lowest reported fruit and vegetable consumption.

Our study focused on the effect of the local environment on fruit and vegetable consumption, rather than overall dietary intake, and this has been a consistent dietary outcome of interest in the literature, partly because of its clear association with health [7, 8, 45]. A recent review found that the majority of studies of the food environment also focused on fruit and vegetable intake but the wide range of methods and approaches makes study comparisons challenging [45]. Positive associations are often identified between perceptions of the food environment and diet [46, 47] but the picture is more mixed when objective assessments of food availability and access are considered, sometimes even within the same study [47]. Interestingly some studies have reported a poor correlation between perceived and objective measures of the food environment [33, 48, 49], suggesting that perception of food access captures different aspects of behaviour than physical proximity to a food outlet [33, 50].

Fruit and vegetable consumption in adults has been associated with proximity to grocery stores in some studies [24, 25, 51] but the picture is mixed [45]. One large multi-centre study reported an association with supermarket density and diet quality (for individuals aged 45-84 years), such that participants with no supermarkets near their homes were 25-46% less likely to have a healthy diet than those with the most stores [29]. Associations between food availability and diet may be more strongly apparent for in-store availability of fruit and vegetables, captured by tools such as the Nutrition Environment Measure Survey in Stores and Restaurants (NEMS) [52] rather than for density of food outlets *per se* [45]. In the UK it has been suggested that proximity to food stores may have less influence on food purchase than in North American settings, which often dominate the literature, as most UK residents in urban areas have reasonable food access [27]. Most studies in this field have relied on cross-sectional design and the few that have incorporated pseudo-experimental approaches, such as the opening of a new supermarket in a previously deprived area, also report mixed results [53, 54]. Despite a growing literature on the influence of different aspects of the neighbourhood food environment on diet, there is little evidence for older adults. One of the only studies to

Table 3 Associations with fruit and vegetable consumption (outcome) and main exposures of interest and confounding variables

	N (%)	N (%) low fruit and veg	N (%) medium fruit and veg	N (%) high fruit and veg	Unadjusted			Confounder adjusted			Mutually adjusted		
					OR	95% CI	*p*-value (trend)	OR	95% CI	*p*-value (trend)	OR	95% CI	*p*-value (trend)
Area-level exposures of interest													
Density of shops selling fruit and vegetables							0.77			0.95			0.84
0 (no shops)	847 (42.2)	280 (33.1)	289 (34.1)	278 (32.8)	1.00	(ref)		1.00	(ref)		1.00	(ref)	
1 (fewer shops)	688 (34.3)	225 (32.7)	209 (30.4)	254 (36.9)	1.05	0.86, 1.27		1.04	0.85, 1.27		0.96	0.74, 1.25	
2 (more shops)	472 (23.5)	163 (34.5)	167 (35.4)	142 (30.1)	0.96	0.78, 1.18		0.98	0.79, 1.22		0.97	0.72, 1.31	
Density of fast food outlets							0.65			0.49			0.25
0 (no fast food outlets)	1193 (59.4)	401 (33.6)	400 (33.5)	392 (32.9)	1.00	0.00, 0.00		1.00	(ref)		1.00	(ref)	
1 (fewer fast food outlets)	503 (25.1)	163 (32.4)	156 (31.0)	184 (36.6)	1.03	0.84, 1.26		1.05	0.86, 1.30		1.08	0.83, 1.41	
2 (more fast food outlets)	311 (15.5)	104 (33.4)	109 (35.1)	98 (31.5)	1.05	0.83, 1.33		1.08	0.85, 1.38		1.22	0.87, 1.72	
Diversity of food retail environment[a]							0.37			0.36			0.34
0 (no food retail outlets present)	437 (21.8)	157 (35.9)	154 (35.2)	126 (28.8)	1.00	(ref)		1.00	(ref)		1.00	(ref)	
1 (low diversity)	904 (45.0)	291 (32.2)	296 (32.7)	317 (35.1)	1.19	0.96, 1.47		1.19	0.96, 1.49		1.31	1.00, 1.71	
2 (high diversity)	666 (33.2)	220 (33.0)	215 (32.3)	231 (34.7)	1.13	0.90, 1.42		1.14	0.90, 1.43		1.22	0.83, 1.79	
Confounders													
Sex (study)							0.49						
Female (BWHHS)	883 (44.0)	293 (33.2)	289 (32.7)	301 (34.1)	1.00	(ref)							
Male (BRHS)	1124 (56.0)	375 (33.4)	376 (33.5)	373 (33.2)	1.06	0.90, 1.26							
Age (years)							0.003						
< 75	646 (32.2)	192 (29.7)	208 (32.2)	246 (38.1)	1.00	(ref)							
75-79	670 (33.4)	230 (34.3)	231 (34.5)	209 (31.2)	0.77	0.63, 0.94							
80-84	480 (23.9)	178 (37.1)	152 (31.7)	150 (31.3)	0.71	0.56, 0.88							
85+	211 (10.5)	68 (32.2)	74 (35.1)	69 (32.7)	0.78	0.58, 1.04							
Adult social class							<0.001						
I (professional)/II (intermediate)	845 (42.1)	232 (27.5)	263 (31.1)	350 (41.4)	1.00	(ref)							
IIInm (skilled non-manual)	348 (17.3)	125 (35.9)	130 (37.4)	93 (26.7)	0.62	0.49, 0.78							
IIIm (skilled manual)	553 (27.6)	197 (35.6)	197 (35.6)	159 (28.8)	0.72	0.59, 0.89							
IV (partially skilled manual)/V (unskilled manual)	261 (13.0)	114 (43.7)	75 (28.7)	72 (27.6)	0.57	0.44, 0.75							

Table 3 Associations with fruit and vegetable consumption (outcome) and main exposures of interest and confounding variables *(Continued)*

Long-standing illness, disability or infirmity							0.07
No	1324 (66.0)	425 (32.1)	431 (32.6)	468 (35.4)	1.00	(ref)	
Yes	683 (34.0)	243 (35.6)	234 (34.3)	206 (30.2)	0.85	0.72, 1.01	
Country							0.03
England	1758 (87.6)	557 (31.7)	584 (33.2)	617 (35.1)	1.00	(ref)	
Scotland	249 (12.4)	111 (44.6)	81 (32.5)	57 (22.9)	0.58	0.35, 0.96	

Multilevel ordinal logistic regression models with random intercepts at the town and LSOA/data zone levels. Restricted to study members non-missing for all variables in the Table (*N* = 2007 (1124 men, 883 women) study members across 740 LSOAs/data zones with median 2 (range 1-20) study members per LSOA/data zone and with median 105 (range 31-158) study members per town)

[a]Diversity of food retail environment calculated using a spatial entropy score taking into account four types of food premises: all food shops, restaurants and cafes, pubs and fast food restaurants

Table 4 Associations with fruit and vegetable consumption (outcome) and additional exposures of interest

	N (%)	N (%) low fruit and veg	N (%) medium fruit and veg	N (%) high fruit and veg	Unadjusted			Confounder adjusted			Mutually adjusted		
					OR	95% CI	*p*-value (trend)	OR	95% CI	*p*-value (trend)	OR	95% CI	*p*-value (trend)
Area-level exposures of interest													
Unhealthy food marketing environment[a]							0.40			0.42			0.27
0 (no adverts present)	1180 (58.8)	382 (32.4)	414 (35.1)	384 (32.5)	1.00	(ref)		1.00	(ref)		1.00	(ref)	
1 (fewer adverts)	481 (24.0)	157 (32.6)	154 (32.0)	170 (35.3)	0.92	0.75, 1.13		0.91	0.74, 1.12		0.84	0.66, 1.06	
2 (more adverts)	346 (17.2)	129 (37.3)	97 (28.0)	120 (34.7)	0.92	0.73, 1.16		0.93	0.73, 1.17		0.89	0.68, 1.17	
Road quality score[b]							0.76			0.91			0.61
0 (worst walking environment)	586 (29.2)	188 (32.1)	183 (31.2)	215 (36.7)	1.00	(ref)		1.00	(ref)		1.00	(ref)	
1	716 (35.7)	262 (36.6)	227 (31.7)	227 (31.7)	0.87	0.71, 1.07		0.89	0.72, 1.10		0.90	0.72, 1.12	
2 (best walking environment)	705 (35.1)	218 (30.9)	255 (36.2)	232 (32.9)	0.96	0.78, 1.20		0.98	0.79, 1.23		1.06	0.84, 1.33	
Transport							0.10			0.26			0.69
0 (fewest bus stops)	620 (30.9)	183 (29.5)	213 (34.4)	224 (36.1)	1.00	(ref)		1.00	(ref)		1.00	(ref)	
1	763 (38.0)	266 (34.9)	234 (30.7)	263 (34.5)	0.87	0.72, 1.07		0.91	0.74, 1.11		0.92	0.72, 1.16	
2 (most bus stops)	624 (31.1)	219 (35.1)	218 (34.9)	187 (30.0)	0.84	0.68, 1.03		0.88	0.71, 1.10		0.94	0.72, 1.24	
Area-level income[c]							<0.001			0.009			0.003
0 (least deprived)	990 (49.3)	289 (29.2)	316 (31.9)	385 (38.9)	1.00	(ref)		1.00	(ref)		1.00	(ref)	
1	598 (29.8)	206 (34.5)	210 (35.1)	182 (30.4)	0.82	0.67, 0.99		0.86	0.71, 1.06		0.82	0.66, 1.01	
2 (most deprived)	419 (20.9)	173 (41.3)	139 (33.2)	107 (25.5)	0.67	0.53, 0.84		0.73	0.58, 0.93		0.69	0.54, 0.89	
Walkability[d]							0.27			0.41			0.52
0 (lowest walkability)	528 (26.3)	158 (29.9)	176 (33.3)	194 (36.7)	1.00	(ref)		1.00	(ref)		1.00	(ref)	
1	772 (38.5)	256 (33.2)	252 (32.6)	264 (34.2)	0.93	0.75, 1.15		0.94	0.76, 1.17		1.09	0.82, 1.46	
2 (highest walkability)	707 (35.2)	254 (35.9)	237 (33.5)	216 (30.6)	0.88	0.71, 1.10		0.91	0.73, 1.14		1.13	0.79, 1.60	
Population density[e]							0.02			0.07			0.20
0 Lowest population density	604 (30.1)	176 (29.1)	197 (32.6)	231 (38.3)	1.00	(ref)		1.00	(ref)		1.00	(ref)	
1	755 (37.6)	256 (33.9)	243 (32.2)	256 (33.9)	0.88	0.72, 1.08		0.89	0.72, 1.09		0.87	0.65, 1.15	
2 Highest population density	648 (32.3)	236 (36.4)	225 (34.7)	187 (28.9)	0.77	0.62, 0.95		0.81	0.66, 1.01		0.79	0.56, 1.13	

Multilevel ordinal logistic regression models with random intercepts at the town and LSOA/data zone levels. Restricted to study members non-missing for all variables in the Table (N = 2007 (1124 men, 883 women) study members across 740 LSOAs/data zones with median 2 (range 1-20) study members per LSOA/data zone and with median 105 (range 31-158) study members per town)

[a]Unhealthy marketing environment defined from a count of unhealthy food and drink adverts within an area including those promoting sugary drinks, unhealthy snacks/junk food and alcohol

[b]Road quality score calculated from latent class analysis including 10 variables: 'quality of pavement'; 'lowered curbs'; 'barriers on pavement'; 'pavement width'; 'pedestrian traffic'; 'road use'; 'road connectivity'; 'traffic calming measures'; 'lamp posts' and 'road crossings' (full details in Additional file 1)

[c]Income deprivation score and crime score generated from the 2010 Index of Multiple Deprivation LSOA rank (IMD: https://www.gov.uk/government/statistics/english-indices-of-deprivation-2010) or the 2009 Scottish Index of Multiple Deprivation datazone rank (SIMD: http://www.gov.scot/Topics/Statistics/SIMD) to define relative deprivation of an area for England and Scotland respectively

[d]Area walkability generated from street connectivity defined as the number of road nodes/interconnections per km^2 within an LSOA/datazone obtained from 2015 Ordinance Survey (Digimap Meridian 2 National)

[e]Population densitiy obtained from mid-year population estimates from 2010 from the Office of National Statistics (www.ons.gov.uk) and the Scottish Neighbourhood Statistics (www.sns.gov.uk). Estimates used to generate population density per km^2 at the area level smoothed using a 5 km radius buffer

focus specifically on the older age group is the NuAge cohort in Montreal where the proportion of stores selling healthful foods (relative to all food stores) was not associated with dietary outcomes [55].

The spatial regulation of fast food or convenience food outlets has recently been seen as a local urban planning policy intervention with the potential to improve population diets [56]. The evidence for neighbourhood influences on availability and consumption of convenience food or fast food amongst older people is also mixed. Again most research has been conducted in the USA. In one study from Portland, Oregon, neighbourhoods with a high density of fast food outlets were associated with a high prevalence of obesity, increases in weight, waist circumference and blood pressure among older residents who reported visiting fast-food restaurants more frequently [57], although this is not a universal finding [47]. In the present analysis, we found no evidence that the density of fast food outlets was associated with fruit and vegetable consumption in older people in the UK, although these findings may reflect the lack of specificity of the outcome measure. In contrast, in the NuAge study of urban-dwelling older adults in Montreal there was evidence that fast food outlets were inversely associated with a more prudent dietary pattern in older people [55].

In agreement with many other studies in the literature, we found an inverse association between area deprivation and fruit and vegetable consumption, although again most of the current evidence base reflects adult populations in the USA [58, 59]. Older residents are often not considered separately in food-environment studies but one recent study from Baltimore found a positive association between neighbourhood SES and serum carotenoid concentrations (reflecting fruit and vegetable consumption) in older individuals (aged 70-79y) [60]. The data are more limited from other settings and a recent cross-country comparison found mixed results between neighbourhood-level SES and fruit and vegetable consumption in adulthood, highlighting the importance of context [61]. One explanation for the link between neighbourhood SES and diet is the 'deprivation amplification' hypothesis that deprived neighbourhoods have poorer access to high-quality food environments [17]. Here we found a relatively poor (r: 0.4) correlation between density of shops and services and area-income deprivation and previous UK studies also suggest a more complex association [62].

People-place interactions for food procurement are important to consider, and that this can be a limitation in this type of study. Hence, multi-dimensional measures of the neighbourhood food environment are likely to be important in understanding links between access and consumption [32]. However, many previous studies have focused solely on proximity to food retail outlets as a measure of food availability. In addition to the density of retail outlets, we considered a novel measure of the diversity of food retail provision in a local neighbourhood but found no clear evidence that this was associated with reported fruit and vegetable consumption. We also considered a number of additional dimensions of the food environment including public transport provision, aspects of the physical urban environment such as the road and path quality and the prevailing marketing environment assessed by the density of advertisements for unhealthy food and drink in the local area. Previous studies of in-store food promotions have highlighted the importance of 'product, price, placement and promotion' in influencing food sales [63], but this is the first study to consider the impact of the neighbourhood advertising environment on dietary patterns for older individuals.

In addition to considering multiple dimensions of the local food environment, we explored potential effect modification by car ownership and found evidence that for individuals who did not own a car a more diverse retail environment was associated with higher fruit and vegetable consumption. This is a potentially interesting finding, suggesting that a diverse local food retail environment may be important for enabling healthier diets in those without access to a car, particularly those that may have mobility constraints, although interpretation should be cautious given the extent of multiple testing. Studies have suggested that individuals will travel to the supermarkets they want to frequent even if these are not the nearest ones to their home, highlighting the importance of a nuanced understanding of how food purchasing behaviour may be influenced by the environment [64]. Previous studies have suggested that vehicle ownership may buffer the effects of limited access to healthy foods although findings are equivocal [65–67]. Such studies have rarely considered the importance of car ownership and food access in older age groups although it could be argued that individuals become more reliant on car use to travel for food shopping as they become less mobile.

This study has a number of strengths. It is the largest study to consider a nationally representative sample of older people outside of the setting of North America. We also considered a wide range of different dimensions of the community food environment and their potential interactions to provide a more comprehensive study of the association between environment and diet than has been done previously. A particular advantage of our study is the fine-detail, national scale of the environmental audit of built environment features; most studies that consider the density of food outlets utilise secondary data, which are prone to error [68–70]. Our analysis utilised multilevel modelling to account for exposures operating at different scales and the resulting confidence intervals around our effect estimates are relatively narrow giving confidence to the null results reported.

We are aware that the study has several limitations that may have affected the results. Although situated within two cohorts, this study uses cross-sectional analysis that has clear limitations when assessing something as dynamic as the local environment. The diet data were collected prior to the environmental audits although this short time-frame is unlikely to have incorporated major changes in environmental exposures [71]. One detailed UK study of food environment changes over 18 years reported a similar distribution pattern to both fast food outlet and supermarket provision even though these had increased over the time period [72]. In addition, no adjustment was possible in the analysis to take account of neighbourhood self-selection. Whilst the measure of diversity of the food environment was detailed, it was novel and was not specific to fruit and vegetable provision as it encompassed all food retail outlets, which may have acted to dilute any association. However, density of all food outlets is often used in the literature as a proxy for the availability of healthy foods such as fruit and vegetables [55]. In addition, distance to, or density of, food retail outlets might be a poor predictor of actual food purchasing behaviour [64]. Multicollinearity between environmental variables also needs to be considered. In the confounder adjusted models there is no evidence of multicollinearity. In the mutually adjusted model there is little evidence of multicollinearity for the majority of exposures of interest and where some evidence exists it makes no difference to our conclusions as the affected exposures were not found to be associated with fruit and vegetable consumption, with the exception of population density. A multicollinearity-inflated *p*-value for the association with population density would mean that we are potentially being conservative in our conclusions. Finally, the study was restricted to urban areas that may not exhibit sufficient variation in food outlet density or diversity to pick up an association with food consumption. A recent study of older individuals residing in rural areas has highlighted the importance that food retail outlets may have in that setting [73].

We looked only at fruit and vegetable consumption as this was the diet component most compatible between the two cohorts and because of the importance of fruit and vegetable intake as a determinant of health. Associations with other dietary patterns cannot therefore be discounted. Finally, we used lower-level administrative boundaries as the unit of analysis that are arbitrary with respect to exposures of interest. Considering exposures within a fixed spatial area may underestimate any associations as individual activity spaces will more accurately capture food access and availability [74, 75]. Our null results may reflect this spatial scale.

Studies suggest older individuals access areas wider than those captured by standard buffer size [76, 77]. To address this we did seek to explore people-place interactions as part of the wider research by conducting a small qualitative GPS sub-study, with a sample of study participants in study towns. This looked in detail at older peoples' activity spaces and reasons for their movement and activities in various places including for food purchase. This study showed that older individuals are often utilising multiple shops, services and social resources at various distances from their home, not just locally [78]. The use of a car, or easy access to public transport, was important to the participants in order for them to access a range of activities including food shops. Lack of transport was a concern for those with less mobility especially as people got older.

Conclusion

The neighbourhood food environment could play an important role in shaping individual dietary behavior, particularly in older age when individuals spend more time locally and may be restricted in their food access through ill health or functional limitations. This is one of the largest studies of food environment influences on diet in older age, and one of the largest to consider such a wide range of dimensions of the neighbourhood food environment. We found no evidence that any of the physical dimensions of the food environment considered were associated with fruit and vegetable consumption in older age within two nationally representative cohorts in 20 UK towns. In contrast, area income-deprivation was inversely associated with fruit and vegetable consumption. Many aspects of aging can impact on food security and nutritional status [79, 80] and older people may be more reliant on immediate neighbourhood resources, which may mean they have reduced access to healthy food [81]. Initiatives such as the WHO Age Friendly Cities recognise the importance of the urban environment for health in older age, and policies that can modify the food environment (such as restricting take away outlets) [56] have received considerable interest despite the limitations of the current evidence base. There is a need to better understand the complex interactions between urban neighbourhood environments and various health behaviours including diet across the life course. This is likely to require new methodological approaches, including those based in systems science, and adoption of standardised metrics, to enable research that is more relevant to policymakers in a rapidly urbanising world.

Acknowledgments
We acknowledge the British Regional Heart Study and British Women's Heart and Health Study teams for collecting the data and the cohort participants for their cooperation with the data collection process. In addition, we acknowledge the assistance of Catherine Bruckner, Marianne Boehme and David Walker for their help with the environmental data collection process.

Funding

This work was supported by the UK Medical Research Council [grant number: MR/J007145/1]. The collection of data on participants and their diet in the BRHS and BWHHS cohorts was supported by grants from the British Heart Foundation [BRHS grant number RG/13/16/30528 and PG/09/024; BWHHS grant number PG/13/66/30442]. The funding bodies played no role in the collection, analysis, and interpretation of data or in writing the manuscript.

Authors' contributions

KL, BA, RM and JPC conceived the study. SH and KL designed and managed the environmental data collection with input from TP and KN. The diet data was processed for the British Regional Heart Study (BRHS) by JA, and for the British Women's Heart and Health Study (BWHHS) by AA. RS conducted the data analysis with input from BA. SH wrote the first draft of the manuscript with input from KL and RS. JPC is Co-Director of the BWHHS; AA is the Study Coordinator and extracted and processed the relevant data. PW and GW are Co-Investigators of the BRHS. All authors contributed to the scientific content of the manuscript and approved the final version for publication.

Competing interests

The authors declare that they have no competing interests.

Author details

[1]Faculty of Public Health and Policy, London School of Hygiene and Tropical Medicine, London WC1E 7HT, UK. [2]Faculty of Epidemiology and Population Health, London School of Hygiene & Tropical Medicine, London WC1E 7HT, UK. [3]UCL Department of Primary Care & Population Health, UCL Medical School, Rowland Hill Street, London NW3 2PF, UK. [4]University of Exeter Medical School, Wonford Barrack Road, Exeter EX2 5DW, UK. [5]Institute of Health & Society, Newcastle University, Newcastle upon Tyne NE2 4AX, UK. [6]Farr Institute of Health Informatics, Faculty of Population Health Sciences, 222 Euston Road, London NW1 2DA, UK. [7]School of Social and Community Medicine, University of Bristol, Bristol BS8 2PS, UK. [8]Population Health Research Institute, St George's, University of London, London SW17 0RE, UK. [9]London School of Hygiene & Tropical Medicine, 15-17 Tavistock Place, London, UK.

References

1. Milte CM, McNaughton SA. Dietary patterns and successful ageing: a systematic review. Eur J Nutr. 2016;55(2):423–50.
2. Myint PK, Smith RD, Luben RN, Surtees PG, Wainwright NW, Wareham NJ, et al. Lifestyle behaviours and quality-adjusted life years in middle and older age. Age Ageing. 2011;40(5):589–95.
3. Vauzour D, Camprubi-Robles M, Miquel-Kergoat S, Andres-Lacueva C, Banati D, Barberger-Gateau P et al: Nutrition for the ageing brain: towards evidence for an optimal diet. Ageing Res Rev. 2017;35:222–40.
4. Chatterji S, Byles J, Cutler D, Seeman T, Verdes E. Health, functioning, and disability in older adults–present status and future implications. Lancet. 2015;385(9967):563–75.
5. Shlisky J, Bloom DE, Beaudreault AR, Tucker KL, Keller HH, Freund-Levi Y, et al. Nutritional considerations for healthy aging and reduction in age-related chronic disease. Adv Nutr. 2017;8(1):17–26.
6. Lock K, Pomerleau J, Causer L, Altmann D, McKee M. The global burden of disease attributable to low consumption of fruit and vegetables: implications for the global strategy on diet. Bull World Health Organ. 2005;83(2):100–8.
7. Wang X, Ouyang Y, Liu J, Zhu M, Zhao G, Bao W, et al. Fruit and vegetable consumption and mortality from all causes, cardiovascular disease, and cancer: systematic review and dose-response meta-analysis of prospective cohort studies. BMJ. 2014;349:g4490.
8. Myint PK, Welch AA, Bingham SA, Surtees PG, Wainwright NW, Luben RN, et al. Fruit and vegetable consumption and self-reported functional health in men and women in the European prospective investigation into cancer-Norfolk (EPIC-Norfolk): a population-based cross-sectional study. Public Health Nutr. 2007;10(1):34–41.
9. Mozaffarian D, Kumanyika SK, Lemaitre RN, Olson JL, Burke GL, Siscovick DS. Cereal, fruit, and vegetable fiber intake and the risk of cardiovascular disease in elderly individuals. JAMA. 2003;289(13):1659–66.
10. Trichopoulou A, Critselis E. Mediterranean diet and longevity. Eur J Cancer Prev. 2004;13(5):453–6.
11. Shepherd A. Nutrition through the life span. Part 3: adults aged 65 years and over. Brit J Nurs. 2009;18:301–7.
12. National Diet and Nutrition Survey. Results from years 1, 2, 3 and 4 (combined) of the rolling Programme (2008/2009 – 2011/2012) [https://www.gov.uk/government/uploads/system/uploads/attachment_data/file/310995/NDNS_Y1_to_4_UK_report.pdf]. Accessed July 2017.
13. Brownie S. Why are elderly individuals at risk of nutritional deficiency? Int J Nurs Pract. 2006;12:110–8.
14. Hanson LC, Ersek M, Gilliam R, Carey TS. Oral feeding options for people with dementia: a systematic review. J Am Geriatr Soc. 2011;59:463–72.
15. Malderen L, Mets T, Gorus T. Gorus.: interventions to enhance the quality of life of older people in residential long-term care: a systematic review. Ageing Res Rev. 2013;12(1):141–50.
16. Cummins S, Macintyre S. Food environments and obesity–neighbourhood or nation? Int J Epidemiol. 2006;35(1):100–4.
17. Macintyre S. Deprivation amplification revisited; or, is it always true that poorer places have poorer access to resources for healthy diets and physical activity? Int J Behav Nutr Phys Activ. 2007;4:32.
18. Swinburn B, Sacks G, Vandevijvere S, Kumanyika S, Lobstein T, Neal B, et al. INFORMAS (international network for food and obesity/non-communicable diseases research, monitoring and action support): overview and key principles. Obes Rev. 2013;14(Suppl 1):1–12.
19. Vandevijvere S, Swinburn B, International Network for F. Obesity/non-communicable diseases research M, action S: towards global benchmarking of food environments and policies to reduce obesity and diet-related non-communicable diseases: design and methods for nation-wide surveys. BMJ Open. 2014;4(5):e005339.
20. Dean WR, Sharkey JR. Rural and urban differences in the associations between characteristics of the community food environment and fruit and vegetable intake. J Nutr Educ Behav. 2011;43(6):426–33.
21. Glanz K, Sallis JF, Saelens BE, Frank LD. Healthy nutrition environments: concepts and measures. Am J Health Promot. 2005;19(5):330–3. ii
22. Kamphuis CB, Giskes K, de Bruijn GJ, Wendel-Vos W, Brug J, van Lenthe FJ. Environmental determinants of fruit and vegetable consumption among adults: a systematic review. Br J Nutr. 2006;96(4):620–35.
23. Larson N, Story M. A review of environmental influences on food choices. Ann Behav Med. 2009;38(Suppl 1):S56–73.
24. Morland K, Wing S, Diez Roux A. The contextual effect of the local food environment on residents' diets: the atherosclerosis risk in communities study. Am J Public Health. 2002;92(11):1761–7.
25. Zenk SN, Lachance LL, Schulz AJ, Mentz G, Kannan S, Ridella W. Neighborhood retail food environment and fruit and vegetable intake in a multiethnic urban population. Am J Health Promot. 2009;23(4):255–64.
26. Bodor JN, Rose D, Farley TA, Swalm C, Scott SK. Neighbourhood fruit and vegetable availability and consumption: the role of small food stores in an urban environment. Public Health Nutr. 2008;11(4):413–20.
27. Macdonald L, Ellaway A, Ball K, Macintyre S. Is proximity to a food retail store associated with diet and BMI in Glasgow, Scotland? BMC Public Health. 2011;11:464.
28. Rantakokko M, Mänty M, Iwarsson S, Törmäkangas T, Leinonen R, Heikkinen E, et al. Fear of moving outdoors and development of outdoor walking difficulty in older people. J Am Geriatr Soc. 2009;57(4):634–40.
29. Moore LVDRA, Nettleton JA, Jacobs DR. Associations of the local food environment with diet quality–a comparison of assessments based on surveys and geographic information systems: the multi-ethnic study of atherosclerosis. Am J Epidemiol. 2008;167(8):917–24.
30. Pearson T, Russell J, Campbell MJ, Barker ME. Do 'food deserts' influence fruit and vegetable consumption?–a cross-sectional study. Appetite. 2005;45(2):195–7.
31. Ball K, Timperio AF, Crawford DA. Understanding environmental influences on nutrition and physical activity behaviors: where should we look and what should we count? Int J Behav Nutr Phys Activ. 2006;3:33.
32. Rose D, Bodor JN, Hutchinson PL, Swalm CM. The importance of a multi-dimensional approach for studying the links between food access and consumption. J Nutr. 2010;140(6):1170–4.

33. Caspi CE, Kawachi I, Subramanian SV, Adamkiewicz G, Sorensen G. The relationship between diet and perceived and objective access to supermarkets among low-income housing residents. Soc Sci Med. 2012;75(7):1254–62.
34. Lennon LT, Ramsay SE, Papacosta O, Shaper AG, Wannamethee SG, Whincup PH. Cohort Profile Update: The British Regional Heart Study 1978-2014: 35 years follow-up of cardiovascular disease and ageing. Int J Epidemiol. 2015; 44(3):826–826g.
35. Lawlor DA, Bedford C, Taylor M, Ebrahim S. Geographical variation in cardiovascular disease, risk factors, and their control in older women: British Women's heart and health study. J Epidemiol Community Health. 2003;57(2):134–40.
36. Pliakas T, Hawkesworth S, Silverwood R, Nanchahal K, Grundy C, Armstrong B, et al. Optimising measurement of health-related characteristics of the built environment: comparing data collected by foot-based street audits, virtual street audits and routine secondary data sources. Health Place. 2017;43:75–84.
37. Super Output Areas [http://www.ons.gov.uk/ons/guide-method/geography/beginner-s-guide/census/super-output-areas%2D-soas-/index.html]. Accessed Sept 2017
38. Scottish Neighbourhood Statistics Guide [http://www.gov.scot/Publications/2005/02/20697/52626]. Accessed Sept 2017.
39. Frank LD, Schmid TL, Sallis JF, Chapman J, Saelens BE. Linking objectively measured physical activity with objectively measured urban form: findings from SMARTRAQ. Am J Prev Med. 2005;28(2 Suppl 2):117–25.
40. Hawkesworth S, Silverwood R, Armstrong B, Pliakas T, Nanchahal K, Jefferis BJ, et al. Investigating associations between the built envrionment and physical activity amongst older people in the UK. JECH. in press September 2017.
41. Office for National Statistics [www.ons.gov.uk]. Accessed Sept 2017.
42. Scottish Neighbourhood Statistics [www.sns.gov.uk]. Accessed Sept 2017.
43. Index of Multiple Deprivation [https://www.gov.uk/government/statistics/english-indices-of-deprivation-2010].
44. Scottish Index of Multiple Deprivation [http://www.gov.scot/Topics/Statistics/SIMD]. Accessed Sept 2017.
45. Rahmanian E, Gasevic D, Vukmirovich I, Lear SA. The association between the built environment and dietary intake - a systematic review. Asia Pac J Clin Nutr. 2014;23(2):183–96.
46. Caldwell EM, Miller Kobayashi M, DuBow WM, Wytinck SM. Perceived access to fruits and vegetables associated with increased consumption. Public Health Nutr. 2009;12(10):1743–50.
47. Moore LV, Diez Roux AV, Nettleton JA, Jacobs DR, M. F: fast-food consumption, diet quality, and neighborhood exposure to fast food: the multi-ethnic study of atherosclerosis. Am J Epidemiol. 2009;170(1):29–36.
48. Williams LK, Thornton L, Ball K, Crawford D. Is the objective food environment associated with perceptions of the food environment? Public Health Nutr. 2012;15(2):291–8.
49. Lucan SC, Hillier A, Schechter CB, Glanz K. Objective and self-reported factors associated with food-environment perceptions and fruit-and-vegetable consumption: a multilevel analysis. Prev Chronic Dis. 2014;11:E47.
50. Caspi CE, Sorensen G, Subramanian SV, Kawachi I. The local food environment and diet: a systematic review. Health Place. 2012;18(5):1172–87.
51. Rose D, Richards R. Food store access and household fruit and vegetable use among participants in the US food stamp program. Public Health Nutr. 2004;7(8):1081–8.
52. Glanz K, Sallis JF, Saelens BE, Frank LD. Nutrition environment measures survey in stores (NEMS-S): development and evaluation. Am J Prev Med. 2007;32(4):282–9.
53. Cummins S, Petticrew M, Higgins C, Findlay A, Sparks L. Large scale food retailing as an intervention for diet and health: quasi-experimental evaluation of a natural experiment. J Epidemiol Community Health. 2005;59(12):1035–40.
54. Wrigley N, Warm D, Margetts B. Deprivation, diet and food retail access: findings from the Leeds "food deserts" study. Environ Plan A. 2003;35:151–88.
55. Mercille G, Richard L, Gauvin L, Kestens Y, Shatenstein B, Daniel M, et al. Associations between residential food environment and dietary patterns in urban-dwelling older adults: results from the VoisiNuAge study. Public Health Nutr. 2012;15(11):2026–39.
56. Takeaways toolkit: tools, interventions and case studies to help local authorities develop a response to the health impacts of fast food takeaways [https://www.london.gov.uk/sites/default/files/takeawaystoolkit.pdf]. Accessed Sept 2017.
57. Li F, Harmer P, Cardinal BJ, Bosworth M, Johnson-Shelton D, Moore JM, et al. Built environment and 1-year change in weight and waist circumference in middle-aged and older adults: Portland neighborhood environment and health study. Am J Epidemiol. 2009;169(4):401–8.
58. Forsyth A, Macintyre S, Anderson A. Diets for disease? Intraurban variation in reported food consumption in Glasgow. Appetite. 1994;22(3):259–74.
59. Black C, Moon G, Baird J. Dietary inequalities: what is the evidence for the effect of the neighbourhood food environment? Health Place. 2014;27:229–42.
60. Nicklett EJ, Szanton S, Sun K, Ferrucci L, Fried LP, Guralnik JM, et al. Neighborhood socioeconomic status is associated with serum carotenoid concentrations in older, community-dwelling women. J Nutr. 2011;141(2):284–9.
61. Ball K, Lamb KE, Costa C, Cutumisu N, Ellaway A, Kamphuis CB, et al. Neighbourhood socioeconomic disadvantage and fruit and vegetable consumption: a seven countries comparison. Int J Behav Nutr Phys Activ. 2015;12:68.
62. Smith DM, Cummins S, Taylor M, Dawson J, Marshall D, Sparks L, et al. Neighbourhood food environment and area deprivation: spatial accessibility to grocery stores selling fresh fruit and vegetables in urban and rural settings. Int J Epidemiol. 2010;39(1):277–84.
63. Glanz K, Bader MD, Iyer S. Retail grocery store marketing strategies and obesity: an integrative review. Am J Prev Med. 2012;42(5):503–12.
64. Aggarwal A, Cook AJ, Jiao J, Seguin RA, Vernez Moudon A, Hurvitz PM, et al. Access to supermarkets and fruit and vegetable consumption. Am J Public Health. 2014;104(5):917–23.
65. Fuller D, Cummins S, Matthews SA. Does transportation mode modify associations between distance to food store, fruit and vegetable consumption, and BMI in low-income neighborhoods? Am J Clin Nutr. 2013;97(1):167–72.
66. Auchincloss AH, Diez Roux AV, Brown DG, Erdmann CA, Bertoni AG. Neighborhood resources for physical activity and healthy foods and their association with insulin resistance. Epidemiology. 2008;19(1):146–57.
67. Burns CM, Inglis AD. Measuring food access in Melbourne: access to healthy and fast foods by car, bus and foot in an urban municipality in Melbourne. Health Place. 2007;13(4):877–85.
68. Liese AD, Colabianchi N, Lamichhane AP, Barnes TL, Hibbert JD, Porter DE, et al. Validation of 3 food outlet databases: completeness and geospatial accuracy in rural and urban food environments. Am J Epidemiol. 2010;172(11):1324–33.
69. Cummins S, Macintyre S. Are secondary data sources on the neighbourhood food environment accurate? Case-study in Glasgow, UK. Prev Med. 2009;49(6):527–8.
70. Powell LM, Han E, Zenk SN, Khan T, Quinn CM, Gibbs KP, et al. Field validation of secondary commercial data sources on the retail food outlet environment in the U.S. Health Place. 2011;17(5):1122–31.
71. Hirsch JA, Grengs J, Schulz A, Adar SD, Rodriguez DA, Brines SJ, et al. How much are built environments changing, and where?: Patterns of change by neighborhood sociodemographic characteristics across seven U.S. metropolitan areas. Soc Sci Med. 2016;169:97–105.
72. Maguire ER, Burgoine T, Monsivais P. Area deprivation and the food environment over time: a repeated cross-sectional study on takeaway outlet density and supermarket presence in Norfolk, UK, 1990-2008. Health Place. 2015;33:142–7.
73. Sharkey JR, Johnson CM, Dean WR. Food access and perceptions of the community and household food environment as correlates of fruit and vegetable intake among rural seniors. BMC Geriatr. 2010;10:32.
74. Cummins S, Curtis S, Diez-Roux AV, Macintyre S. Understanding and representing 'place' in health research: a relational approach. Soc Sci Med. 2007;65(9):1825–38.
75. Kestens Y, Lebel A, Chaix B, Clary C, Daniel M, Pampalon R, et al. Association between activity space exposure to food establishments and individual risk of overweight. PLoS One. 2012;7(8):e41418.
76. Prins RG, Pierik F, Etman A, Sterkenburg RP, Kamphuis CB, van Lenthe FJ. How many walking and cycling trips made by elderly are beyond commonly used buffer sizes: results from a GPS study. Health Place. 2014;27:127–33.
77. Villanueva K, Knuiman M, Nathan A, Giles-Corti B, Christian H, Foster S, et al. The impact of neighborhood walkability on walking: does it differ across adult life stage and does neighborhood buffer size matter? Health Place. 2014;25:43–6.
78. Milton S, Pliakas T, Hawkesworth S, Nanchahal K, Grundy C, Amuzu A, et al. A qualitative geographical information systems approach to explore how older people interact with and define their neighbourhood environment. Health Place. 2015;36:127–33.

7

Randomized trial comparing group size of periodic in-person sessions in a remotely delivered weight loss intervention

Deborah F. Tate[1*], Carmina G. Valle[2], Melissa M. Crane[3], Brooke T. Nezami[4], Carmen D. Samuel-Hodge[5], Karen E. Hatley[6], Molly Diamond[6] and Kristen Polzien[6]

Abstract

Background: Few randomized studies have examined differential effects of group size in behavioral weight control, especially in hybrid programs that include Internet treatment approaches.

Methods: Randomized controlled trial (n = 195) comparing a 4 month hybrid internet weight loss program coupled with monthly face to face groups of 100 persons (Large Group, LG; 1 group) or to the same approach with monthly groups of 20 persons (Small Group, SG; 4 groups). Repeated-measures mixed-model analysis with age and race as covariates were used to estimate primary (weight) and secondary outcomes, and to test group differences in change over time.

Results: The sample was 46.3 years old ±10.4, 90.3% female, and 51.9% non-white, with BMI 37.9 ± 8.4 kg/m^2. Participants in the LG were more likely to return for the 4-month assessment visit than those in the SG (p = 0.04). Participants randomized to both the LG and SG conditions experienced significant WL over time (no between group difference: −4.1 kg and −3.7 kg, respectively) and weight loss was positively associated with attendance at monthly meetings and logins to the website. Satisfaction with the program was high and similar in both groups (94.4% reported that they were "satisfied" or "very satisfied").

Conclusions: Using a hybrid approach of in-person and online weight loss interventions may be an effective way to reach larger and more diverse populations. Delivering the face to face component of the intervention in groups larger than those traditionally delivered (20–25 people) could increase the cost-effectiveness of group-based behavioral weight loss interventions.

Clinical trials registration number: NCT01615471. Registered June 6, 2012. Registered retrospectively.

Keywords: Hybrid internet plus in-person groups, Large group, Behavioral weight loss

Background

The majority of US adults are overweight and obese [1], and studies show that even modest weight loss of approximately 5% of initial body weight can improve health parameters like cholesterol, blood glucose, and blood pressure, and reduce risk for chronic diseases like diabetes and cardiovascular disease [2, 3]. More recent evidence links obesity to progression and recurrence of some cancers [2–4]. Therefore, for the majority of US adults, risk reduction through modest weight loss is a public health priority.

Intensive behavioral lifestyle interventions have been developed and are proven to reduce weight in clinical trials at levels that are beneficial for health [5–8]. The 2014 American Heart Association evidence-based guidelines on the treatment of obesity suggest that lifestyle interventions are most successful when they include face-to-face sessions [6]. Research also suggests that both individual and group sessions are effective delivery formats for face-to-face sessions in behavioral lifestyle interventions [6–8], and that group format may be more effective and cost-effective for delivery of comprehensive treatment [9].

* Correspondence: dtate@unc.edu
[1]Department of Health Behavior, Department of Nutrition, The University of North Carolina at Chapel Hill, Chapel Hill, NC 27599-7440, USA
Full list of author information is available at the end of the article

Other than the comparison of individual with group delivery formats, little research has examined the effect of group size on weight loss. The Look Ahead study delivered 3 of 4 sessions per month in group format with an average group size of 11 participants; groups ranged from 6 to 21 participants over the 209 groups delivered across the 15 sites [10]. In an analysis controlling for site differences, group size was not found to be associated with mean weight loss [10]. In the single randomized trial conducted to date on this topic in obesity, Dutton and colleagues examined the effects of group size on engagement and weight loss [5]. Sixty-six participants were randomized to one group of 30 or to one of three smaller groups of 12 members. Behavioral weight loss treatment was delivered with 24 weekly groups (months 1–6) followed by 6 monthly sessions (months 7–12). Weight losses were over 3 kg and 4 kg greater in the smaller groups versus larger group at 6 and 12 months respectively. Participants in the smaller groups completed significantly more self-monitoring records ($p < .01$) than the larger group, and there was a trend for smaller group participants to attend more sessions ($p = .09$), at least partially explaining the differences in weight loss between groups. Thus, the limited available evidence is mixed regarding group size and weight loss outcomes and no data exists on group sizes above 20–25 persons. With dissemination of group based treatment in mind, examination of larger group sizes is needed as the cost of in-person treatment delivery is affected by the number of sessions needed and also the number of individuals who can be treated in each group session.

The cost, logistics and accessibility of comprehensive group behavioral lifestyle interventions have resulted in much research over the past decade on alternative delivery formats and locations for weight loss interventions. One promising alternative has been delivery via technology, including Internet interventions accessed via computer and mobile devices. In general, weight losses of approximately 4–6 kg can be reliably achieved with Internet programs that involve some form of weekly human e-counseling or ongoing feedback from behavioral lifestyle counselors (email, group chat, etc.) [11–16]. Research also suggests the efficacy of weekly professionally led group chat visits as part of an internet program [17, 18] but less is known about periodic human support delivered either in person or online.

The combination of periodic face-to-face visits and internet delivery might be appealing for several reasons: it retains some of the benefits of face-to-face delivery through participant interaction and modeling; it provides opportunity for greater accountability with periodic in-person weigh-ins; and using Internet intervention components has the potential to reduce labor costs in program delivery, allows constant access to ongoing treatment components, and increased convenience for participants. One study examined a hybrid approach delivered predominantly via weekly Internet chat groups (15–20 individuals), coupled with individual sessions once per month with a dietitian. Results suggested no additional benefit from the monthly individual face-to-face sessions, given an effective Internet program that included participant-provider interaction and participant-participant interaction within the online treatment [13]. Another study by Leahey and colleagues [19] added optional weekly group-delivered weight loss sessions to a 3-month online behavioral weight loss program and demonstrated no differences at the end of treatment (5.8% vs. 4.3% loss), but significantly greater weight losses were maintained 1 year after baseline (9 months post-treatment: optional groups 4.5% loss vs. 1.2% for internet only).

Given that individual treatment is more costly to deliver than group treatment [9], and that Internet delivered programs are largely accessed by individuals on their own, we reasoned that an Internet- and mobile-delivered program could be combined with periodic group treatment and that it might promote ongoing engagement with the program when delivered in a community setting. Another reason for offering a hybrid program in a community setting was to increase potential to appeal to a broader audience since treatment was delivered via multiple formats. Since little data existed on group size, we also sought to explore the feasibility of delivering the face-to-face component of the hybrid program in a larger group of 100 compared with more traditional large group sizes of 25. Therefore, the objective of this study was to evaluate the feasibility and preliminary efficacy of a 4-month Internet- and mobile-delivered weight loss program with monthly face-to-face group sessions delivered in a large group format (approximately 100 person group) compared with the Internet and mobile program delivered via a smaller group format (20 person groups).

Methods

Recruitment of intervention participants

We recruited and enrolled participants between April and June 2012 in Kannapolis, NC and the surrounding area, beginning the intervention in mid-June. A comprehensive recruitment website was developed to provide details about the study, eligibility, a video of a former research participant (African American female) talking about study participation, general information about participating in a research study and frequently asked questions. Potential participants were recruited through television advertisements, flyers and word of mouth and directed to the recruitment website, which linked to an online eligibility screener. Individuals were eligible if they met the following criteria: overweight and obese

(BMI ≥25 kg/m^2); aged 18–65 years old; living or working within 30 miles of Kannapolis; able to attend 4 monthly Saturday group sessions and 2 assessment visits at the Nutrition Research Institute in Kannapolis; had access to the Internet on at least a weekly basis; and had an email address or were willing to sign up for a free account (e.g., gmail). Participants were excluded if they were unable to read and write English, taking insulin, pregnant during the previous 3 months or planning pregnancy in the following 6 months, participating in another weight loss program, or were taking weight loss medications. Though no upper BMI limit was set, physician consent was required for individuals with BMI > 50, previous history of heart attack or stroke, or current treatment for cancer. To ensure participant safety, The Physical Activity Readiness Questionnaires (PAR-Q) was administered at the baseline assessment visit, and those endorsing any item on the PAR-Q were encouraged to consult their primary care physician prior to making any changes to their exercise routine.

To aid with recruitment into a study where participants could be randomized to come to a large treatment group with 100 people, participants could join the study alone but were encouraged to enroll in the study with up to three friends or family members who also met eligibility criteria. Participants were oriented (video), provided informed consent, and enrolled online. A paper copy of the consent was provided to the participant at the baseline assessment visit. This study was approved by and was in accordance with the ethical standards of the UNC Chapel Hill Institutional Review Board.

Randomization

Participants in the Lose Now NC intervention trial were randomized to one of 2 intervention groups: a "large group format" (LG) in which monthly sessions would include up to 100 participants, or a "small group format" (SG) in which monthly sessions would include approximately 20 participants. Randomization was stratified on the size of the "friends or family" social group joining together (1 = joining alone, 2, 3, or 4). Eligible participants were randomized following baseline measures, using a computer generated random numbers method by the project coordinator with allocation concealed to participants until randomization was revealed at the initial group session.

Intervention

A standard behavioral intervention based on the DPP, and adapted for use by our research team in other internet and face-to-face delivered studies [11, 12, 20–23] was adapted for this protocol. Behavioral weight control approaches are founded on teaching self-regulatory and behavioral skills (self-monitoring, goal setting, problem solving, stimulus control, etc.) and providing the support necessary to enable participants to adopt lower calorie diets (e.g., 1500–2000 kcals per day based on starting weight) and moderate physical activity (e.g., walking) to produce energy deficits necessary to produce modest weight losses of 1–2 lbs. per week. Both treatment groups attended four monthly group sessions and had access to an identical Internet program in between sessions. The main difference between the two study groups was the size of the monthly group sessions.

Monthly Treatment Groups: Treatment group sessions were held in a community facility equipped with a large room with chairs, a podium, and audio-visual equipment, which would accommodate 150 people. Smaller rooms with conference style tables and audio-visual equipment were also used. At the beginning of the program, all participants were provided with a "weight loss toolkit" to encourage evidence-based weight loss behaviors and for retention purposes. The kit included a 16 oz. water cup, Meal Measure portion control plate, and a Calorie King calorie counting guide [24]. They also were given a pedometer (PE-330 Step Tri-Axis Pocket Pedometer) at the second group session to correspond with the lifestyle physical activity lesson topic. Group sessions were held once a month on a Saturday and were approximately 90 min in duration. Over the 4 months, the same interventionists co-led the large group and individually led the small groups. Interventionists were from a multi-disciplinary team of dietitians, psychologists, exercise physiologists and health behavior experts and were trained at the Master's or PhD level. The monthly sessions began with an individual, semi-private weigh-in, followed by a group session. Both groups received the same paper copy of the 'lesson' for the session, but delivery of the content followed a slightly different format. In the LG, there were interactive features such as group text polling, cooking and exercise demonstrations, information tables for browsing before and after the session, and audience participation using a microphone. The SG sessions followed traditional behavioral weight control group session protocol with groups sitting in a small group or circle format with a table and allowing for more interaction and discussion between members and with the leader.

Internet and Mobile Program: Between face-to-face sessions, participants were asked to log into a comprehensive Internet program adapted from those tested previously by Tate et al. [11, 12, 22] that provides the self-monitoring tools, tailored automated behavioral feedback, tailored lifestyle content resources (lessons and a problem solving tool to help overcome barriers to diet and exercise change), and social support (e.g., online message board). New lesson content was posted weekly, and included information on making dietary changes, goal setting, exercise barriers, and problem solving. Presentation of the content included text, videos and interactive questionnaires. The expected frequency of Internet use was at least once a week in order to report weight, diet and exercise, and to use the program tools.

Weighing, Diet, and Exercise Recommendations and Self-Monitoring Options: Participants were instructed to weigh daily and to report weight on the study website. At session one, participants were given calorie goals designed to produce 1–2 lb. weight loss per week based on starting weight. They were given three "plans" designed to help them meet their prescribed weight loss calorie goal. The first plan offered was to self-select their diet and use the website diary to monitor all calories consumed and meet the calorie goal. The website diary used the Calorie King database and was fashioned after many commercial online diet self-monitoring tools. The second was to use an external diary (commercial smartphone app, other web-based diary or paper diary), and to enter total daily calories and fat to the website at the end of the week. The third option was to follow a study-provided meal plan at the recommended reduced calorie level and indicate only deviations to the meal plan on the study website diary. No preference was proposed for the three plans, however, the "pros" and "cons" to each were presented at the first session, and participants were encouraged to select the plan that fit best with their lifestyle and preferences for self-monitoring.

Participants also were asked to select a physical activity progression plan that took into account their baseline level of activity and progressed gradually towards an increased goal during the intervention. Plans for baseline "low active" (<60 min/week), "somewhat active" (60–150 min/week), and "highly active" (>150 min/week) levels recommended a progression over the 16-week intervention that increased the weekly minutes to 175, 200, and 250, respectively. Participants were asked to report their exercise minutes on the website. An online exercise scheduler and exercise barrier problem solving tool were provided to promote adherence to the recommendations. The pedometer was provided, after one month, as an additional tool for monitoring total activity and reporting steps on the study website was optional.

Measures

Assessments occurred at baseline and 4 months in person and using online questionnaires. Basic demographic information, including age, sex, race, education level, and income, was assessed at baseline only. Body weight was measured in lightweight street clothes, without shoes, on a calibrated digital scale (Tanita BWB 800) by blinded assessors. Height was measured at baseline using a portable stadiometer (Seca). Resting blood pressure was measured in seated position using a GE Dinamap ProCare 100 after 5 min rest; the average of two measures was used [25]. If there was a discrepancy of >10 mmHg systolic or >6 mmHg diastolic, a third measure was taken and the average of the three measures was used. Non-fasting blood samples were collected by fingerstick according to standard protocol. Hemoglobin A1C (HgA1C) was analyzed using an Alere Afinion (Orlando, Florida) point of care analyzer. Blood lipids (triglycerides, total cholesterol, HDL and LDL) were analyzed using the Alere Cholestech LDX point of care analyzer.

Dietary intake was measured via two 24-h dietary recalls conducted at each assessment time point using the Automated Self-Administered 24-Hour Dietary Recall (ASA-24) from the National Cancer Institute [26]. Participants were provided with pre-established logins and prompted to log in to the ASA-24 website at an unscheduled time and complete a 24-h recall on one weekday and one weekend day, at which time they reported everything they had to eat and drink in the 24 h on the day prior.

Physical activity was measured using a staff-administered version of the Paffenbarger Physical Activity Questionnaire (PAQ) at each assessment period [27]. Using a guided-interview format, this measure assesses leisure-time physical activity, walking, and stair-climbing over the previous week. Although originally developed as a self-report measure, the interview format allows for clarification of the activities and activity intensity unavailable when using the questionnaire alone.

Participants also completed a measure of quality of life at baseline and 4 months using the CDC Health-Related Quality of Life scale [28]. This is a 4-item measure that assesses perceptions of general health, including self-reported ratings of number of unhealthy physical and mental health days in the last 30 days. In this study the measure had acceptable internal consistency (α = .70). The Physical Activity Group Environment Questionnaire (PAGEQ) is a 26-item measure that assessed group cohesion at 4 months (α = .96) [29]. The measure assessed individuals' perceptions of the cohesiveness of the group sessions and was modified for this study to assess a weight loss group. Program adherence was measured by recording attendance at face-to-face group sessions and logins to the study website. Participants also completed a study-developed program satisfaction questionnaire at 4 months.

Statistical methods

The primary outcome of change in weight, as well as secondary outcomes of percent weight loss, change in blood pressure, cholesterol, HbA1c, general health, calorie intake, and calorie expenditure, were analyzed using intent-to-treat methodology. Multiple imputation using Markov chain Monte Carlo (MCMC) method was used to replace missing values. PROC MI and PROC MIANALYZE in

SAS 9.3 were used to conduct repeated-measures mixed-model analysis with age and race as covariates to estimate primary and secondary outcomes and to test group differences in change over time [9, 30]. Race and age were included as covariates in our analysis as they have been shown in prior studies to be associated with weight loss [31, 32]. Individuals who reported using medication for hypertension were censored for analyses of change in blood pressure. Similar methodology was used for analyses of total cholesterol and HbA1c. This program was designed to be inclusive (i.e., did not include an upper BMI cut off) and included a participant with a weight that was a statistical outlier located six standard deviations above the mean. Analyses were conducted both with and without this case (data not shown) and were similar. The results presented follow intention to treat and include the outlying case.

Given the pilot nature of this study, analyses presented here were conducted using the individual as the unit of analysis. Sensitivity analyses were also conducted considering the social grouping of participants with their friend and family. These were unadjusted analyses that used the average weight loss of the social group (containing between 1 and 4 individuals) as the unit of analysis with baseline observations carried forward for any missing data at 4 months. Analyses conducted considering the clustering of participants yielded results for weight and secondary outcomes that were similar to those when using the individual as the unit of analysis. Therefore, we subsequently present the results of the sensitivity analyses for the primary outcome of weight in the text, but not for the remaining outcomes.

Program retention, adherence, and satisfaction measures were compared using t-tests and chi-squared tests. Group comparisons with skewed distributions were analyzed using Wilcoxon-Mann-Whitney tests and are reported with medians and interquartile ranges. Relationships between program participation and weight loss were assessed with Spearman correlations. Finally, logistic regressions were used to test baseline characteristics as predictors of achieving a five-percent weight loss.

Results

Table 1 describes the baseline characteristics of participants in the Lose Now NC program ($N = 195$). Participant flow is shown on Fig. 1 [33]. Overall, 75% of participants returned for the 4 month follow-up visit. Participants in the LG were more likely to return for the 4-month assessment visit than those in the SG (80.4% vs. 67.5%, $\chi^2 = 4.21$, $p = 0.04$). Individuals who reported taking medications for hypertension, hyperlipidemia, or oral medications for diabetes were more likely to complete the 4-month assessment than those not reporting medication use at baseline (82.9% vs. 69.0%, $\chi^2 = 4.88$, $p = 0.03$). There were no other differences on baseline characteristics

Table 1 Baseline characteristics by treatment group

	Total Sample (N = 195)	Large Group (N = 112)	Small Group (N = 83)
Age (y) [m ± sd]	46.3 ± 10.8	45.0 ± 10.4	48.2 ± 11.1
Female [n (%)]	176 (90.3%)	102 (91.1)	74 (89.2)
Education[1]			
High school or less	19 (9.8)	12 (10.8)	7 (8.4)
Some college	80 (41.2)	39 (35.1)	41 (49.4)
College graduate or beyond	95 (49.0)	60 (54.1)	35 (42.2)
Race or ethnic group			
White	88 (45.1)	58 (51.8)	30 (36.1)
Black	101 (51.8)	52 (46.4)	49 (59.0)
Other	6 (3.1)	2 (1.8)	4 (4.8)
Married or living with partner	124 (63.6)	70 (62.5)	54 (65.1)
Current smoker	15 (7.7)	7 (6.3)	8 (9.6)
Medications[2]	82 (42.1)	44 (39.3)	38 (45.8)
Weight (kg)	103.7 ± 27.1	102.7 ± 23.7	105.0 ± 31.3
BMI (kg/m^2)	37.9 ± 8.4	37.6 ± 8.0	38.3 ± 8.9
Systolic blood pressure (mm Hg)	127.4 ± 14.7	126.5 ± 14.6	128.6 ± 15.0
Diastolic blood pressure (mm Hg)	75.1 ± 10.7	74.0 ± 11.1	76.5 ± 9.9
Total cholesterol (mg/dL)	188.0 ± 35.1	186.0 ± 34.8	190.8 ± 35.7
HbA1c	5.6 ± 0.6	5.6 ± 0.7	5.7 ± 0.6
Enrolled with friends/family	134 (68.7)	75 (67.0)	59 (71.1)

Notes. [1]n = 194; [2]Medications for hypertension, hyperlipidemia, or oral medications for diabetes

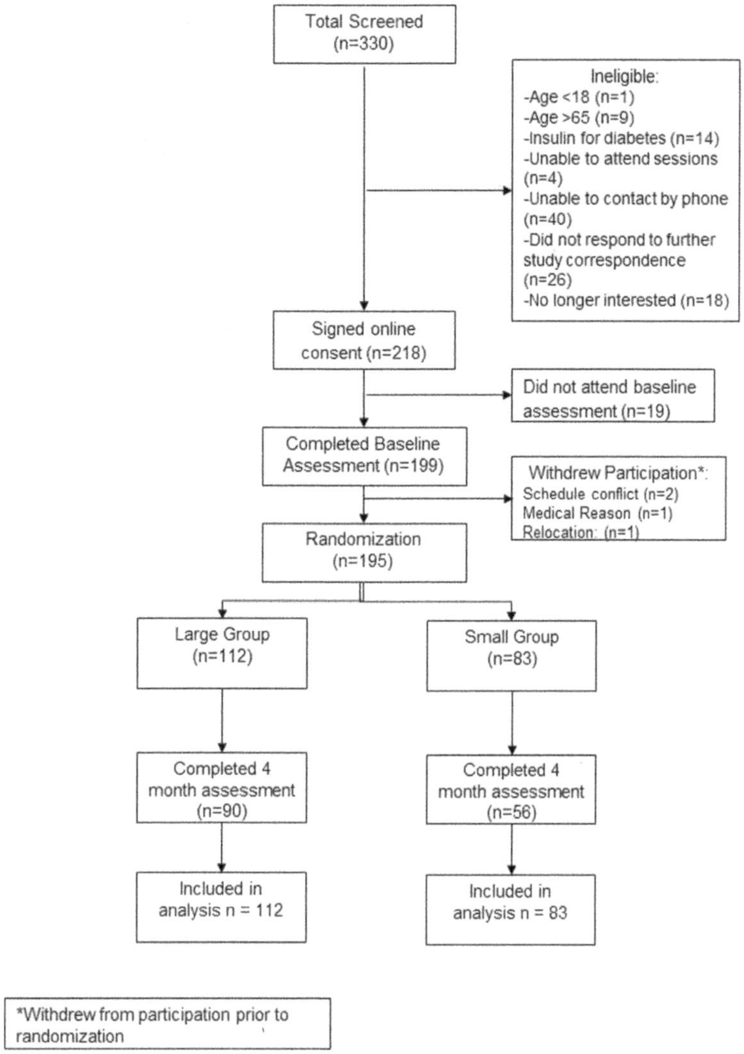

Fig. 1 CONSORT Diagram

between those who completed the study and those who did not (all p's > 0.17).

Intervention adherence

Attendance at the 4 monthly treatment group meetings did not differ by group. LG and SG participants did not differ in the number of sessions attended (median, interquartile range (IQR); LG: 3, 1–4; SG: 2, 1–4; z = −1.00, p = 0.32) nor number of times they logged into the study website (LG: 22, 3.5–56.5; SG: 9, 2–47, z = −1.44, p = 0.15). Figure 2 shows the percentage of participants who attended each group session, logged into the website during each month of the program, and the percentage who either attended the session or logged into the website. The only significant difference between groups was that a greater percentage of participants in LG attended the final group session compared to SG (χ^2 = 5.83, p = 0.02). Thirteen participants (6 LG, 7 SG) participants never logged into the website and attended no sessions; there was no difference between groups (χ^2 = 0.73, p = 0.39). Participants monitored their dietary intake on the website on average 26.4 days (SD = 31.5), with no difference between treatment groups. More participants used the web diary (n = 73) than tracking on their own and manually entering their total calories (n = 19), while 61 participants used a combination of both. Forty-two participants did not use either form of monitoring. There were no differences in type of monitoring used between groups.

Weight loss and secondary outcomes

As shown in Table 2, both groups in the study experienced significant weight losses (LG: −4.1 kg, 95% CI: -5.1, −3.0; SG: -3.7 kg, 95% CI: -5.0, −2.4) at the 4-month assessment, however, there was no difference between groups (p = 0.67). Sensitivity analyses using average weight loss of each social group as the unit of

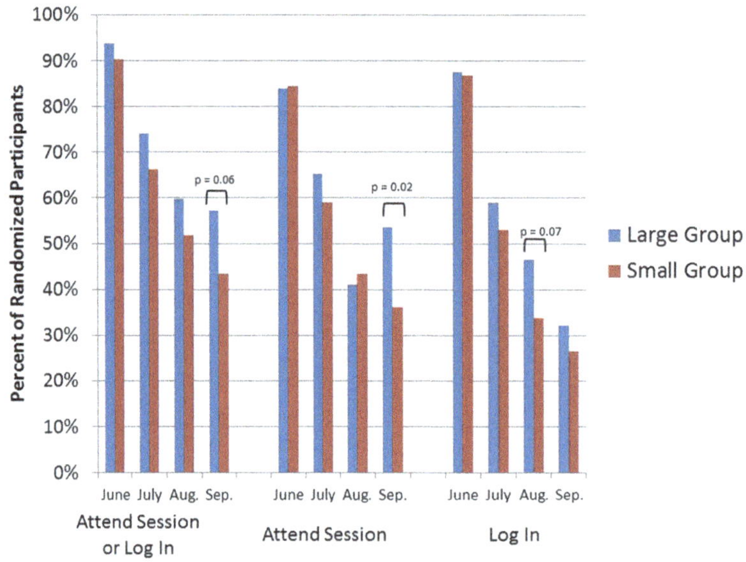

Fig. 2 Session attendance and online program use by treatment group and program month

analysis had similar results, with no difference between groups ($p = .20$). There were no differences in completion of the follow-up assessment by those who enrolled with friends and family (71.2%) or alone (65.3%; $p = 0.43$). Among those who completed the assessment, there were no differences in weight loss based on enrollment status (friends/family: –3.7 kg ± 5.2; alone –4.2 kg ± 4.2; $p = 0.56$).) A similar proportion of participants in each treatment group who returned for the follow-up visit lost at least 5% of their initial body weight during the program (LG: 35.6%, SG: 28.6%, $\chi^2 = 0.76$, $p = 0.38$). Weight loss was associated with sessions attended (Spearman's rho = –0.25, $p = 0.002$), and logins to the study website (rho = –0.50, $p < 0.001$). Participants who lost at least 5% of their initial body weight were more likely to be white (OR = 2.28; 95% CI: 1.17, 4.43) and older (OR = 1.03; 95% CI 1.00, 1.07) than participants who did not reach this goal. No other baseline characteristics were associated with achieving a 5% weight loss.

There were improvements in systolic BP, HbA1c, and self-reported health ratings over time (p's < 0.01); however, there were no differences by group (p's > 0.18). There were no significant changes to total cholesterol or diastolic BP over time (p's > .15). Participants in both groups reported decreased caloric intake at 4 months and increased caloric expenditure in leisure time physical activity (p's < 0.005), with no difference in the magnitude of the dietary and activity changes made by treatment group.

Among those who completed the 4-month assessment, weight loss was associated with change in calorie intake (rho = 0.26, $p = 0.004$), self-reported ratings of general health (rho = 0.18, $p = 0.04$), and change in HbA1c (rho = 0.38, $p < 0.001$). Weight loss was not associated with change in self-reported physical activity (rho = –0.15, $p = 0.06$), change in blood pressure (systolic, rho = 0.18, $p = 0.10$; diastolic rho = 0.05, $p = 0.66$) or change in cholesterol (rho = 0.08, $p = 0.36$).

Satisfaction with program

Seventy-three percent (142 out of 195) of participants completed questions focused on program satisfaction. Mirroring the overall completion rate of the assessment visit, somewhat more participants in the LG completed the survey than the SG (78.6% vs. 65.1%, $\chi^2 = 4.40$, p = 0.06). Among those who completed the survey, 94.4% reported they were "satisfied" or "very satisfied" with the program they received (no difference between groups $\chi^2 = 0.61$, $p = 0.43$). Nearly all participants reported that they would recommend the program to a friend; however, this was slightly lower among participants in the SG than in the LG (92.6% vs. 98.9%, $\chi^2 = 3.82$, $p = 0.05$). In ratings of individual components of the face-to-face and online program, the groups reported similar levels of satisfaction with the group meetings (97.5% satisfaction), weigh-in process (98.4%), and session topics (96.7%). These measures did not differ between groups (p's > 0.37). As shown in Table 3, group cohesion measures indicated that the LG and SG participants reported similar attraction to the group they were assigned to and felt similar levels of integration with the group members (all p's > 0.19).

Discussion

The objective of the present study was to compare the effects of treatment group size in the context of a hybrid program using the Internet and monthly face-to-face

Table 2 Anthropometric, diet, physical activity, and cardiometabolic changes[a]

			p-values		
	Baseline[b]	Change at 4-months	Time	Group	Time x Group
Weight (kg)			**<0.001**	0.50	0.67
Large group	102.5 (97.6, 107.5)	−4.1 (−5.1, −3.0)			
Small group	105.2 (99.5, 111.0)	−3.7 (−5.0, −2.4)			
Weight (%)			**<0.001**	0.72	0.52
Large group	0	−4.0 (−5.0, −3.0)			
Small group	0	−3.5 (−4.7, −2.3)			
Systolic Blood Pressure (mm Hg)			**<0.001**	0.63	0.77
Large group	123.9 (120.7, 127.1)	−5.9 (−8.8, −3.0)			
Small group	125.2 (121.2, 129.1)	−5.1 (−10.8, 0.7)			
Diastolic Blood Pressure (mm Hg)			0.25	**0.02**	0.56
Large group	72.0 (69.6, 74.3)	−1.5 (−4.0, 1.0)			
Small group	76.5 (73.6, 79.4)	0.02 (−4.9, 5.0)			
Total Cholesterol (mg/dL)			0.15	0.07	0.29
Large group	183.6 (177.2, 189.9)	−3.3 (−7.9, 1.2)			
Small group	192.8 (185.0, 200.6)	−7.9 (−15.3, −0.6)			
HbA1c [e]			**<0.001**	0.16	0.18
Large group	5.5 (5.4, 5.6)	−0.1 (−0.2, −0.1)			
Small group	5.6 (5.5, 5.7)	−0.2 (−0.2, −0.1)			
General health rating			**0.01**	0.94	0.95
Large group	2.9 (2.7, 3.0)	−0.2 (−0.4, −0.04)			
Small group	2.9 (2.7, 3.0)	−0.2 (−0.4, −0.00)			
Caloric Intake (kcal)			**<0.001**	0.14	0.69
Large group	1985 (1866, 2105)	−316 (−492, −139)			
Small group	1844 (1705, 1984)	−378 (−621, −136)			
Caloric Expenditure (kcal)[c]			**0.005**	0.79	0.67
Large group	278 (194, 780)	254			
Small group	299 (197, 456)	191			

[a]Intention-to-treat with multiple imputation repeated-measures mixed-model analysis with age and race as covariates. n = 112 for LG and n = 83 for SG for all analyses except those for BP, total cholesterol and HbA1c. Adjustments were made to the sample to exclude for BP, lipid lowering, and diabetes medication use. For BP: $n = 71$ for LG and $n = 47$ for SG. For total cholesterol: $n = 97$ for LG and $n = 65$ for SG. For HbA1c: $n = 101$ for LG and $n = 80$ for SG. Statistically significant *P* values are shown in bold
[b]All values are model predicted means; 95% CIs in parentheses
[c]Analyses conducted using log-transformed values

Table 3 Group Cohesion at 4 months[a]

	Large Group	Small Group	*p*-value
N	88	54	
Attraction to group-Task[b]	7.0 ± 1.2	6.8 ± 1.4	0.31
Attraction to group- Social	5.6 ± 1.9	6.0 ± 1.6	0.21
Integration with group- Task	6.3 ± 1.2	6.1 ± 1.5	0.41
Integration with group- Social	5.4 ± 1.3	5.1 ± 1.4	0.19
Attraction to group leader	6.1 ± 1.5	6.6 ± 1.6	0.08

[a]Difference between means tested using independent t-tests. Values are mean ± standard deviation
[b]Subscale scores range from 1 to 9 with higher scores indicating greater attraction/integration

groups. The study delivered treatment using an Internet program coupled with either monthly large group (100 persons) or smaller groups (20 persons). Participants in both large and small treatment group formats showed significant weight loss over the 4 month intervention (approximately 4 kg) and weight losses did not differ significantly between groups. Weight losses were approximately 4% at 4 months and were associated with reduction in HbA1c.

This study is among the first to investigate delivering behavioral weight loss in a group of more than 100 individuals and to examine group size in the context of supplementing a primarily Internet delivered program. Though other studies examining group size used large groups of a similar size to the "small" groups used here (approximately 20–30), our results are similar to the Look Ahead findings where group size was not related to weight loss [10]. In contrast, Dutton et al. [5] found weight losses to be 3–4 kg better in smaller groups (8–10 participants) compared to larger groups (30 participants), and this was partially explained by adherence such that small group participants showed better self-monitoring and a trend toward better session attendance. Participants in the current study were encouraged to join the study with friends or family members, so it is possible that participating in a large group was less overwhelming with existing social support members than participating alone. Moreover, because much of the treatment was actually delivered online, it may be that more than four in-person treatment sessions are needed to see an effect of group size, as found in the Dutton study with 24 weekly sessions. Finally, it may be necessary to use much smaller groups of approximately 10 individuals to see the benefits of small group size.

We have previously reported on a Stepped Care model for delivering behavioral weight loss that began with monthly group contact (groups of approximately 25) and utilized postal mail for lesson and diary exchange between monthly sessions [20]. At 3 months, weight losses averaged 5.9% in the group receiving monthly group treatment, somewhat better than reported here; however participants in that study had to agree to be randomized to receive either weekly or monthly group treatment sessions which may reflect a different study sample. The weight losses achieved in this study were similar to those in Leahey et al. [19]. The Leahey study reported average weight losses of approximately 5% after 4 months using a hybrid in-person and online approach, however the in-person meetings were more frequent (weekly versus monthly) and were optional. Interestingly, the hybrid approach produced better maintenance in that study; our study did not have a longer term follow-up visit. Though few studies have examined ways to augment remotely delivered treatments with in-person sessions, future research might examine the size, frequency, and timing of face-to-face interaction that produce the best outcomes.

Though not statistically significant, it is worth noting that the direction of the observed means in this study were in a direction favoring the LG (weight loss, attendance, logins etc.). LG participants attended 25% more treatment sessions compared with small group participants (3 vs. 2). They also logged into the study website twice as many times over the 4 months (22 vs. 9 times), on average. Retention was significantly greater in the LG compared with SG ($p < .05$). When we designed the study we were unsure whether the large group might lead to greater feelings of anonymity, and if so, whether this would be beneficial or detrimental for attendance. Our measure of group cohesion did not show differences on feelings of integration with group members, and while program satisfaction was high in both groups, 99% of LG participants would recommend the program to a friend. Taken together, these metrics suggest that engagement and satisfaction was not worse, and may have been somewhat better in the LG participants compared with the SG.

To control for potential effects of treatment group leaders, all four SG treatment leaders participated as leaders in various sessions in the LG. However, to encourage participation with the large number of people necessitated conducting the LG in a somewhat different manner than the SG. For example, text message/internet polling were used during the sessions to allow participants to express how they had done the previous week, amount of weight lost, etc. and view group level feedback instantaneously. Similarly, participants could text in questions or problems at any time and the treatment providers address questions during the session. These aspects may have created a fun and engaging atmosphere. Future research might examine approaches to interaction in groups in addition to group size.

This study was not designed to study non-inferiority, however, future well powered studies might include careful cost tracking to determine the cost-effectiveness of behavioral weight loss delivered in substantially larger groups. Similarly, we employed a novel method of recruiting in a community setting - encouraging enrollment with family or friends. This study was also not designed to examine the effects of enrolling with others on weight loss but this method of delivering treatment in a large group may be of interest to those seeking to study social influences on weight loss.

One of the notable strengths of this study is the diversity represented in the sample. Prior to recruitment for the randomized intervention trial, we conducted focus groups of men (any race) and African American women to gather feedback on recruitment messages and message placement that would maximize recruitment of groups that are typically underrepresented in behavioral weight loss trials. Consensus from participants was that joining a weight loss program as part of a research study would be highly favorable and most were likely to attend the monthly visits and use the web-based program, suggesting feasibility of our approach. Sample recruitment flyers with images, taglines and a brief description of the program were also presented to the groups. The results of the focus groups were summarized in a report and provided to a marketing company for finalization of the study recruitment website and advertisements. Our recruitment approach also utilized a community member who was a Black male. These combined approaches resulted in a yield of 50% of the participants self-identifying as African American and fewer than 50% reporting a college degree which lends to the generalizability of the findings. Despite these efforts, men were underrepresented in our sample, indicating a need for further study of how men can be recruited to participate in weight loss programs [34]. A further strength of this study was that weight was measured objectively by blinded assessors. The weight losses were modest, 3–4%, however the study was 4 rather than 6 months duration, as is commonly reported in the literature and used tailored, automated feedback rather than human email counseling; thus the human counseling support was limited to the monthly face-to-face group sessions. The study is also limited by the short duration, modest follow-up rates (75%), self-report measures of diet and activity, and our ability to study only a single large group. Furthermore, we are unable to separate group size from other aspects of treatment delivery as noted above. Future trials should control for this.

Conclusions

The results of this study suggest that using a hybrid approach of in-person and online weight loss interventions may be an effective way to reach larger and more diverse populations. While a fully-powered study with multiple large groups is needed to confirm this initial finding, this study provides preliminary evidence that moving beyond modest-sized treatment groups (20 people) may be a worthwhile direction for increasing the cost-effectiveness of group-based behavioral weight loss interventions. Further, it will be important for future studies to investigate the mechanisms through which larger versus smaller groups operate and perhaps whether smaller versus larger groups may be more appropriate for use with mobile technologies, specific demographic subgroups, or phases of treatment.

Acknowledgements

The study team would like to acknowledge the Nutrition Research Institute for hosting study assessments and group sessions and the NC SPEED team for their contributions to the formative work and community recruitment efforts. We also acknowledge the efforts of Graduate Research Assistants Candice Alick, Loneke Blackman, Jennifer Frank and Mary Shen.

Funding

Funding for this study was provided by the Lineberger Comprehensive Cancer Center and the University Cancer Research Fund at the University of North Carolina at Chapel Hill.

Authors' contributions

DT was the Principal Investigator on the study and was responsible for the study design, overall direction, data analysis and manuscript development. CV, BN and MC contributed to the study design, implementation, data analysis and manuscript development. CSH contributed to the study design and manuscript development. KH contributed to the study design, intervention development, management of the day to day implementation of the study, and manuscript development. KP and MD contributed to the intervention development, intervention implementation and manuscript development. All authors read and approved the final manuscript.

Competing interests

DT is a member of the Scientific Advisory Board for Weight Watchers International.

Author details

[1]Department of Health Behavior, Department of Nutrition, The University of North Carolina at Chapel Hill, Chapel Hill, NC 27599-7440, USA. [2]Department of Nutrition, The University of North Carolina at Chapel Hill, Chapel Hill, NC 27599-7294, USA. [3]Department of Preventive Medicine, Rush University Medical Center, 1700 W. Van Buren St., Suite 470, Chicago, IL 60612, USA. [4]Lineberger Comprehensive Cancer Center, The University of North Carolina at Chapel Hill, Chapel Hill, NC 27599-7294, USA. [5]Department of Nutrition, The University of North Carolina at Chapel Hill, Chapel Hill, NC 27599-7426, USA. [6]Lineberger Comprehensive Cancer Center, The University of North Carolina at Chapel Hill, Chapel Hill, NC 27599-7294, USA.

References

1. Ogden CL, Carroll MD, Kit BK, Flegal KM. Prevalence of childhood and adult obesity in the United States, 2011-2012. JAMA. 2014;311:806–14.
2. Renehan AG, Tyson M, Egger M, Heller RF, Zwahlen M. Body-mass index and incidence of cancer: a systematic review and meta-analysis of prospective observational studies. Lancet. 2008;371:569–78.
3. The Role of Cancer Survival and Recurrence - Workshop Summary. https://iom.nationalacademies.org/Reports/2012/The-Role-of-Obesity-in-Cancer-Survival-and-Recurrence.aspx. Accessed 30 May 2017.
4. What you need to know about Cancer and Obesity. http://www.aicr.org/learn-more-about-cancer/infographics/infographic-obesity-and-cancer.html.
5. Dutton GR, Nackers LM, Dubyak PJ, Rushing NC, Huynh TV, Tan F, Anton SD, Perri MG. A randomized trial comparing weight loss treatment delivered in large versus small groups. Int J Behav Nutr Phys Act. 2014;11:123.
6. Jensen MD, Ryan DH, Apovian CM, Ard JD, Comuzzie AG, Donato KA, Hu FB, Hubbard VS, Jakicic JM, Kushner RF, et al. AHA/ACC/TOS guideline for the management of overweight and obesity in adults: a report of the American College of Cardiology/American Heart Association task force on practice guidelines and the Obesity Society. Circulation 2014. 2013;129:S102–38.
7. Diabetes Prevention Program Research G. Reduction in the incidence of type 2 diabetes with lifestyle intervention or Metformin. N Engl J Med. 2002;346:393–403.
8. Delahanty LM, Nathan DM. Implications of the diabetes prevention program and look AHEAD clinical trials for lifestyle interventions. J Am Diet Assoc. 2008;108:S66–72.
9. Befort CA, Donnelly JE, Sullivan DK, Ellerbeck EF, Perri MG. Group versus individual phone-based obesity treatment for rural women. Eat Behav. 2010;11:11–7.
10. Wing RR, Leahey T, Jeffery R, Johnson KC, Hill JO, Coday M, Espeland MA. Do weight loss and adherence cluster within behavioral treatment groups? Obesity (Silver Spring). 2014;22:638–44.
11. Tate DF, Jackvony EH, Wing RR. Effects of internet behavioral counseling on weight loss in adults at risk for type 2 diabetes: a randomized trial. JAMA. 2003;289:1833–6.
12. Tate DF, Jackvony EH, Wing RR. A randomized trial comparing human e-mail counseling, computer-automated tailored counseling, and no counseling in an internet weight loss program. Arch Intern Med. 2006;166:1620–5.
13. Harvey-Berino J, West D, Krukowski R, Prewitt E, VanBiervliet A, Ashikaga T, Skelly J. Internet delivered behavioral obesity treatment. Prev Med. 2010;51:123–8.
14. Gold BC, Burke S, Pintauro S, Buzzell P, Harvey-Berino J. Weight loss on the web: a pilot study comparing a structured behavioral intervention to a commercial program. Obesity (Silver Spring). 2007;15:155–64.
15. Crane MM, Lutes LD, Ward DS, Bowling JM, Tate DF. A randomized trial testing the efficacy of a novel approach to weight loss among men with overweight and obesity. Obesity (Silver Spring). 2015;23:2398–405.
16. Steinberg DM, Tate DF, Bennett GG, Ennett S, Samuel-Hodge C, Ward DS. The efficacy of a daily self-weighing weight loss intervention using smart scales and e-mail. Obesity (Silver Spring). 2013;21:1789–97.
17. West DS, Harvey JR, Krukowski RA, Prewitt TE, Priest J, Ashikaga T. Do individual, online motivational interviewing chat sessions enhance weight loss in a group-based, online weight control program? Obesity (Silver Spring). 2016;24:2334–40.

18. Harvey-Berino J, Pope L, Gold BC, Leonard H, Belliveau C. Undergrad and overweight: an online behavioral weight management program for college students. J Nutr Educ Behav. 2012;44:604–8.
19. Leahey TM, Subak LL, Fava J, Schembri M, Thomas G, Xu X, Krupel K, Kent K, Boguszewski K, Kumar R, et al. Benefits of adding small financial incentives or optional group meetings to a web-based statewide obesity initiative. Obesity (Silver Spring). 2015;23:70–6.
20. Jakicic JM, Tate DF, Lang W, Davis KK, Polzien K, Rickman AD, Erickson K, Neiberg RH, Finkelstein EA. Effect of a stepped-care intervention approach on weight loss in adults: a randomized clinical trial. JAMA. 2012;307:2617–26.
21. Phelan S, Brannen A, Erickson K, Diamond M, Schaffner A, Munoz-Christian K, Stewart A, Sanchez T, Rodriguez VC, Ramos DI, et al. 'Fit moms/mamas Activas' internet-based weight control program with group support to reduce postpartum weight retention in low-income women: study protocol for a randomized controlled trial. Trials. 2015;16:59.
22. Tate DF, Wing RR, Winett RA. Using internet technology to deliver a behavioral weight loss program. JAMA. 2001;285:1172–7.
23. Webber KH, Tate DF, Michael BJ. A randomized comparison of two motivationally enhanced internet behavioral weight loss programs. Behav Res Ther. 2008;46:1090–5.
24. Borushek A. The CalorieKing calorie, fat & Carbohydrate Counter 2012 edn. Huntington Beach: Family Health Publications.
25. National Institutes of Health NH, Lung, and Blood Institute, Joint National Committee on Prevention D, Evaluation, and, the ToHBPNAAf, Obesity. So. The practical guide: identification, evaluation, and treatment of overweight and obesity in adults. Bethesda: NIH; 2000.
26. Automated Self-Administered 24-Hour (ASA24®) Dietary Assessment Tool. http://riskfactor.cancer.gov/tools/instruments/asa24/. 30 May 2017.
27. Paffenbarger RS Jr, Wing AL, Hyde RT. Physical activity as an index of heart attack risk in college alumni. 1978. Am J Epidemiol. 1995;142:889–903. discussion 887-888
28. Measuring Healthy Days: Population Assessment of Health-Related Quality of Life. https://www.cdc.gov/hrqol/pdfs/mhd.pdf. Accessed 30 May 2017.
29. Estabrooks PA, Carron AV. The physical activity group environment questionnaire: an instrument for the assessment of cohesion in exercise classes. Group Dynamics. 2000;4:240–3.
30. Gadbury GL, Coffey CS, Allison DB. Modern statistical methods for handling missing repeated measurements in obesity trial data: beyond LOCF. Obes Rev. 2003;4:175–84.
31. Gokee-LaRose J, Gorin AA, Raynor HA, Laska MN, Jeffery RW, Levy RL, Wing RR. Are standard behavioral weight loss programs effective for young adults? Int J Obes. 2009;33:1374–80.
32. Wingo BC, Carson TL, Ard J. Differences in weight loss and health outcomes among African Americans and whites in multicentre trials. Obes Rev. 2014;15(Suppl 4):46–61.
33. Moher D, Hopewell S, Schulz KF, Montori V, Gotzsche PC, Devereaux PJ, Elbourne D, Egger M, Altman DG. CONSORT 2010 explanation and elaboration: updated guidelines for reporting parallel group randomised trials. J Clin Epidemiol. 2010;63:e1–37.
34. Crane MM, LaRose JG, Espeland MA, Wing RR, Tate DF. Recruitment of young adults for weight gain prevention: randomized comparison of direct mail strategies. Trials. 2016;17:282.

8

Obstacles to preventing obesity in children aged 2 to 5 years: Latino mothers' and fathers' experiences and perceptions of their urban environments

Carlos Penilla[1*], Jeanne M. Tschann[2], Emma V. Sanchez-Vaznaugh[3], Elena Flores[4] and Emily J. Ozer[1]

Abstract

Background: The prevalence of obesity among Latino children is alarmingly high, when compared to non-Latino White children. Low-income Latino parents living in urban areas, even if they are well-educated, face obstacles that shape familial health behaviors. This study used qualitative methods to explore parents' experiences in providing meals and opportunities to play to their children aged 2 to 5 years. In contrast to most prior studies, this study examined perceptions of familial behaviors among both mothers and fathers.

Methods: An ecological framework for exploring the associations of parental feeding behaviors and children's weight informed this study. An interview guide was developed to explore parents' experiences and perceptions about children's eating and physical activity and administered to six focus groups in a community-based organization in the Mission District of San Francisco. Transcripts were coded and analyzed. Twenty seven mothers and 22 fathers of Latino children ages 2 to 5 participated.

Results: Mothers, fathers, and couples reported that employment, day care, neighborhood environments and community relationships were experienced, and perceived as obstacles to promoting health behavior among their children, including drinking water instead of soda and participating in organized playtime with other preschool-age children.

Conclusions: Results from this study suggest that the parents' demographic, social and community characteristics influence what and how they feed their children, as well as how often and the types of opportunities they provide for physical activity, providing further evidence that an ecological framework is useful for guiding research with both mothers and fathers. Mothers and fathers identified numerous community and society-level constraints in their urban environments. The results point to the importance of standardized work hours, resources for day care providers, clean and safe streets and parks, strong community relationships, and reduced access to sugar-sweetened beverages in preventing the development of obesity in preschool-age Latino children.

Keywords: Latino, Childhood obesity, Parent feeding behavior, Urban environments, Fathers

* Correspondence: cpenilla@berkeley.edu
[1]School of Public Health, University of California, Berkeley, 50 University Hall, Berkeley, CA 94720-7360, USA
Full list of author information is available at the end of the article

Background

Addressing childhood obesity is an urgent public health concern. In the United States, the prevalence of overweight and obesity among children is especially high in the Latino population [1]. In 2011–2012, 17% of Latino children ages 2 to 5 were considered obese, as defined by a body mass index (BMI) greater than or equal to the 95th percentile, compared to 4% of non-Latino White children of similar ages [1]. In the short term, obese children are at higher risk for health problems such as hypertension, type 2 diabetes, sleep disordered breathing and asthma, fatty liver disease, and abnormalities in menstruation and early menarche [2]. Obesity research and interventions with preschool-age Latino children have primarily focused on mother-child dyads [3]. While these interventions can be beneficial, an unintended negative consequence is the potential blaming of mothers for their children's overweight without considering key factors beyond the dyad. Empirical evidence suggests that structural and environmental factors such as the cost of food, junk food advertising, the abundance of fast food, lack of places to exercise, and traffic or crime-related safety may be associated with obesity-related health disparities, especially among disadvantaged populations [4, 5]. No previous research has explored structural and environmental factors as related to parent-child relationships and how these factors may shape both mothers' and fathers' decisions and behaviors about what preschool-age Latino children eat or how they play.

Framework

Using a socioecological approach to understanding familial health behaviors, we conceptualized children's eating and physical activity routines as shaped by parents' experiences and cultural traditions, as well as by environmental conditions outside of the parents' control [6, 7]. These environmental conditions may support and or constrain parental goals of raising healthy children [8, 9]. A growing body of research has linked healthy behaviors with built, social and socioeconomic environmental assets (access to parks, social ties, affluence); similarly, unhealthy behaviors have been linked with built environmental obstacles (access to fast food outlets), suggesting that neighborhood environments are an important level at which to intervene to prevent childhood obesity [5, 10]. For example, a recent study of racial/ethnic and socioeconomic characteristics in urban environments suggests that Latino families may not have access to either supermarkets or grocery stores [11, 12]. These factors and other features, such as accessibility to high-density fast food, may create obesogenic environments that influence parents' decisions and behaviors.

This qualitative study was informed by Davison and Birch's (2001) ecological framework of childhood obesity, which poses that three contextual layers influence the development of overweight: 1) child's characteristics and risk factors, 2) parenting practices and family characteristics, and 3) demographic, social and community characteristics (see Fig. 1). This study focused on the broader social and environmental influences, namely, how urban neighborhoods influence children's weight status through parents' child-feeding and physical activity routines.

Why explore both mothers' and fathers' child-feeding behaviors?

While mothers can play a dominant role in child feeding, fathers play a role as well [13–15]. Nevertheless, fathers are seldom included in pediatric obesity research [16, 17]. The U.S. Department of Labor reported that mothers spend more time on childcare tasks than fathers do, but the time gap between full-time working mothers and full-time working fathers continues to narrow [18]. Because the majority (66%) of Latino children live in two-parent families [19], Latino fathers play a role in two-parent households. Moreover, nationally, the share of Latino single-mother households (22%) and Latino single-father households (24%) is similar, and part of a growing national trend in single-parent households [20].

Studies conducted with Latino mothers about their role in feeding have primarily focused on the needs of mother-child dyads within the home and school environments [21]. Results from these studies generally indicate that mothers describe their primary responsibility as feeding the family, but that in addition to the cost of food, mothers may experience various obstacles outside the home, such as unappealing lunches provided to children at school, proximity to grocery stores, junk food advertising, busy schedules, and in some low-income neighborhoods, unsafe streets and parks [22–26]. A qualitative study with Latino mothers reported that some children come home and request specific foods they perceive as healthy and/or refuse foods that parents offer if they perceive them as unhealthy, because of what they are taught in school about nutrition, as well as what they are offered for school lunch [23]. Unfortunately, some children may come home hungry from school because they did not get enough to eat at lunch or found the lunch choices unappealing. Results from a recent study exploring obstacles to low-income Latino and African American mothers' preferred child feeding indicated that parents in neighborhoods without grocery stores take public transportation and/or carpool to other neighborhoods to buy healthful food, making it challenging to offer healthful food [24]. For immigrant mothers, the feeling of isolation that develops as a result of cultural differences between their country of origin and the U.S. and loss of social support were also reported as obstacles to feeding children healthful foods. When these

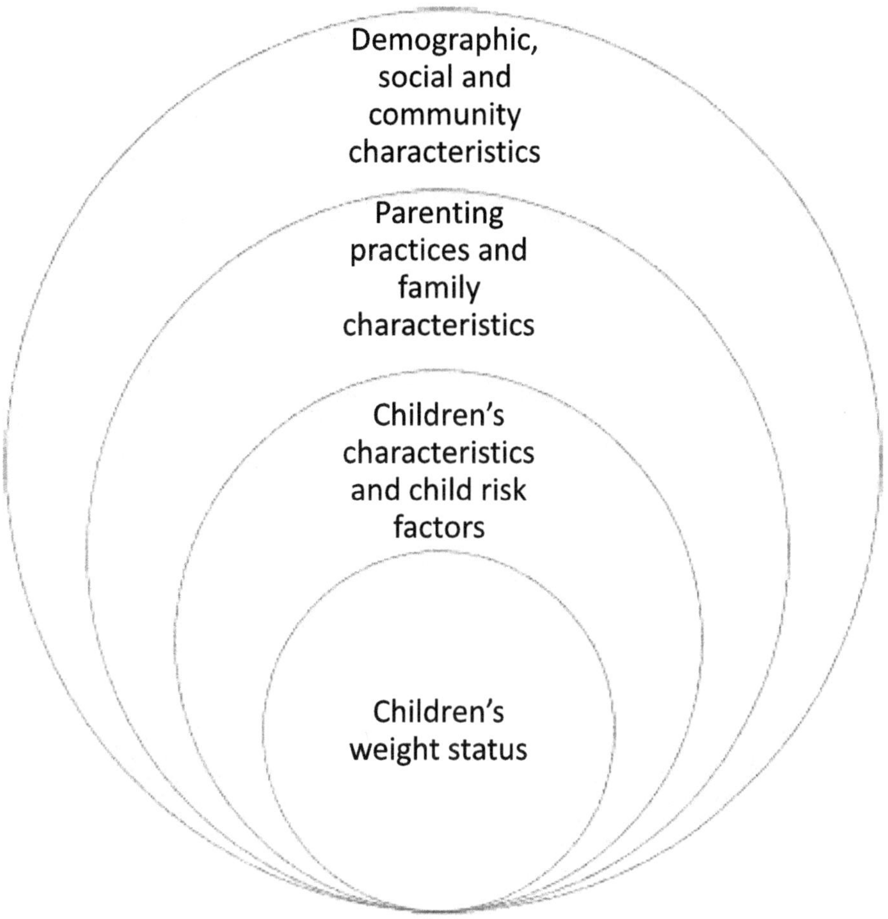

Fig. 1 Graphic based on Davison and Birch's (2001) ecological framework for exploring factors associated with children's weight status

factors interact, they may limit newly immigrated mothers' opportunities to adapt to the local community and navigate through its resources. There is extensive research on obstacles to feeding children healthful food within the home and school environment, but there is a dearth of research about how community, demographic and social characteristics in underserved urban communities influence eating and drinking, especially among Latino children.

Although research with mothers has helped our understanding of some of the factors that influence parents' behavior, studies have often not included fathers. In order to inform effective obesity prevention interventions among preschool-age Latino children, research is needed that moves beyond mother-child dyads at home and school. To our knowledge, no qualitative studies on broader environmental obstacles to preventing childhood obesity have reported on the experiences and perspectives of both mothers and fathers of preschool-age Latino children. This study addresses this gap by investigating Latino mothers' and fathers' experiences and their perceptions about the ways in which community and environmental factors influence the development of obesity among children aged 2 to 5 years. The overall research question was: What social and environmental characteristics in urban neighborhoods influence familial relationships and make it harder for children to eat healthful food and stay physically active, and how do these characteristics operate?

With the goal of informing future community-level research aimed at preventing obesity among preschool-age children living in low-income urban neighborhoods, this research used focus group methodology to examine mothers' and fathers' perceived environmental obstacles to preventing obesity and the influence of these obstacles on children's eating and physical activity. A major aim of focus group methodology is to shed new light on a group of people's understanding of a phenomenon, such as the eating behavior of children living in urban environments, by using group interaction to produce data and insights that might otherwise not emerge in individual interviews [27]. Focus group interviews with Latino parents living in urban areas allowed for in-depth group discussion of unique and shared experiences and perceptions. Another benefit of focus groups is that it helps prevent the power dynamics between interviewer and interviewee that can emerge in one-to-one interviews, and encourages a freer flow of communication among the members in the group. For example, having the parents talk amongst themselves about healthy eating allowed freer dynamics to emerge and gave space for parents to agree and disagree with each other; thus, deepening the discussion.

Methods

Participants

Using a purposive approach to sample selection [28, 29], the present study recruited 49 Latino parents (27 mothers and 22 fathers) to participate in six focus groups. Parents were recruited from throughout San Francisco, with emphasis on the Mission District, because it has the largest Latino population in the city (approximately 38% of local residents are Latino) [30], and has multiple organizations that serve low-income Latino families with preschool-age children. Most referrals to the focus groups were provided by personnel working at community-based health centers and immigrant resource centers, who distributed study flyers to their clients with children. Trained bilingual research assistants screened potential participants who called the research offices in response to recruitment efforts. Eligible participants were the parent/guardian of a child between ages 2 to 5, spoke English or Spanish and were of Mexican, Guatemalan or Salvadoran descent (see Table 1). These three major ethnic groups make up over 82% of the Latino population in the San Francisco area [31]. This research was approved by the university's institutional review board.

Table 1 Characteristics of Mexican, Guatemalan and Salvadorian origin parents who participated in child obesity focus groups

	Mothers (n = 27) % or M (SD)	Fathers (n = 22) % or M (SD)
Country of birth[a]		
USA	19%	23%
Mexico	37%	41%
El Salvador	19%	9%
Guatemala	15%	9%
Honduras	7%	5%
Nicaragua	4%	14%
Spanish is primary language	59%	46%
# of years lived in the US	16 (11.2)	19 (8.0)
Age (years)	30 (5.8)	35 (9.1)
Currently employed	33%	68%
Years of education	12 (3.7)	11 (2.3)
Relationship status		
Single/Divorced	34%	32%
Married/Living with sig. other	66%	68%

[a]Though a few participants were born in Honduras and Nicaragua, they reported that they were of Mexican, Guatemalan or Salvadoran descent

Focus groups

The focus groups were conducted in the conference room of a community-based organization in San Francisco in 2011 and 2012. This organization was chosen for its central and accessible location in a neighborhood with a high concentration of Latino families [25]. A total of six focus groups were conducted, two with mothers-only (English, $n = 7$; Spanish, $n = 12$), two with fathers-only (English, $n = 8$; Spanish, $n = 6$), and two with couples (English, $n = 8$; Spanish, $n = 8$). We included both single and married mothers and fathers in order to obtain a broader view on preventing obesity. Focus group facilitators were matched by gender. Couples focus groups were co-led by a female and male facilitator. The first author participated as facilitator in the two fathers-only and two couples focus groups. Three focus groups were conducted in English and three were conducted in Spanish. The focus groups lasted approximately two hours and were audiotaped. Focus group participants were given $50 for their participation and $30 to assist with childcare while attending the focus groups.

A focus group guide was developed to help obtain information on promoting healthful food and healthy weight in urban areas. The initial questions and probes were used to explore parental concerns about childhood obesity and how parents determine the type and amount of food to offer children on a daily basis. For example, "In your neighborhood, how much do parents with Latino children ages 2 to 5 talk about concerns about childhood overweight or eating better?" and "How do parents figure out how much to feed their children as

Table 2 Focus group guide

1. Overweight: In your neighborhood, how much do parents with Latino children ages 2 to 5 talk about concerns about childhood overweight or eating better? What do they say?
2. Children's meals: How do parents figure out how much to feed their children as the children grow older?

   Probe: a) If some days family members, or another person feeds the child, how do parents figure out how much their child has eaten that day?
3. Soda: If a family likes to drink soda, what would make it harder for them to drink less soda?

   Probes: a) What would make it easier for a family to drink less soda?
4. Physical activity: How much do parents with Latino children ages 2 to 5 talk about physical activity?

   Probes: a) Is there anything that makes it easier for families to do physical activity with their children?; b) Is there anything that could be done in neighborhoods to make it easier for families to do physical activity?

they grow older?" (see Table 2). The remaining three questions and probes were used to explore parents' perceptions of factors that are highly correlated with child weight such as soda consumption, physical activity routines and sedentary behavior including questions about experiences related to maintaining healthful behavior [32]. For example, "If a family likes to drink soda, what would make it harder to drink less?" and "Is there anything that makes it easier for families to do physical activity with their children?" (see Table 2). The focus group guide was translated side-by-side for accuracy. The audiotapes of the groups were transcribed in their original language and checked for accuracy against original recordings.

Qualitative analysis

Consistent with guidelines for qualitative analysis described by Miles and Huberman (1994), we used a multi-stage analytic process that combined deductive, inductive and verification techniques to strengthen the reliability of the coding system and validity of the findings. In the initial stage, the authors read the transcripts and summary notes to generate an initial set of descriptive phrases that would be used to code the transcript text. In order to establish consistent application of codes to text, two trained Spanish-bilingual research assistants coded the six transcripts. Using an iterative process to strengthen the reliability of the coding system [28, 29], the first two transcripts of two focus groups (one in English and one in Spanish) were coded in increments of about 10 pages at a time and immediately reviewed to examine closely the agreement between the two research assistants. Any inconsistencies in the coded text were discussed and resolved by the authors at each interval, to ensure clear inclusion and exclusion criteria. This process resulted in changes to the initial codes, such as expanding on initial two-word themes, and in changes to how the remaining four transcripts were coded by the two research assistants.

With respect to the deductive process, some codes were developed based on focus group questions reflecting the conceptual framework, such as environmental features including liquor stores and fast food availability. In terms of the inductive process, we developed codes to reflect new themes that emerged from the focus group discussions, such as emigrating to the U.S. and fears of deportation. In the next stage, transcripts with coded text were uploaded into QSR NVivo in order to generate groupings of coded passages and to facilitate further analysis and interpretation. Software was used to connect relevant data segments with each other, forming new categories, clusters and networks of information for analysis in order to draw new conclusions [28, 29, 33]. The coded transcript data from the six focus groups were then sorted by codes and analyzed by the authors to identify the larger emergent themes and to organize the results. In the verification stage, all transcripts and resultant data analyses were reviewed by the authors to confirm accuracy of reported conceptual relationships between the themes.

Results

Most participants were born outside the U.S. (81% of mothers and 77% of fathers; see Table 1). Generally, mothers had lived in the U.S. for 16 years (SD = 11.2) and had completed 12 years of education (SD = 3.7). Fathers had lived in the U.S. for an average of 19 years (SD = 8.0) and had completed an average of 11 years of education (SD = 2.3). Most mothers were unemployed (67%), while most fathers were employed (68%).

Results are presented following the ecological framework of childhood obesity [9], from individual to community levels, but organized according to broader social and environmental characteristics. This study reports on four structural categories relevant to the ecological framework of childhood obesity which guides this study: employment, day care, neighborhood environments and community relationships (see Table 3). Except for employment, which was not mentioned by mothers in the English-language mothers-only group, all themes were mentioned in all groups so results are presented together. The relative emphasis of themes by group type is described at the end of the results section (see Fig. 2). The results from the Spanish and English-language focus groups were similar and are presented together (all quotes have been translated into English).

Structural obstacle 1: Employment

Discussions in this category included work as the highest priority, exhausting work schedules, a bad economy, and sensitivity to food and drink prices. Parents reported that spending time with their children was key to getting them to eat healthful food and to participate in physical activity. However, a bad economy and insufficient income were obstacles.

Work is a parent's highest priority

When asked about concerns about childhood overweight, parents reported that their highest priority is to provide for the family: for example, "Where I work there is a big Latin community, and it's a lot of single mothers, or single fathers who come in and they have children that are very obese, and their thing is, 'We work all day.'" Parents reported that work is a higher priority than their health. One father stated, "One thing I've learned is that the working man....won't take time off to spend with his family unless he's hurt, or sick... You see them working, he'll get two jobs and work."

Table 3 Eleven themes and three subthemes from focus groups

Employment

1. Work is a parent's highest priority.
2. Exhausting work schedules make it hard to prevent childhood overweight.
3. A bad economy, insufficient income and food price sensitivity influence parents' ability to promote their preferred home and food environment.

Day care

1. Preschool policy influences what children ate at home.
2. Preschools can do more to help parents keep their children at a healthy weight.
   a. Food provided to children in family-based day care is often unhealthy.
3. Schools should provide more opportunities for children to participate in physical activity.

Neighborhood environments

1. Liquor stores, fast food and soda are everywhere and influence what children eat.
   a. Soda is addictive.
2. Advertisements influence what children want to consume and ultimately what they eat.
3. Dirty, unsafe neighborhood streets and parks are obstacles to children's health.
   a. Relatives help by providing children opportunities for physical activity.

Community relationships

1. Neighborhood structural factors influence community relationships.
2. Compared to their country of origin, parents experience a lack of social support from neighbors in the U.S., which limits children's access to healthful food and physical activity.

Exhausting work schedules make it hard to prevent childhood overweight

Parents reported that exhausting work schedules reduced parenting time, which in turn put their children at risk for obesity. One mother stated, "In the United States...people go to work, they have their own problems, the rent, the bills, the telephone, as a result, sometimes we don't have time for our children, what we do is place them in day care or with the baby sitter." Parents reported that work schedules disrupted child-feeding routines, and that having two jobs limited playtime with children. One mother stated, "But also because of the lifestyle that I have had, I am a salesperson...I have to leave for work, all of this creates a nutritional imbalance." One father stated, "It's all the Latinos, they got two jobs, so as long the kid is fed they're fine, but if their kid is not doing anything athletic then the little kid is going to get chubby, he is just going to be bored watching TV, being on the computer and eating."

A bad economy, insufficient income and food price sensitivity influence parents' ability to promote their preferred home and food environment

When discussing childhood overweight, parents reported that the high cost of food can lead to the purchase of unhealthy food, especially since quantity matters to big families. One parent stated, "It's hard to...move towards healthy living when their environment...you go to McDonalds, buy a meal, $4 compared to making, buying a healthy meal will cost $10, they [parents] know it's healthier for their kids, but...how is it going to hurt me financially?" Parents also indicated that a bad economy meant parents were experiencing increased financial and time constraints on their parenting practices. One father

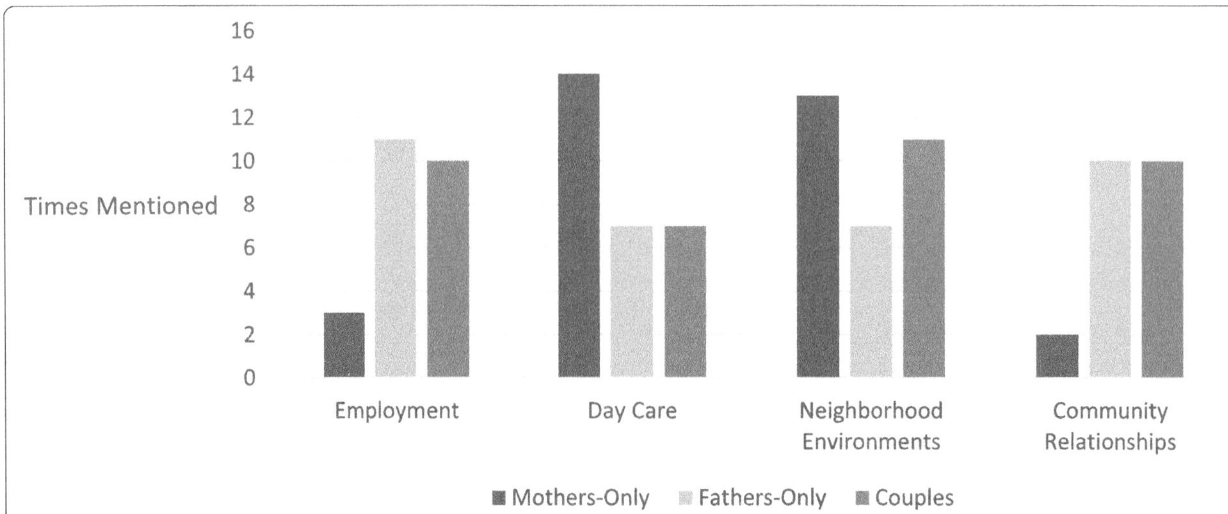

Fig. 2 Frequency of four structural themes (employment, day care, neighborhood environments and community relationships) by mothers-only, fathers-only and couples focus groups

stated, "We are in a bad economy, you are either trying to get your kid to day care, rushing to find a job, or going to work. It's kind of rough right now, I don't think anybody...is talking about [childhood overweight]."

Structural obstacle 2: Day care

Discussion in this category included preschool policy and family-based day care. Parents reported that they used multiple types of day care and that providers often differed from parents, as well as other providers, in terms of child-feeding behaviors, including the types of foods and drinks given to children. Someone other than a parent routinely helped feed young children.

Preschool policy influences what children ate at home

When asked about children's meals, parents reported that preschool health and food policy had both good and bad influences on what and how much their children ate at home. One mother stated, "Well, my son goes to a preschool that's in my neighborhood and they have a... healthy snack policy... So for me sometimes it is really difficult because sometimes when I make their lunch with a fruit snack, which are like gummy bears, they... don't allow that." Conversely, parents reported that preschool feeding schedules included up to five meals per day, in addition to food eaten at home. One mother stated, "My child is two years old, weighs 40 pounds and eats five times per day because of the routine at day care, they [children] eat breakfast, a snack, lunch, a snack, an afternoon meal, and they eat a little bit of everything, when they are at home." Parents explained that sometimes children came home hungry, because they did not like the school food. One parent stated, "Our daughter also goes to preschool and we always ask her when we pick her up, we pick her up after lunchtime, at noon, so I ask 'What did you eat?', and she says 'I did not eat because I did not like the food.'"

Preschools can do more to help parents keep their children at a healthy weight

Parents commented that preschools offered processed high fat foods to children and wanted preschools to provide all healthy food options. One father stated, "Food in schools and high schools, to be honest, has been bad, with high fat content and carbohydrates, very bad." Parents said that preschool staff should give parents more information: for example, "I believe that parents are unaware of what they [children] ate...they [preschool personnel] tell you either that your child ate or that they ate well, but...parents don't know what they ate if they are not with them."

Food provided to children in family-based day care is often unhealthy

Parents were aware and worried that grandmothers and/or eldest children, while valued as child care providers, were often an unhealthy influence on what children ate. One mother stated, "When I'm not at my house he asks, 'Where's mommy?' and my parents are like, 'She's at work' and he's like, 'Yay, I get to eat ice cream for breakfast.'" One father stated, "My grandma watches my kid sometimes...she gives them whatever they ask for, which is not good, but, it's like other people that are not your parents, they tend to show a little more leniency on them, 'Oh you want ice cream? Okay, go ahead.'"

Schools should provide more opportunities for children to participate in physical activity

When discussing day care, parents added that they wanted schools to provide more opportunities for preschool-age children to participate in physical activity. One father stated, "A lot of teachers will just throw them the ball and say, 'go have fun at recess.' You got to be creative and make it fun, so everybody participates and nobody feels like they are better than the other." Another parent stated, "It's really hard for the Hispanic community since sometimes parents work 16-18 hours a day and don't have time after they get home, tired, but one thing that we can do as a community is to push our schools, so they can have physical education."

Structural obstacle 3: Neighborhood environments

Discussion in this category included the abundance of liquor stores, fast food and soda, and dirty, unsafe parks. Parents reported that society, and neighborhood stores and restaurants in particular, influences what their children consume. They also said that soda was unhealthy, addictive and everywhere.

Liquor stores, fast food and soda are everywhere and influence what children eat

When asked about soda, parents reported that not all neighborhoods were the same and that their neighborhoods had an over-abundance of liquor stores, fast food and soda. One parent stated, "Every corner store is a liquor store, or fast food, and it's hard when your kids leave the house, you don't know what they are going to be exposed to, when a lot of kids come back home, they want a can of coke, cause all day that's what we see in the streets." Parents reported soda was common at parties. One mother stated, "I try to tell the kids no soda, no soda, but then we go to a party and there's nothing but soda and there's nothing else to drink. We'll drink water. So it's hard."

Soda is addictive

Parents reported that soda was unhealthy and addictive and it was hard to stop drinking it. One father stated, "I'm going to stop drinking soda, but then my family member is constantly drinking soda, it's just like an addict, you try to quit a drug, but your best friend that you're with all the time is constantly doing it, so you can't give up that addiction." To emphasize this point, one parent suggested putting limits on the amount of soda that can be purchased and consumed at one time, "This is going to sound crazy, but there are limits for wines, there are limits for beer, there are limits for almost everything, but except for soda. Like in my country, in Mexico they drink 10 beers and that's all you can have...it's almost the same like here, DUI or whatever."

Advertisements influence what children want to consume and ultimately what they eat

Parents reported that there are more advertisements for processed food and sugar-sweetened beverages than for free options, such as tap water, which in turn impacted what children consumed at home. One mother stated, "Because advertisements are everywhere, stores and restaurants. They don't say have a Big Mac and some water, they say have a Big Mac and a coke." Parents reported that TV ads targeted children and that they had a strong influence on what their children wanted to consume. One father stated, "You see all these messages on TV, like McDonalds get a 32 ounce coke, but you don't see any bad commercials about soda, what it does." To emphasize this point, parents suggested that soda marketing to children should be stopped: for example, "Talk to the Coca-Cola factories and tell them to stop promoting it."

Dirty, unsafe neighborhood streets and parks are obstacles to children's health

When asked about physical activity, parents reported that cities like San Francisco have many resources, but obstacles such as high participation fees prevented family participation. Parents also said that they wanted structural changes such as more clean and safe parks in order to prevent childhood obesity. Parents reported that under-policing and park conditions require additional vigilance if and while their children use a park: for example, "You see broken glass, you see a basketball, but no rims, the parks are empty...they [parents] just rather keep their kids at home because of gang violence, drugs...they buy them a TV, play station, Xbox, or computer, as long as they don't bother nobody." Another parent stated, "Sometimes when we go to the park, we are there for like two to three hours and we never see a policeman, like coming around and checking, you know, 'How's everything?' never, we have been living there for almost two years."

Parents added that small apartments and small yards limit their children's ability to do sufficient physical activity, which in turn increased their stress level and reduced their desire to eat. One mother stated, "It is very small where I live...not much space for playing, I am constantly tripping on a toy car or a shoe, boy does it get me upset."

Relatives help by providing children opportunities for physical activity

Parents reported that relatives and friends increased opportunities for their children's physical activity. One mother stated, "Well my five-year old, there's in-laws downstairs, so they play a lot, because the other kids are his age, so they are always playing on their scooters and their go-carts. My oldest takes them out and they go walk the dog."

Structural obstacle 4: Community relationships

Discussion in this category included the importance of neighborhood structural factors for building community relationships and a lack of social support from neighbors. Parents reported that they wanted help to improve community relationships, which in turn would help improve the environment for their children to grow up healthily.

Neighborhood structural factors influence community relationships

Parents shared that families fought over limited public spaces, which in turn hurt rapport with neighbors. One parent stated, "My brother used to work at the Boys and Girls Club...that place got so packed with different nationalities and there became like racial fights...they stopped taking their kids, so it's real limited, you know, resources for kids to play." Parents reported that neighbors had different physical activity preferences, which made it hard to build rapport. One mother stated, "People [in my neighborhood]...don't really go outside and play, they go to a school or a park."

Parents expressed that a bad economy influenced community relationships, because it placed much stress and time-constraints on their social lives. One father stated, "I mean there is no work, so people are out there looking for jobs, you don't have time to be socializing about stuff like this [childhood overweight]."

Compared to their country of origin, parents experience a lack of social support from neighbors in the U.S., which limits children's access to healthful food and physical activity

Parents who immigrated to the U.S. reported that neighborhoods in their country of origin were often places where everyone knew each other and where they had a feeling of belonging to a community, which in turn strengthened their family. One father stated, "In our countries, children played together, the neighbors' doors were always open and we didn't have any problems... Here...I don't feel safe letting my daughter play outside, because I don't know the neighbors." In contrast to their country of origin, immigrant parents reported that neighborhoods in the U.S. are not built for developing community relationships: for example, "We can't let our kids go out, because they're going to get kidnapped. In our country, our kids could run up and down...everybody knew each other...over here, you see somebody coming, they lock the door, shut their shades." Immigrant parents reported that fears of deportation narrowed their family's ability to open up to other parents and fully engage in the community with their children. One father stated, "A large part of the city, the people, Latinos, many of them are here, let's say undocumented, they live here in a state of fear which prevents them from relating with others, they live in a world with fewer options, a world that is more closed off."

Differences between mothers-only, fathers-only and couples focus groups

Based on focus groups with mothers-only, fathers-only and couples, we found that all categories of themes were discussed in all three types of groups, but the frequency with which some categories were discussed varied somewhat (see Fig. 2). We were unable to separate out mothers and fathers in the couples focus groups. As illustrated in Fig. 2, overall, mothers in the mothers-only focus groups raised themes of day care and neighborhood environments more than fathers, and fathers in the fathers-only focus groups reported employment and community relationships more than mothers. Fathers and couples mentioned employment more than mothers. We note that mothers in the English-language mothers-only group did not discuss employment. Mothers had twice as much to say about day care compared to both fathers and couples. Mothers also talked about neighborhood environments more than fathers and couples, while fathers and couples had the most to say about community relationships.

Discussion

Results from this study suggest that community, demographic and social characteristics influence what parents feed their children and opportunities for physical activity, providing evidence that an ecological framework is useful for guiding research with both mothers and fathers. Moreover, study results illuminate the processes within parent-child relationships that may be related to child feeding in the context of these broader environmental factors. In contrast to an individual-level interpretation, the study findings shed light on Latino parents' child-feeding decisions in environments that parents identify as lacking options for fresh food, having an overabundance of processed food, and an absence of clean and safe recreational areas. For many Latino families in urban areas, such structural factors are likely to undermine healthful decisions and behaviors, by creating chronic barriers to feeding children healthful food and keeping them active. These results point to Latino parents' awareness of environmental factors, which can help in the development of obesity interventions addressing these issues. The study also reinforces the need for an ecological perspective on obesity prevention, as well as the need for interventions that target multiple factors that influence children's health, including parents' work structure, the varying quality of day care, unsafe neighborhood environments, and poor community relationships. Latino populations tend to live in neighborhood environments with fewer supermarkets, recreational opportunities, and these families typically have fewer socioeconomic resources; thus, compared to non-Latino populations, Latino families are likely to be disproportionately affected by the barriers identified in this study. On average, our study sample had resided in the U.S. for more than 15 years; thus, we would expect the structural obstacles we identified to be worse for less educated and recent immigrant families. Future research should examine environmental factors that may affect more recent immigrants. Furthermore, additional research is needed to identify new strategies for overcoming structural risk factors for obesity and supporting parents' child-feeding behaviors in urban environments.

Employment. Our findings suggest that working multiple jobs influence what and how parents feed their children as well as reduce the time available for modeling their behaviors. Similar to some studies conducted with mothers, work schedules are exhausting and place time constraints on both mothers' and fathers' ability to provide healthful meals on a daily basis for their children. Lower wages require that parents take on more than one job to meet financial obligations, which reduces their personal time and prevents them from spending more time with their children. These findings have important implications for research and interventions related to the role of parental employment in childhood obesity prevention overall, such as addressing the impact of work schedule instability and unpredictability, especially among populations that work two or more jobs.

Day care. Additionally, our study suggests that day care influences what and how children are fed and that these factors are typically out of the parents' control. For example, parents employ day care, neighbors and relatives to provide child care, which involves providing meals during the day, but feeding behaviors differ among providers. Furthermore, children's meals away from home are not always healthy. These results imply that over time, preschool-age children who are fed by various providers may develop poor eating habits that may lead to the development of obesity by the time they enter school. Because many children are routinely fed outside of the home and typically not by a parent, future interventions in day care settings should consider partnering with parents to determine menus and eating schedules. Future research could explore methods for helping busy parents monitor their children's meals for the entire day, every day during this critical developmental time.

Neighborhood environments. Liquor stores, fast food and soda were easily accessible and influenced parents' decisions and behavior regarding what children ate. Additionally, dirty, unsafe parks in their neighborhoods restricted parents' ability to offer opportunities for play and were barriers to children's overall health. These findings are consistent with existing research indicating that behavioral targets for childhood interventions should continue to include avoiding sugar-sweetened beverages, reducing exposure to food marketing by decreasing screen time, and replacing sugar, and fried and empty-calorie foods with fruit, and vegetables at all meals and all snacks [34]. In order to encourage families to be physically active in urban areas, cities, parks and police departments should coordinate resources to provide children with safe environments when not at home or at school, such as providing clean sand boxes and regular police patrolling at public recreation areas.

Community Relationships. Parents not born in the US highlighted that they have lost social support as a result of migration and struggle with building new social support networks in their current neighborhoods. This loss of social support networks, plus fears of deportation among some family members leads parents to feel isolated and alone, and may have a negative effect on their parenting practices, including feeding practices. Similar to studies conducted with mothers who immigrated to the U.S. [24], these factors are perceived by immigrant parents in our study as limiting opportunities to develop relationships with other families; thus, making it challenging to fully adapt to the local culture and to successfully navigate through the local resources, including stores and organized sports programs. Local events that encourage both mothers and fathers to meet might influence family decisions about allowing children to go outside and play with the neighbors' kids. Future research could explore how events such as school, park and community fairs could help create safe places for mothers and fathers to enhance social support focused on obesity prevention.

This is the first qualitative study conducted with both mothers and fathers of preschool-age Latino children to investigate their experiences and perceptions about feeding children healthy food, providing opportunities for physical activity and keeping them at a healthy weight. By including both mothers and fathers, this research contributes to the literature by illuminating parents' beliefs and behaviors that could be targets of interventions to reduce the health risks associated with obesity, and improve the health status of Latino children regarding food, healthy feeding and opportunities to play. The themes from the mothers-only, fathers-only, and couples focus groups had some overlap and also some unique contributions. The frequency with which each type of focus group mentioned each theme suggests that all parents face similar obstacles, but that their influence is perceived to be more or less critical, depending on a parent's role in the family. When examining the focus group themes by parents' gender, it appears that mothers and fathers each have a somewhat distinct perspective and role in helping children stay at a healthy weight. While mothers mainly perceived structural characteristics, such as day care and neighborhood environment as obstacles to preventing obesity, fathers perceived employment and community relationships as the main obstacles. Future research could examine more closely why and how unpredictable work shifts and community relationships influence the child-feeding behaviors of fathers, especially single fathers and couples in order to understand their role, and to potentially identify new pathways for improving the socio-cultural and physical environment in urban areas to change the risk status of Latino children.

Strengths of this study include a methodological approach well-suited to providing a contextualized understanding of both Latino mothers' and fathers' experiences with raising preschool-age children in urban environments, and rigorous attention to increasing the trustworthiness of our findings by taking systematic steps to establish the reliability of the analysis among coders and the validity of our interpretation of data [29]. Focus groups have some potential disadvantages, such as the possibility that some parents may not have felt comfortable sharing their experiences in a group setting, or that some participants can take on more dominating roles and influence the expression of others in the group. It should be noted that we did not detect such occurrences in our reading of the transcripts. Consent to conduct follow-up interviews was not obtained so we were not able to assess whether the identified themes resonated with focus group participants. Qualitative data helps to capture some, but not all contextual information that helps explain the influences of neighborhood and familial resources on the meals and physical activity provided to Latino children ages 2 to 5 [35]. Other qualitative methods such as participant observation could help further explain how broader environmental factors influence eating and playing. Using different techniques such as surveys or individual interviews and controlling for neighborhoods with different socioeconomic characteristics could offer new, complementary results that could be useful in identifying factors that may influence obesity in preschool-age Latino children [36]. Our qualitative approach to discovering parents' experiences and perspectives about children's eating and physical activity offers important information that can be used to design future research and inform obesity prevention interventions in this population.

Conclusions

Results from this study suggest that both mothers and fathers perceive that what Latino preschool-age children are fed, as well as their physical activity opportunities are influenced by their community, demographic and social characteristics. Parents often know what to do, but the results of this study point to the importance of critical structural factors such as standardized work hours and increased resources for day care providers to supporting their cultural practices to promote child health overall. Moreover, urban communities need clean, safe streets and parks, plus strong community relationships so that parents can feed children healthful food and provide physical activity opportunities. While most research on childhood obesity has focused on the child or mother-child dyads, this study found that mothers, fathers, and couples identified numerous community and society-level constraints on their ability to promote their preferred health behaviors and prevent obesity in children aged 2 to 5 years.

Acknowledgements
The authors wish to thank the 49 parents who participated in the focus groups, and Karla Henriquez and Elizabeth Vergara for their assistance with coding transcripts. We thank Deborah Lustig and David Minkus, Graduate Fellows Program, Institute for the Study of Societal Issues, for their invaluable consultation. We also thank Julianna Deardorff and Kurt Organista for mentoring provided to the first author on this research study. We acknowledge salary support from the National Institutes of Health (K01HL115471) to Dr. Sanchez-Vaznaugh. The content in this paper is solely the responsibility of the authors and does not necessarily represent the official views of the funding institution.

Funding
This study was supported by a grant from the Robert Wood Johnson Health Disparities Fund (Tschann, J., Ph.D., P.I.).

Authors' contributions
CP and JT were responsible for the study design including questionnaire development and conceptualization of the manuscript. CP was responsible for study implementation, oversaw the Spanish-language translation of the questionnaire and drafted the manuscript. All authors contributed to the analyses, CP provided guidance on the analyses and wrote much of the analysis section. All authors contributed to the writing and interpretation of the results and approved the final manuscript.

Competing interests
The authors declare that they have no competing interests.

Author details
[1]School of Public Health, University of California, Berkeley, 50 University Hall, Berkeley, CA 94720-7360, USA. [2]Department of Psychiatry, University of California, San Francisco, Box 0848, San Francisco, CA 94143-0848, USA. [3]Health Education Department, San Francisco State University, 1600 Holloway Ave, San Francisco, CA 94132, USA. [4]Department of Counseling, University of San Francisco, 2130 Fulton St., San Francisco, CA 94118, USA.

References
1. Ogden C, Carroll M, Kit B, Flegal K. Prevalence of childhood and adult obesity in the United States, 2011-2012. JAMA. 2014;311:806–14.
2. Lobstein T, Baur L, Uauy R. Obesity in children and young people: a crisis in public health. Obes Rev. 2004;5(Suppl 1):4–104.
3. Power T, O'Connor T, Fisher J, Hughes S. Obesity risk in children: the role of acculturation in the feeding practices and styles of low-income Hispanic families. Child Obes. 2015;11:715–21.
4. Lovasi GS, Hutson MA, Guerra M, Neckerman KM. Built environments and obesity in disadvantaged populations. Epidemiol Rev. 2009;31:7–20.
5. Mazarello Paes V, Ong KK, Lakshman R. Factors influencing obesogenic dietary intake in young children (0-6 years): systematic review of qualitative evidence. BMJ Open. 2015;5:e007396.
6. Bronfenbrenner U. Ecology of the family as a context for human development: research perspectives. Dev Psychol. 1986;22:723–42.
7. Krieger N. Theories for social epidemiology in the 21st century: an ecosocial perspective. Int J Epidemiol. 2001;30:668–77.
8. Smedley BD, Syme SL. Committee on capitalizing on social science and behavioral research to improve the Public's health. Promoting health: intervention strategies from social and behavioral research. Am J Health Promot. 2001;15:149–66.
9. Davison KK, Birch LL. Childhood overweight: a contextual model and recommendations for future research. Obes Rev. 2001;2:159–71.
10. Carroll-Scott A, Gilstad-Hayden K, Rosenthal L, Peters SM, McCaslin C, Joyce R, et al. Disentangling neighborhood contextual associations with child body mass index, diet, and physical activity: the role of built, socioeconomic, and social environments. Soc Sci Med. 2013;95:106–14.
11. Moore LV, Diez Roux AV. Associations of neighborhood characteristics with the location and type of food stores. Am J Public Health. 2006;96:325–31.
12. Powell LM, Slater S, Mirtcheva D, Bao Y, Chaloupka FJ. Food store availability and neighborhood characteristics in the United States. Prev Med. 2007;44:189–95.
13. Davis RE, Cole SM, Blake CE, McKenney-Shubert SJ, Peterson KE. Eat, play, view, sleep: exploring Mexican American mothers' perceptions of decision making for four behaviors associated with childhood obesity risk. Appetite. 2016;101:104–13.
14. Martinez SM, Rhee K, Blanco E, Boutelle K. Maternal attitudes and behaviors regarding feeding practices in elementary school-aged Latino children: a pilot qualitative study on the impact of the cultural role of mothers in the US-Mexican border region of San Diego. California J Acad Nutr Diet. 2014;114:230–7.
15. Mena NZ, Gorman K, Dickin K, Greene G, Tovar A. Contextual and cultural influences on parental feeding practices and involvement in child care centers among Hispanic parents. Child Obes. 2015;11:347–54.
16. Davison KK, Gicevic S, Aftosmes-Tobio A, Ganter C, Simon CL, Newlan S, et al. Fathers' representation in observational studies on parenting and childhood obesity: a systematic review and content analysis. Am J Public Health. 2016;106:1980.
17. Morgan PJ, Young MD, Lloyd AB, Wang ML, Eather N, Miller A, et al. Involvement of fathers in pediatric obesity treatment and prevention trials: a systematic review. Pediatrics. 2017;139:1–11.
18. Drago R. The parenting of infants: a time-use study [Internet]. Bureau of labor statistics. 2009 [cited 2015 Nov 9]. Available from: https://www.bls.gov/opub/mlr/2009/10/art3full.pdf. Accessed 9 Nov 2015.
19. Children who live in two-parent families, by race ethnicity | KIDS COUNT Data Center [Internet]. 2016 [cited 2016 Feb 15]. Available from: http://datacenter.kidscount.org/data/Tables/8053-children-who-live-in-two-parent-families-by-race-ethnicity. Accessed 15 Feb 2016.
20. Livingston G. The rise of single father [Internet]. Pew social & demographic trends. 2013 [cited 2013 Aug 7]. Available from: http://www.pewsocialtrends.org/2013/07/02/the-rise-of-single-fathers/. Accessed 7 Aug 2013.

21. Ochoa A, Berge JM. Home environmental influences on childhood obesity in the Latino population: a decade review of literature. J Immigr Minor Health. 2017;19:430–47.
22. Crawford PB, Gosliner W, Anderson C, Strode P, Becerra-Jones Y, Samuels S, et al. Counseling Latina mothers of preschool children about weight issues: suggestions for a new framework. J Am Diet Assoc. 2004;104:387–94.
23. Evans A, Chow S, Jennings R, Dave J, Scoblick K, Sterba KR, et al. Traditional foods and practices of Spanish-speaking Latina mothers influence the home food environment: implications for future interventions. J Am Diet Assoc. 2011;111:1031–8.
24. Showell NN, Cole KW, Johnson K, DeCamp LR, Bair-Merritt M, Thornton RLJ. Neighborhood and parental influences on diet and physical activity behaviors in young low-income pediatric patients. Clin Pediatr. 2016;56(13): 1235-1243.
25. Small L, Melnyk BM, Anderson-Gifford D, Hampl JS. Exploring the meaning of excess child weight and health: shared viewpoints of Mexican parents of preschool children. Pediatr Nurs. 2009;35:357–66.
26. Torres ME, Meetze EG, Smithwick-Leone J. Latina voices in childhood obesity: a pilot study using Photovoice in South Carolina. Am J Prev Med. 2013;44:S225–31.
27. Tolley EE, Ulin PR, Mack N, Succop SM, Robinson ET. Collecting qualitative data the science and the art. Qualitative methods in public health: a field guide for applied research. Second. San Francisco: John Wiley & Sons; 2016. p. 85–142.
28. Miles MB, Huberman AM. Qualitative data analysis: an expanded sourcebook. 2nd ed. Thousand Oaks: SAGE Publications, Inc; 1994.
29. Miles MB, Huberman AM, Saldaña J. Qualitative data analysis: a methods sourcebook. Thousand Oaks, Califorinia: SAGE Publications, Inc.; 2014.
30. Vital Signs. Wall Street Journal [Internet]. 2011 Sep 8 [cited 2013 May 14]; Available from: http://online.wsj.com/article/SB10001424053111904537404576554763763815664.html. Accessed 14 May 2013.
31. Motel S, Patten E. Characteristics of the 60 largest metropolitan areas by Hispanic population [Internet]. Pew Hispanic Center. 2012 [cited 2013 May 14]. Available from: http://www.pewhispanic.org/2012/09/19/characteristics-of-the-60-largest-metropolitan-areas-by-hispanic-population/. Accessed 14 May 2013.
32. Flores G, Lin H. Factors predicting overweight in US kindergartners. Am J Clin Nutr. 2013;97:1178–87.
33. Maxwell JA. Qualitative research design: an interactive approach. Thousand Oaks: SAGE; 2012.
34. Baidal JAW, Taveras EM. Childhood obesity: shifting the focus to early prevention. Arch Pediatr Adolesc Med. 2012;166:1179–81.
35. Smith JA. Qualitative psychology: a practical guide to research methods. Thousand Oaks: SAGE Publications; 2003.
36. Ryan GW, Bernard HR. Techniques to identify themes. Field Methods. 2003;15:85–109.

9

Developing a systems-based framework of the factors influencing dietary and physical activity behaviours in ethnic minority populations living in Europe - a DEDIPAC study

Michelle Holdsworth[1*], Mary Nicolaou[2], Lars Jørun Langøien[3], Hibbah Araba Osei-Kwasi[1], Sebastien F. M. Chastin[4], F. Marijn Stok[5], Laura Capranica[6], Nanna Lien[7], Laura Terragni[8], Pablo Monsivais[9,10], Mario Mazzocchi[11], Lea Maes[12], Gun Roos[13], Caroline Mejean[14], Katie Powell[1] and Karien Stronks[2]

Abstract

Background: Some ethnic minority populations have a higher risk of non-communicable diseases than the majority European population. Diet and physical activity behaviours contribute to this risk, shaped by a system of inter-related factors. This study mapped a systems-based framework of the factors influencing dietary and physical activity behaviours in ethnic minority populations living in Europe, to inform research prioritisation and intervention development.

Methods: A concept mapping approach guided by systems thinking was used: i. Preparation (protocol and terminology); ii. Generating a list of factors influencing dietary and physical activity behaviours in ethnic minority populations living in Europe from evidence (systematic mapping reviews) and 'eminence' (89 participants from 24 academic disciplines via brainstorming, an international symposium and expert review) and; iii. Seeking consensus on structuring, rating and clustering factors, based on how they relate to each other; and iv. Interpreting/utilising the framework for research and interventions. Similar steps were undertaken for frameworks developed for the majority European population.

Results: Seven distinct clusters emerged for dietary behaviour (containing 85 factors) and 8 for physical activity behaviours (containing 183 factors). Four clusters were similar across behaviours: Social and cultural environment; Social and material resources; Psychosocial; and Migration context. Similar clusters of factors emerged in the frameworks for diet and physical activity behaviours of the majority European population, except for 'migration context'. The importance of factors across all clusters was acknowledged, but their relative importance differed for ethnic minority populations compared with the majority population.
(Continued on next page)

* Correspondence: michelle.holdsworth@sheffield.ac.uk
[1]Public Health Section, School of Health and Related Research-ScHARR, The University of Sheffield, Sheffield, UK
Full list of author information is available at the end of the article

(Continued from previous page)

Conclusions: This systems-based framework integrates evidence from both expert opinion and published literature, to map the factors influencing dietary and physical activity behaviours in ethnic minority groups. Our findings illustrate that innovative research and complex interventions need to be developed that are sensitive to the needs of ethnic minority populations. A systems approach that encompasses the complexity of the inter-related factors that drive behaviours may inform a more holistic public health paradigm to more effectively reach ethnic minorities living in Europe, as well as the majority host population.

Keywords: Minority populations, Europe, Migrants, Immigrants, Physical activity, Sedentary behaviour, Diet, Framework, Systems

Background

Some ethnic minority groups living in Europe have a high prevalence of preventable non-communicable diseases (NCDs), such as obesity, type 2 diabetes and cardiovascular diseases [1–4]. Diet and physical activity behaviours are likely to play a role in their aetiology and differences in these behaviours compared with host populations are well documented [4–10]. However, there are fewer studies of the differences in the underlying factors influencing these behaviours [11–13]. Most studies have focused either on a small number of minority groups or are limited to specific European countries, which makes it challenging to generalise about the nature of any differences [14–20]. It could be argued that the variation between ethnic groups is as great as that between the general European population. Nonetheless, it could be expected that there are commonalities in people's lives who are either first or second generation migrants, which are distinct from the general population [11–13]. Thus, understanding the factors underlying diet and physical activity behaviours in ethnic minority groups is a first step to informing the development of public health interventions that are successful in reaching minority ethnic populations in Europe.

Existing frameworks are insufficient for prioritising research or interventions development, as they either focus on migration and dietary acculturation processes [13] or on a specific health outcome, such as obesity in the whole population [21, 22]. Alternatively, they are based on evidence of ethnic minority populations living outside of Europe, for example, of African descent in the US [21] or Iranians living in Australia [23]. This may offer useful insights, even though contextual differences limit their transferability to Europe. Likewise, focusing only on obesity has the potential to ignore important drivers of the complex system of factors influencing dietary and physical activity behaviours.

A system-based approach has the potential to cast a holistic analytic lens [24] to developing interventions, because it is based on the interrelationship of clusters within a dynamic system. Systems thinking can simply be defined as *'looking at things in terms of the bigger picture'* [25]. Dietary and physical activity behaviours therefore emerge as a property, which cannot be resolved from simple, uni-faceted interventions [26]. Shifts are likely to be required within multiple clusters of factors, even though some of these may only have small effects on individuals, they have the potential to stimulate population changes when combined [26]. Therefore, the aim of the current study was to develop a systems-based framework of the factors influencing dietary and physical activity behaviours in ethnic minority populations living in Europe, to be able to inform research prioritisation and the development of interventions to reach these groups.

Methods

The framework was constructed as part of the DEDIPAC-KH (DEterminants of DIet and Physical ACtivity Knowledge Hub) [27] for European populations. Within the DEDIPAC-KH, an inter-disciplinary group focused on the determinants of dietary and physical activity/sedentary behaviours. The task was undertaken at several steps involving scholars with varying academic backgrounds and from different countries (Table 1 for more details).

A total of 89 participants contributed to at least one step of the creation of the framework. This comprised a team focusing on the factors influencing the behaviours of ethnic minority populations ('DEDIPAC ethnic minority team'). Other teams in the DEDIPAC-KH focussed on the factors influencing dietary [28] and physical activity/sedentary behaviours [29, 30] of the general European population ('DEDIPAC general population team'). This approach followed earlier successful examples of multidisciplinary partnerships that comprehensively described the factors influencing obesity-related behaviours [31].

The method was guided by concept mapping; drawing on both quantitative [32], and qualitative [33] approaches. Traditionally, quantitative concept maps have been used in health research, yet the case for flexible use of concepts maps has been advocated for, requiring a less rigid and more qualitative approach [33, 34]. Concept mapping is influenced by systems thinking and involves gathering and analysing different types of data

Table 1 Characteristics of participants in the different concept mapping stages to develop the framework

	Stage i, ii: Preparation and generation of factors	Stage iii: Structuring, rating and producing cluster map	Stage iv: Interpretation and utilisation
Participant numbers	n = 12 ethnic minorities DEDIPAC team n = 21 DEDIPAC general population team	n = 12 ethnic minorities DEDIPAC team n = 21 DEDIPAC general population team	International symposium: n = 44 delegates and n = 2 invited experts Finalisation n = 18 members of DEDIPAC ethnic minorities and general population teams
Fields of expertise	Agricultural economics Behavioural economics Behavioural nutrition Consumer science Dietary inequalities Dietetics Epidemiology Exercise physiology Health inequalities Medicine Migrant health Nutritional epidemiology Physical activity Psychology (health, cognitive and social) Public health nutrition Social anthropology Social demography Social inequalities Sociology of health	Agricultural economics Behavioural economics Behavioural nutrition Consumer science Dietary inequalities Dietetics Epidemiology Exercise physiology Health inequalities Medicine Migrant health Nutritional epidemiology Physical activity Psychology (health, cognitive and social) Public health nutrition Social anthropology Social demography Social inequalities Sociology of health	Agricultural economics Behavioural economics Behavioural nutrition Behavioural sciences Consumer science Dietary inequalities Dietetics Epidemiology Exercise physiology Food engineering Health inequalities Medicine Migrant health Nutritional epidemiology Nutrition science Physical activity Physical education and physiotherapy Physical anthropology Psychology (health, cognitive and social) Public health nutrition Social anthropology Social demography Social inequalities Sociology of health
Countries	Belgium France Germany Ireland Italy Netherlands Norway UK	Belgium France Germany Ireland Italy Netherlands Norway UK	Australia Belgium Denmark France Germany Ireland Italy Netherlands Norway Poland Spain Sweden UK

and integrating these with prior research/experience [35]. Concept mapping was selected because it can illustrate how people visualize relationships between concepts within a map [34] and it can be used for research prioritisation [30]. The approach was structured around the four main phases proposed in quantitative concept mapping [32], but a more flexible mixed methodology was employed [34]: i. preparation; ii. generation of factors; iii. Structuring and rating factors into clusters; and iv. interpretation and utilisation of the framework.

Preparation (terminology, protocol)

The scope and purpose of the study protocol was developed (Fig. 1- step 1) by the DEDIPAC ethnic minority team, in consultation with the DEDIPAC general population team. Consensus was reached on the terminology for the different behaviours and for defining factors/correlates/determinants, so that there was a common understanding across the DEDIPAC-KH. Minority ethnic populations were defined as *'immigrants/populations of immigrant background from low and middle income countries, population groups from the former Eastern Bloc countries who migrate to other parts of Europe and minority indigenous populations in Europe'*.

Three criteria were selected to score each factor, for its priority for future research ('research priority') and for how useful it would be in developing interventions ('expected modifiability'; 'potential effect size on behaviour').

It was also decided how consultation outside of the DEDIPAC network could be undertaken, to ensure that a wide range of viewpoints were considered from diverse disciplines to encourage 'buy in' to the resulting framework [32]. The concept mapping process does not stipulate that

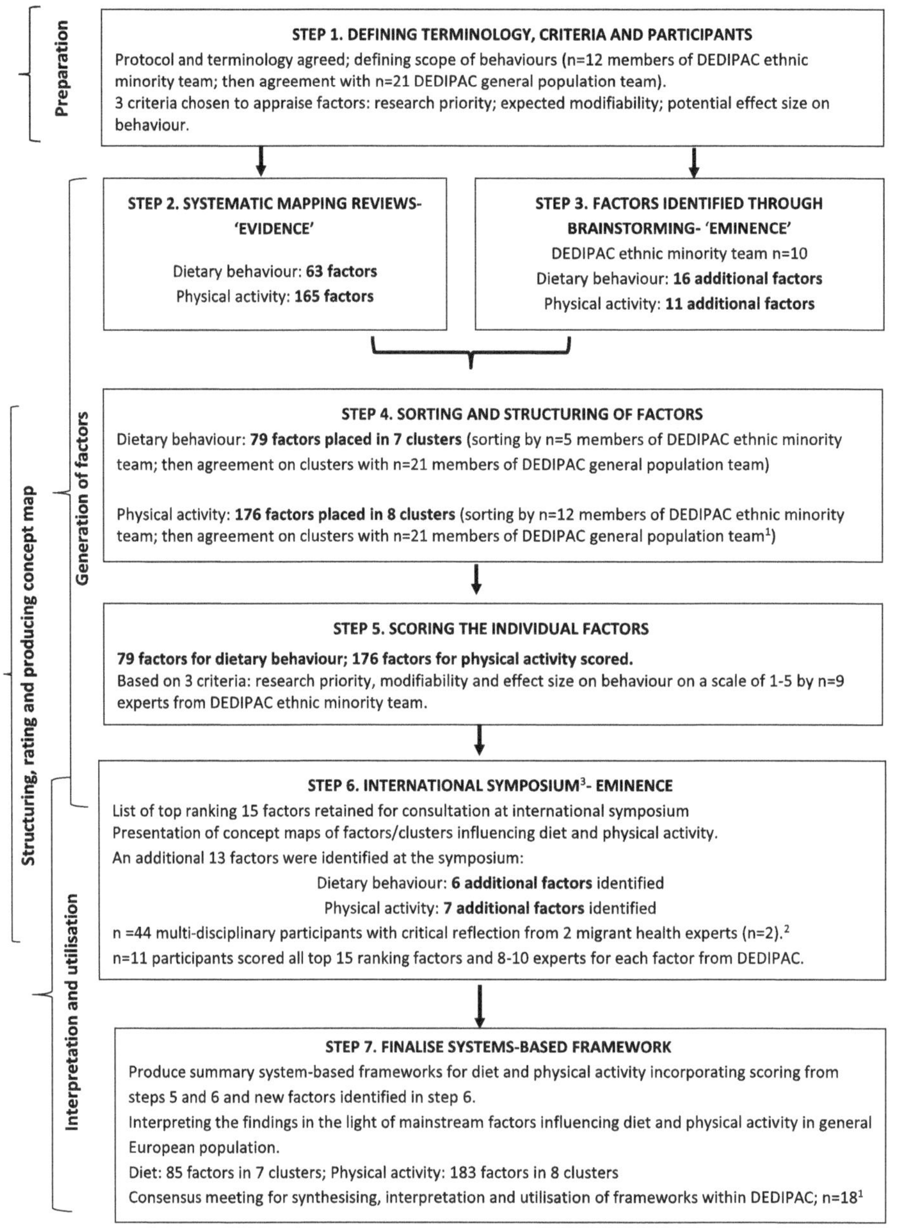

Fig. 1 [1]Areas of expertise that were represented in the process are summarised in Table 1. [2]Holdsworth M, Nicolaou M, Araba Saeed H, Jørun Langøien L, Powell K, Terragni L et al. (2015) Developing a framework map of the major determinants of dietary behaviour and physical activity/ sedentary behaviour in minority ethnic groups living in Europe. International Society for Behavioral Nutrition and Physical Activity, June, Edinburgh (UK), abstract book p107, S6.73. https://eventmobi.com/api/events/7231/documents/download/596c6adb-ef0f-4695-be2c-8a1927877d2c.pdf/as/ISBNPA%202015%20bstract%20Book.pdf. Concept mapping process for developing the systems-based framework for dietary and physical activity behaviours in ethnic minority populations

all participants have to be involved in every step [32], so it was agreed that a small group would generate the factors and a larger group would sort and rate them.

Generation of factors

The next phase (Fig. 1- steps 2 and 3; then steps 4 and 6) involved generating a set of factors to represent the entire conceptual domain of the topic area, i.e. the factors that influence diet and physical activity (incorporating sedentary behaviours) of ethnic minority populations living in Europe. This was conducted in parallel for diet and physical activity behaviours from published 'evidence' and expert opinion ('eminence'). The aim was to develop wording that was detailed enough to convey the underlying meaning for each factor without requiring further explanation.

Published evidence (systematic mapping reviews)

Factors were generated from published 'evidence' by conducting systematic mapping reviews (Fig. 1- step 2) of the factors influencing dietary behaviours [36] and physical activity behaviours (incorporating sedentary behaviours) [37] among minority groups living in Europe. The review methods and protocols were published elsewhere [PROSPERO database #CRD42014013549/ #CRD42014014575], but essentially primary data from quantitative and qualitative studies published over the 15 year period preceding data searching (1999–2014) were extracted. In synthesizing the findings, all of the factors (63 factors for diet; 165 factors for physical activity) were listed [36, 37]. Physical activity and sedentary behaviours were integrated together, as there was a lack of published research on sedentary behaviours of ethnic minority populations.

Expert opinion ('eminence')

Expert opinion was sought from three sources: brainstorming within the DEDIPAC ethnic minority team (Fig. 1- step 3) and by members of the DEDIPAC general population team (Fig. 1- step 4); and later by consultation with external experts during an international symposium (Fig. 1- step 6). Participants (n = 89 in total throughout the process) were from a range of disciplines (Table 1), but they were not all involved at every step.

Factors that had not emerged from the reviews, but could be important, were generated by the DEDIPAC ethnic minority team (Fig. 1- step 3). Existing frameworks were also used to extract additional factors [13, 21, 23, 38]. An additional 40 factors (to those from the systematic mapping reviews) were identified at steps 3 and 6 combined (22 for diet and 18 for physical activity).

Structuring, rating and producing a concept map

Sorting and structuring of factors

The emerging factors from the systematic mapping reviews and expertise within the DEDIPAC-KH were grouped into clusters, according to how they were seen to relate to each other. This resulted in 7 dietary behaviour clusters containing 79 factors and 8 physical activity clusters containing 176 factors (Additional file 1: Tables S1 and S2). This process was undertaken in two ways (Fig. 1- step 4). Firstly, during meetings of the DEDIPAC ethnic minority team, when the relationships between factors were collectively debated. Secondly, during a confirmatory stage involving members of the DEDIPAC ethnic minority and the general population teams. The concept map that emerged was discussed collectively, which led to some changes in wording of the clusters to enhance clarity and some factors were moved into different clusters (Fig. 1- step 4).

Scoring the individual factors

All of the factors were scored individually (Fig. 1- step 5) by DEDIPAC ethnic minority team members and some general population team members (Table 1) using the three criteria identified in the preparation phase, i.e. 'research priority', 'expected modifiability' and 'potential effect size on behaviour'. When scoring, individuals were asked to provide their scores based on their own professional judgments. The rating focus statement selected was: 'Score the *following factors* for their importance on a scale of 1 to 5 for dietary behaviour [or physical activity and sedentary behaviour] in ethnic minority groups', where 1 = the lowest importance and 5 = the highest. These three criteria were added together as a total measure of the perceived importance of individual factors for research and interventions. Individuals rated the factors separately and these scores were subsequently collated to develop the ranking of factors within clusters. The mean is the total sum divided by the number of factors, so a maximum of 15 could be gained for the three criteria on a Likert scale of 1–5, with 5 as most modifiable, strongest effect, largest priority. The position that the factors were ranked in was based on the overall sum divided by the number of factors in each cluster (Table 4).

International symposium- eminence

Consultation took place during a dedicated symposium at an international conference (Fig. 1- step 6) [39]. Symposium participants scored the top 15 factors that had emerged from step 5 (Fig. 1) using the same three criteria. The decision to only request scoring of the top 15 factors was for pragmatic reasons as the symposium was time limited. The symposium also allowed reflection on the next phase of 'Interpretation and utilisation' of the framework.

Interpretation and utilisation

International symposium- eminence

Two invited experts (external to DEDIPAC) in migrant health gave their views about the draft concept map, particularly where there were gaps in published literature and key research challenges for the future. This was followed by a short interactive discussion drawing on experiences and views from the audience (n = 44), during which, ideas were captured from symposium participants. The discussion resulted in the identification of a further 13 factors (6 for diet, 7 for physical activity), which were subsequently incorporated into the framework. This process led to a summary of the research challenges and knowledge gaps identified (Fig. 1- step 6).

Finalise systems-based framework

The rating of individual factors and clusters were assembled for the separate diet and physical activity frameworks.

A face-to-face meeting of the DEDIPAC ethnic minority and general population teams was held to discuss the integrated framework (Fig. 1- step 7) and consensus was sought at the cluster level. It was the final step in the framework development process to compare the scoring of factors and ranking of clusters across minority ethnic populations with the general European population and to discuss the implications for research and interventions of the factors and clusters in the final framework.

Frameworks in the general population of factors influencing physical activity [29] and sedentary behaviour [30] separately, as well as for dietary behaviour [28] were developed in parallel by the general population teams in the DEDIPAC-KH. While the factors for ethnic minority populations fed into these general population frameworks, they were developed in separate processes [28–30]. This allowed for a post-hoc comparison of clusters identified in the general population with those identified in the ethnic minority framework.

Results

Emerging clusters for dietary and physical activity behaviours

Seven distinct clusters (containing 85 factors) were identified for dietary behaviour of ethnic minority populations (Additional file 1: Table S1): 'migration context'; 'social and cultural environment'; 'food beliefs and perceptions'; 'accessibility of food'; 'the body'; 'psychosocial'; and 'social and material resources'. The highest number of factors were identified in the 'social and cultural environment' cluster (20 factors), followed by 'food beliefs and perceptions' (13 factors). The 'psychosocial' and 'accessibility of foods' clusters had an equal number of factors (12 factors each). Only five factors were identified for 'the body' cluster.

Eight distinct clusters (containing 183 factors) were identified for physical activity behaviours (Additional file 1: Table S2): health and health communication; political environment; social and cultural environment; psychosocial; institutional environment; physical environment and opportunity; social and material resources; and migration context. The highest number of factors were identified in the social and cultural environment cluster (53 factors), followed by the psychosocial cluster (38 factors). Whilst the lowest number was identified for the political environment cluster (3 factors).

Priority ranking of factors for dietary behaviour

One-third of the top rated 15 factors for diet were related to food accessibility (Table 2). These factors scored highly in all criteria; and three of these factors (food availability, food policy, food price) were in the top five overall; indeed food price scored highest for its likely impact on population behaviour.

The factors in the 'food beliefs and perceptions' cluster that scored highly related to children's food preferences and the social role of food and food beliefs; although the latter two did not score well for modifiability, as they were seen as difficult to change, presumably because of their socially engrained nature. The psychosocial cluster of factors that reached the top 15 were related to perceived barriers, psychosocial stress and subjective norms influencing dietary behaviours. Perceived barriers in particular scored well for modifiability, suggesting barriers could be targeted in subsequent interventions. Even though so many factors emerged in the social and cultural cluster (Additional file 1: Table S1), only two of these were ranked highly enough across all criteria to be included in the final list of 15 factors (social networks; level of acculturation).

Only 'nutrition knowledge' scored well amongst the 'material and social resources' cluster (Table 2); the other factors in this cluster scored low on modifiability and therefore were not seen as imperative to study, e.g. income. Only 'immigrant related policy' in the host country scored well amongst the 'migration context' cluster, but even then it did not score well as a research priority. Others in this cluster had low scores for modifiability, such as the political context in the host country. No factors in 'the body' cluster emerged in the top 15.

Priority ranking of factors for physical activity

Almost one-third of the top rated 15 physical activity factors were related to the 'physical environment and opportunity' cluster (Table 3). Two factors related to provision of culturally sensitive and/or women only facilities (Table 3). Four psychosocial factors were ranked highly overall, scoring well for modifiability (knowledge of physical activity, lack of physical activity skills, expectations of physical activity, attitudes).

'Physical activity at school' was ranked first, performing well in terms of its likely impact on population health, due to the potential reach that school based interventions can have, suggesting schools could be a priority setting in subsequent interventions. Only 'area deprivation' scored highly amongst the 'material and social resources' cluster, as it was seen to have an important impact on behaviours, but it scored less well for modifiability. Other factors related to material and social resources, such as income, scored less well, as they were seen as hard to modify.

Only three factors ranked highly (Table 2) amongst the 53 factors that emerged in the 'Social and cultural environment' cluster (Additional file 1: Table S2). Two of these appeared closely inter-related (social influence, habitus), where habitus was seen as how individuals perceive and react to the social world around them. The third factor (parental attitudes) reflects the high ranking given to children's physical activity behaviours. Of the 12

Table 2 Ranking of top 15 dietary factors (presented in table are mean (SD))

Rank[a]	Factor	Modifiability	Priority for research	Effect on Behaviour	SUM	Cluster name
1	Food availability	3.37 (1.18)	3.50 (1.00)	3.93 (1.10)	10.80	Accessibility of food
2	Food policy	3.27 (0.96)	3.95 (0.94)	3.57 (1.19)	10.78	Accessibility of food
3	Perceived barriers	3.82 (0.75)	3.43 (1.27)	3.52 (0.99)	10.77	Psychosocial
4	Nutrition knowledge	4.23 (0.73)	3.20 (1.20)	3.22 (0.89)	10.65	Resources/social capital
5	Food prices	2.68 (1.33)	3.72 (1.17)	4.20 (0.77)	10.60	Accessibility of food
6	Children's food preferences	3.43 (0.75)	3.35 (0.93)	3.72 (0.91)	10.50	Food beliefs & perceptions
7	Food-related life-style	2.95 (1.00)	3.70 (0.98)	3.77 (1.11)	10.42	Accessibility of food
8	Social role of food	2.23 (0.88)	3.85 (0.81)	3.98 (0.80)	10.07	Food beliefs & perceptions
9	Psycho-social stress	2.95 (1.00)	3.65 (1.09)	3.45 (0.94)	10.05	Psychosocial
10	Food beliefs	2.93 (0.81)	3.42 (0.82)	3.68 (0.92)	10.03	Food beliefs & perceptions
11	Social networks	2.55 (0.83)	3.62 (0.59)	3.68 (0.73)	9.85	Social and cultural
12	Subjective norms	2.87 (1.05)	3.33 (0.87)	3.52 (0.94)	9.72	Psychosocial
13	Accessibility of traditional foods	3.32 (1.08)	3.08 (1.06)	3.05 (1.19)	9.45	Accessibility of food
14	Immigrant related policy	3.05 (1.05)	3.52 (1.14)	2.85 (1.18)	9.42	Migration context
15	Level of acculturation	2.62 (1.20)	3.32 (0.98)	3.28 (0.91)	9.22	Social and cultural

All scores on a scale of 1–5, with 5 as most modifiable, strongest effect, largest priority
[a]Position that the factors were ranked in from the 79 diet factors based on 3 criteria of 'research priority', 'expected modifiability' and 'potential effect size on behaviour'; factors were scored by 20 people for all 3 criteria

factors in the 'health and health communication' cluster, only 'primary health care' was ranked highly. The high rating of primary health care in part stems from the central role of health professionals conveying the importance of physical activity, as it was seen as modifiable, with potential to reach many people through interventions. Only 'lack of knowledge of host culture' scored well in 'migration status', as it was seen as modifiable, whereas the other factors in this cluster were perceived as difficult to change. No factors in 'the political environment' emerged amongst those in the top 15.

Cluster ranking for factors influencing dietary and physical activity behaviours

For both diet and physical activity, 'psychosocial' factors was the top ranking cluster, which scored highly on all

Table 3 Ranking of top 15 factors related to physical activity behaviours (presented in table are mean (SD))

Rank[a]	Factor	Modifiability	Priority for research	Effect on Behaviour	SUM	Cluster name
1	Lack of physical activity at school	3.82 (1.10)	3.53 (0.86)	3.67 (0.77)	11.02	Institutional environment
2	Knowledge of physical activity	4.11 (0.96)	3.08 (1.37)	3.15 (1.10)	10.35	Psychosocial
3	Social influence	2.86 (1.02)	3.60 (1.09)	3.78 (0.88)	10.25	Social and cultural environment
4	Lack of physical activity skills	3.61 (1.04)	3.14 (0.86)	3.39 (0.98)	10.14	Psychosocial
5	Parental attitudes	3.10 (0.68)	3.38 (1.09)	3.61 (0.92)	10.08	Social and cultural environment
6	Lack of culturally sensitive facilities	3.28 (1.07)	3.44 (0.92)	3.33 (0.84)	10.05	Physical environment and opportunity
7	Expectations of physical activity	3.33 (1.08)	3.22 (1.06)	3.45 (1.10)	10.00	Psychosocial
8	Attitudes	3.38 (0.98)	3.27 (1.07)	3.35 (1.03)	10.00	Psychosocial
9	Facilities available	3.05 (1.06)	3.38 (0.78)	3.50 (0.96)	9.94	Physical environment and opportunity
10	Access to a play area	3.23 (0.94)	3.26 (0.89)	3.44 (0.78)	9.93	Physical environment and opportunity
11	Lack of knowledge of host culture	3.72 (0.96)	2.94 (0.87)	3.12 (0.68)	9.78	Migration context
12	Area deprivation	2.50 (0.86)	3.50 (0.92)	3.72 (0.83)	9.71	Social and material resources
13	Lack of women only facilities	3.25 (1.00)	3.20 (1.11)	3.22 (1.00)	9.66	Physical environment and opportunity
14	Primary health care	3.36 (1.14)	3.23 (1.11)	3.05 (1.00)	9.64	Health and health communication
15	Habitus	2.60 (1.14)	3.23 (1.40)	3.63 (1.29)	9.46	Social and cultural environment

All scores on a scale of 1–5, with 5 as most modifiable, strongest effect, largest priority
[a]Position that the factors were ranked in from the 183 Physical activity/Sedentary behaviour factors based on the overall scores of the 3 criteria of 'research priority', 'expected modifiability' and 'potential effect size on behaviour'; factors were scored by 20 people for all 3 criteria

three criteria, but particularly as a priority for research and its likely impact on behaviour (Table 4). The scores for the remaining clusters were ranked closely behind. The 'migration context' cluster of factors scored lowest, mainly because it had a low score for modifiability. Social and material resources were seen to have an important impact on behaviour, but scored less for modifiability. Overall, the relatively close ranking of the clusters for both behaviours suggested that all could have a part to play in developing interventions and research.

A systems-based framework – A tool for prioritising research and interventions

Figures 2 and 3 summarise the clusters that emerged and their priority ranking. The top scoring five factors in each cluster are highlighted.

An integrated framework for the major clusters of factors influencing both dietary and physical activity behaviours and the overlap between them is illustrated in the overall framework (Fig. 4).

The clusters of factors influencing the different behaviours were integrated to illustrate both similar and distinct clusters of factors. Four of the clusters were similar (psychosocial; social and cultural; social and material resources; and migration context) for diet and physical activity behaviours.

Research priorities for ethnic minorities compared with those for the general host population

Some similarities and differences were observed between ethnic minorities and general host populations. Similar sub-categories of clusters of factors emerged in the general population frameworks for diet [28], physical activity [29] and sedentary behaviours [30] combined, except for those in the migration context (Table 5).

The clusters of 'health and health communication' and 'institutional environment' did not emerge in the general population for physical activity; and 'material and social resources' did not emerge as a distinct cluster of factors influencing sedentary behaviours in the general population.

Table 4 Ranking of clusters for dietary and physical activity behaviour factors

Cluster	Number of factors[a]	Mean Modifiability max score 5	Mean Priority for research max score 5	Mean effect on behaviour max score 5	SUM of raw scores	Mean score/factor[b] max score 15	Cluster rank[c]
Dietary behaviour							
Psychosocial	12	3.07	3.10	3.69	108.43	9.04	1
Food beliefs and perceptions	11	2.73	2.88	3.34	98.50	8.96	2
Social and material resources	10	2.36	3.04	3.51	89.03	8.90	3
Accessibility of food	12	2.46	3.02	3.31	105.57	8.80	4
The body	5	2.87	2.54	3.14	42.75	8.55	5
Social and cultural environment	18	1.99	2.84	3.19	144.27	8.02	6
Migration context	13	1.47	2.51	3.08	91.70	7.05	7
Physical activity behaviours							
Psychosocial	38	2.70	2.64	3.17	323.62	8.52	1
Institutional environment	14	2.68	2.29	3.00	114.73	8.20	2
Political environment	3	2.14	2.95	3.05	24.44	8.15	3
Social and cultural environment	49	2.13	2.64	3.12	394.32	8.05	4
Physical environment and opportunity	31	2.45	2.47	3.08	247.81	7.99	5
Social and material resources	12	1.83	2.66	3.41	94.71	7.89	6
Health and health communication	12	2.29	2.35	3.22	94.34	7.86	7
Migration context	17	1.76	2.31	2.70	121.90	7.17	8

[a]The number of factors here does not include those 6 factors identified at the ISBNPA symposium, as they were not scored. The full list is in Tables 1 and 3
[b]Mean is the total sum divided by the number of factors- so a maximum of 15 could be gained as 3 criteria on a Likert scale of 1–5, with 5 as most modifiable, strongest effect, largest priority
[c]Position that the factors were ranked in based on overall SUM/number of factors in each cluster

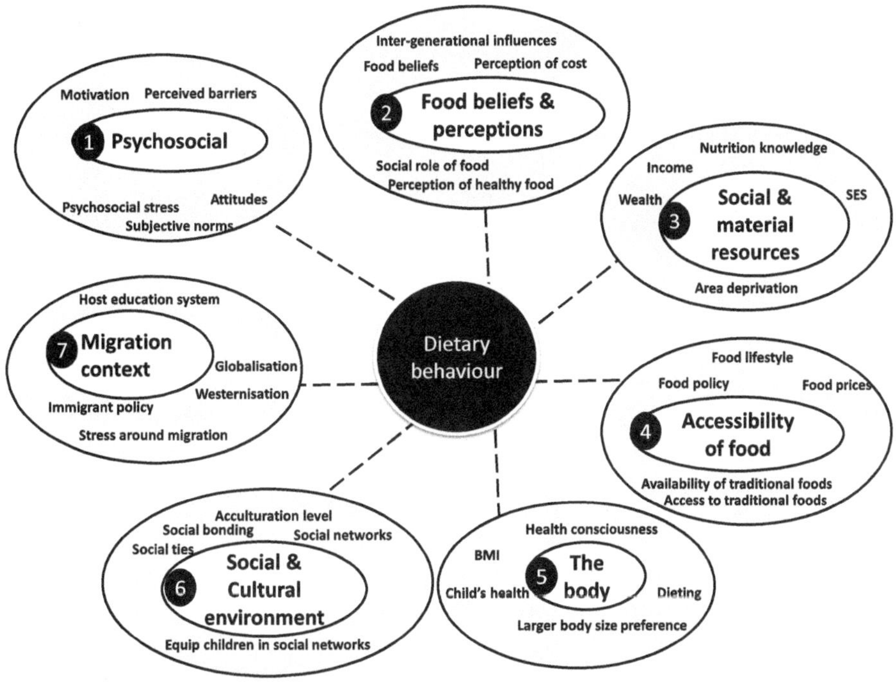

Fig. 2 A systems-based framework of the priority factors and clusters influencing dietary behaviours in ethnic minority populations living in Europe. The numbers represent the order of ranking of the clusters. The factors listed under each cluster are the top 5 factors ranked by a range of experts from a wide array of disciplines for their importance based on 3 criteria of 'research priority', 'expected modifiability' and 'potential effect size on behaviour'. Dotted lines indicate that factors in the cluster are associated with behaviours, but they do not indicate evidence for causation

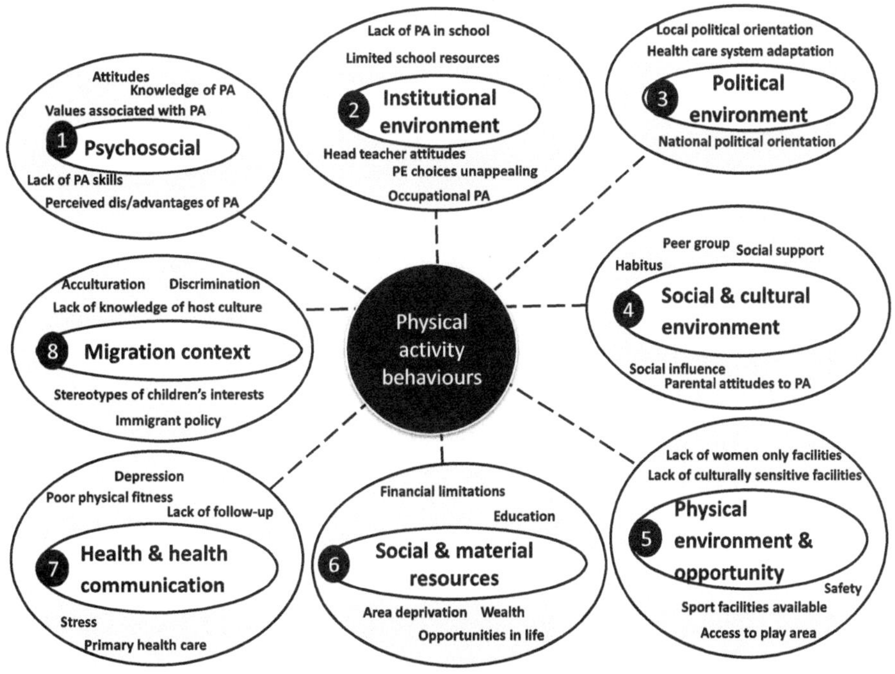

Fig. 3 A systems-based framework of the priority factors and clusters influencing physical activity behaviours in ethnic minority populations living in Europe. The numbers represent the order of ranking of the clusters. The factors listed under each cluster are the top 5 factors ranked by a range of experts from a wide array of disciplines for their importance based on 3 criteria of 'research priority', 'expected modifiability' and 'potential effect size on behaviour'. Dotted lines indicate that factors in the cluster are associated with behaviours, but they do not indicate evidence for causation

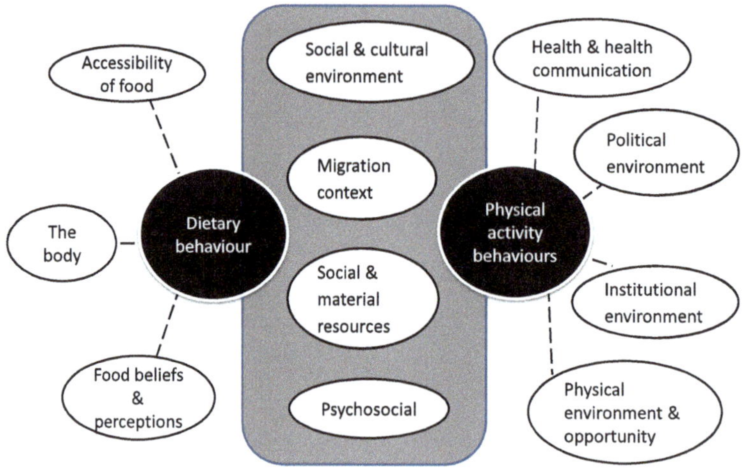

Fig. 4 A systems-based integrated framework of the clusters influencing dietary and physical activity behaviours in ethnic minority populations living in Europe. Dotted lines indicate that factors in the cluster are associated with behaviours, but they do not indicate evidence for causation

The 'social and cultural' cluster was ranked first for overall importance for its influence on physical activity amongst ethnic minority populations. Even though social and cultural factors emerged in the general population, the overall cluster was ranked lower for physical activity and sedentary behaviour (Table 5). The importance of psychosocial factors in the general population was ranked slightly less than for ethnic minority groups, as they were ranked in second and third position for sedentary behaviour and physical activity respectively. The political environment was ranked higher for its importance in influencing physical activity in ethnic minority populations than in the general population, where it was ranked last (sedentary behaviour) or next to last (physical activity) (Table 5).

For diet, the importance of 'psychosocial' factors, 'food beliefs and perceptions', 'social and material resources', and the 'social and cultural environment' were all ranked

Table 5 Comparing emerging clusters and their overall ranking in ethnic minorities with sub-categories in the general European population for dietary and physical activity behaviours

Dietary behaviours			Physical activity behaviours			
	Cluster Rank			Cluster Rank		
Cluster name	Ethnic minorities	General population[a]	Cluster name	Ethnic minorities (PA/SB)	General population (PA)[b]	General population (SB)[c]
Psychosocial	1	7	Psychosocial	1	3	2
Food beliefs and perceptions	2	17	Institutional environment	2	–	1
Social and material resources	3	18	Political environment	3	5	6
Accessibility of food	4	2	Social and cultural environment	4	2 and 4	5
The body	5	30	Physical environment and opportunity	5	1	3
Social and cultural environment	6	20	Social and material resources	6	6	-
Migration context	7	–	Health and health communication	7	–	4
			Migration context	8	–	-

Matches here are based on overlap of the individual factors included in each sub-category[a] or cluster but it should be noted that overlap may only be partial. All scores were ranked based on criteria including priority for research, modifiability and population-level effect (and relationship strength[a])
There are a total of 51 sub-categories in the general population diet framework[a] [31], 6 clusters in both the physical activity framework[b] [32] and sedentary behaviour framework[c] [33]
[PA = physical activity and SB = sedentary behaviour]

lower in the general population than for ethnic minority groups (Table 5). However, the importance of the cluster of factors relating to the 'accessibility of food' emerged as important across all populations.

Discussion

A system-based framework was established in this study to summarise the factors influencing dietary and physical activity behaviours in ethnic minority populations living in Europe. This is the first framework developed using a formal consensus methodology, drawing upon wide transdisciplinary evidence and eminence. It is envisaged that the framework will primarily be used as a tool to stimulate operationalisation and contextualisation for research and interventions.

There was insufficient evidence from specific ethnic minority groups, so therefore they were treated together, as there are shared experiences in the lives of people from ethnic minority populations that justify grouping them together. However, as with majority host populations, it is important to acknowledge the heterogeneity of ethnic minority populations living in Europe [36]. The different clusters are likely to interact, implying that factors in a specific cluster operate differently, depending on the factors in other clusters. In addition, clusters are highly dynamic, and might change over time as populations evolve, as the needs of ethnic minority populations are not static.

Implications for *research priorities* for ethnic minority populations

The framework highlights key research priorities for ethnic minority populations. For instance, addressing the highest rated factors associated with dietary behaviour would involve consideration of several clusters including 'accessibility of food', 'psychosocial' and 'resources/social capital'. The clustering of factors in this way might precipitate a shift in the way complex behaviours are viewed; from a simple approach focusing on individual level factors, to a more holistic systems approach. In our study, psychosocial factors were ranked highly overall, particularly as they were seen as modifiable, which probably explains why research and interventions tend to focus on individual psychosocial factors [26].

The lack of evidence to attribute causation and effect strength is a major gap and research on causal models and pathways needs developing. Identifying and visualising inter-connections between factors remains difficult to do without data on their relationships, which requires more research taking a systems approach [22, 24, 26]. Both qualitative and longitudinal quantitative research provide useful insights for these inter-linkages and pathways that lead to dietary and physical activity behaviours [36, 40].

Practical considerations include the need for multidisciplinary researchers involved in understanding and changing behaviours to develop skills to evaluate the impact of complex, upstream, population-level interventions on the underlying clusters of factors [26], as well developing skills in cultural adaptation. Furthermore, in light of the peak migration in 2015–16 to Europe [41], new research regarding the impact of dietary behaviours on health for these populations is required, particularly amongst vulnerable migrant populations, including refugees, unaccompanied children and illegal migrants.

Research on ethnic minority populations often look through a lens of difference [36], i.e. focussing on what is different rather than similar with the general population, which may explain the wealth of social and cultural factors identified through this process. Although important, there is also scope for investigating commonalities, for example, how factors that drive dietary and physical activity behaviours in the majority population influence these behaviours amongst ethnic minority populations, which emphasises the needs for a systems approach across all populations. For example, one-third of the top rated 15 factors for diet were related to food accessibility, including food availability, how food policy shapes access to food and the price of food, which all emerged as important areas for research for the general population too. Interventions targeting these factors will require a whole population approach.

Most of the factors specific to the 'migration context' were not seen as a research priority, possibly because they would require studies involving several countries to research populations in different countries, and the context was seen as hard to change. The converse is also true, as research in the majority population seldom sheds light on how social and cultural factors influence behaviours, which may explain why they were ranked lower in the general population framework. The importance of research on collective behaviours, especially on the social practices that shape social habits and therefore practices around diet and physical activity is key for all population groups [40, 42], regardless of their ethnicity.

Implications for developing *interventions* for ethnic minority populations

The study's findings have highlighted that there are unlikely to be quick fixes or tipping points that can be isolated to change behaviours, rather, several factors could be targeted to improve diet and/or physical activity behaviours across the inter-related system of clusters. This reinforces the need for a systems approach in planning multifaceted interventions in order to account for the (sometimes unexpected) interaction between the factors influencing behaviour. Conventional approaches focusing on individual level behaviour change are insufficient [26].

The contextualisation for interventions is crucial too, which is in contrast with the high priority given to the individual level psychosocial factors in this study. This finding is largely a reflection of prevailing perceptions that these are easy to change. However, changing individual level factors, whilst the context remains the same, is insufficient to drive behaviour change, in view of the socially and culturally embedded nature of dietary [43] and physical activity behaviours.

This study's findings have highlighted much commonality between the factors influencing the behaviours in ethnic minority groups and the majority population. This begs the question of whether interventions are needed that address factors that are specific to ethnic minority groups, or whether mainstream interventions should be encouraged that can reach all groups. The study suggests that 'mainstream' interventions targeting the general population could address many factors identified as there was much in common between minority and host populations, such as food policy, food pricing, physical activity at school, access to play areas, area-level deprivation and so forth. However, even if factors are shared, their importance and focus might differ, e.g. the need for women only facilities, the social role of food might be stronger in more collective cultures. There are specific factors in the context of migration that will need to be addressed at a higher policy level, including policies encouraging integration.

Two different approaches for developing interventions that can reach ethnic minority populations are advocated for [44]. These consist of either adapting mainstream interventions for the majority population to be 'diversity sensitive', so that they can be equally effective for all citizens regardless of their cultural, religious or ethnic background, or alternatively developing 'migrant-specific' interventions by culturally adapting services and interventions to individual backgrounds of specific minority ethnic groups. The framework developed could be used to develop either approach, as well as encourage new approaches. Most of the evaluations of culturally sensitive interventions have been conducted in the US [45, 46] and may not be transferable. Additionally, evidence has indicated that evaluations lack explicit information about the components of cultural adaptation, and little or no detail is provided regarding how interventions are cultural adapted [47]. Evaluating interventions in a way that goes beyond 'what works', but also identifies 'for whom it works and in what context', such as realist approaches [48] would be well adapted to unravel the underlying processes. It should also be emphasised that this framework does not provide ready-made answers for intervention development. As for the case for 'majority' populations, a needs assessment will remain a necessary part of the process [49].

Methodological limitations

An important limitation was that whilst the frameworks for physical activity and sedentary behaviour followed a very similar concept mapping approach to determining clusters of factors, the framework for dietary behaviours did not include emerging clusters [28]. The dietary behaviour framework was developed by sorting individual factors into pre-defined categories with a positivist top-down process, using a socio-ecological approach [31]. Whereas a constructivist approach was taken in the development of the other frameworks, as clusters emerged from the data. However, both approaches are holistic, given that the clusters that emerged were so similar with the different approaches. In addition, factors were rated in a different manner in the general population's dietary behaviour framework as the overall priority for research was based on a weighted average of ratings for their modifiability, relationship strength and population-level effect [28].

Another limitation is that research participants did not cluster factors as individuals, but collectively as a group, meaning that clusters could not be created mathematically using cluster analysis [32]. This approach was decided against due to time limitations during data collection for individuals to cluster factors together separately. Even in the case of individual clustering, the results of cluster analysis often require visible adjustment to make them meaningful [32].

The decision to only request scoring of the top 15 ranking factors in the international symposium may have introduced bias, as it is unknown if these factors would be different if other people from within the broader DEDIPAC-KH or from outside it had participated in the rating of all factors. However, new/additional factors were explicitly sought from external participants, in order to compensate for this limitation.

The concept mapping exercise led to a hypothesised ranking of factors within clusters, while the systems approach implies that the interaction of context and interrelated factors is what influences behaviour [26]. However, evidence for links between factors was not found, due to a lack of research on the underlying mechanisms. Given this, there remains uncertainty about the specific factors that are a priority for research. A further limitation was the profile of participants. The framework was informed by academic researchers and although some have extensive experience with ethnic minority and migrant origin populations, input from individuals from agencies who work closely with different populations would have improved its completeness. Academic specialists in migrant health were invited as experts, enhancing confidence in the potential utility of the framework presented.

Other limitations included the lack of research highlighting the drivers of dietary and physical activity behaviours across the life-course, as most research targeted adults. There were insufficient studies to differentiate by age or life-course and further research is particularly required on children and adolescents, as they clearly have a role in influencing behaviours of the whole family. There was limited research on sedentary behaviour among ethnic minorities. Some ethnic minority groups were under-represented, particularly recent migrant populations to Europe, which should also be a priority for research.

Conclusions

This is the first systems-based framework to be developed that sheds light on dietary and physical activity behaviours of ethnic minority populations living in Europe, drawing on both evidence and eminence. Distinct clusters emerged for both dietary and physical activity behaviours, of which four clusters were similar across behaviours (social and cultural environment; social and material resources; psychosocial; and migration context), suggesting that an integrated approach for interventions across behaviours in these clusters of factors could bring maximum benefit. Similar clusters of factors emerged in the majority population frameworks for diet and physical activity behaviours, but their relative importance differed for ethnic minority populations, compared with the majority population.

Our findings illustrate that innovative research and interventions need to be developed that are sensitive to the needs of ethnic minority populations. Dietary and physical activity behaviours are intransigent and addressing them will require enormous innovation. A systems approach may help in shifting the current public health paradigm towards a more holistic approach that considers what works for whom and in what context, in order to ensure that ethnic minorities are included, alongside mainstream European populations.

Abbreviations

BMI: Body mass index; DEDIPAC: DEterminants of DIet and Physical ACtivity; PA: Physical activity; SB: Sedentary behaviour; SES: Socioeconomic status

Acknowledgements

Not applicable.

Funding

The preparation of this paper was supported by the Determinants of Diet and Physical ACtivity (DEDIPAC) knowledge hub. This work is supported by the Joint Programming Initiative 'Healthy Diet for a Healthy Life'. The funding agencies supporting this work are (in alphabetical order of participating Member State in this paper): Belgium: Research Foundation – Flanders; France: Institut National de la Recherche Agronomique (INRA); Germany: Federal Ministry of Education and Research; Italy: Ministero dell'Istruzione, Università e Ricerca, Italy; Norway: The Research Council of Norway; The Netherlands: The Netherlands Organisation for Health Research and Development (ZonMw); The UK: The Medical Research Council (MRC). The authors would like to thank the entire thematic area 2 of the DEDIPAC project.

Authors' contributions

All authors conceptualized and designed the study. MH drafted the manuscript. All authors reviewed draft versions of the manuscript and provided suggestions and critical feedback. All authors have made a significant contribution to this manuscript and approved the final manuscript.

Competing interests

The authors declare that they have no competing interests.

Author details

[1]Public Health Section, School of Health and Related Research-ScHARR, The University of Sheffield, Sheffield, UK. [2]Academic Medical Centre, University of Amsterdam, Department of Public Health, Amsterdam Public Health research Institute, Amsterdam, The Netherlands. [3]Department of Physical Education, Norwegian School of Sport Sciences, Oslo, Norway. [4]Institute for Applied Health Research, School of Health and Life Science, Glasgow Caledonian University, Glasgow, UK. [5]Department of Psychological Assessment and Health Psychology, University of Konstanz, Constance, Germany. [6]Department of Movement, Human and Health Sciences, University of Rome Foro Italico, Rome, Italy. [7]Department of Nutrition, University of Oslo, Oslo, Norway. [8]Department of Nursing and Health Promotion Faculty of Health Sciences, Oslo and Akershus University College of Applied Sciences, Oslo, Norway. [9]UKCRC Centre for Diet and Activity Research, MRC Epidemiology Unit, University of Cambridge School of Clinical Medicine, Box 285, Institute of Metabolic Science, Cambridge Biomedical Campus, Cambridge CB2 0QQ, UK. [10]Present address: Department of Nutrition and Exercise Physiology, Elson S Floyd College of Medicine, Washington State University, Spokane WA 99210-1495, USA. [11]Department of Public Health, Ghent University, Ghent, Belgium. [12]Department of Public Health, Ghent University, Ghent, Belgium. [13]Consumption Research Norway SIFO, Oslo and Akershus University College of Applied Sciences, Oslo, Norway. [14]UMR MOISA, Campus INRA-SupAgro de la Gaillarde, Montpellier, France.

References

1. Faskunger J, Eriksson U, Johansson SE, Sundquist K, Sundquist J. Risk of obesity in immigrants compared with swedes in two deprived neighbourhoods. BMC Public Health. 2009;9(1):304.
2. Patel J, Vyas A, Cruickshank J, Prabhakaran D, Hughes E, Reddy K, et al. Impact of migration on coronary heart disease risk factors: comparison of Gujaratis in Britain and their contemporaries in villages of origin in India. Atherosclerosis. 2006;185(2):297–306.
3. Leung G, Stanner S. Diets of minority ethnic groups in the UK: influence on chronic disease risk and implications for prevention. Nutr Bull. 2011;36(2):161–98.
4. Hayes L, White M, Unwin N, Bhopal R, Fischbacher C, Harland J, et al. Patterns of physical activity and relationship with risk markers for cardiovascular disease and diabetes in Indian, Pakistani, Bangladeshi and European adults in a UK population. J Public Health. 2002;24(3):170–8.
5. Babakus WS, Thompson JL. Physical activity among south Asian women: a systematic, mixed-methods review. Int J Behav Nutr Phys Act. 2012;9(1):1.
6. Besharat Pour M, Bergström A, Bottai M, Kull I, Wickman M, Håkansson N, et al. Effect of parental migration background on childhood nutrition, physical activity, and body mass index. J Obes. 2014; https://doi.org/10.1155/2014/406529.
7. De Munter JS, Agyemang C, Van Valkengoed IG, Bhopal R, Zaninotto P, Nazroo J, et al. Cross national study of leisure-time physical activity in Dutch and English populations with ethnic group comparisons. Eur J Pub Health. 2013;23(3):440–6.
8. Hansen AR, Ekholm O, Kjøller M. Health behaviour among non-western immigrants with Danish citizenship. Scandinavian Journal of Public Health. 2008;36(2):205–10.
9. Hornby-Turner YC, Hampshire KR, Pollard TMA. Comparison of physical activity and sedentary behaviour in 9–11 year old British Pakistani and white British girls: a mixed methods study. Int J Behav Nutr Phys Act. 2014;11(1):1.
10. Dagkas S, Benn T. Young Muslim women's experiences of Islam and physical education in Greece and Britain: a comparative study. Sport Educ Soc. 2006;11(1):21–38.

11. Södergren M, Hylander I, Törnkvist L, Sundquist J, Sundquist K. Arranging appropriate activities: immigrant women's ideas of enabling exercise. Womens Health Issues. 2008;18(5):413–22.
12. Rawlins E, Baker G, Maynard M, Harding S. Perceptions of healthy eating and physical activity in an ethnically diverse sample of young children and their parents: the DEAL prevention of obesity study. J Hum Nutr Diet. 2013; 26(2):132–44.
13. Satia-About a J, Patterson RE, Neuhouser ML, Elder J. Dietary acculturation: applications to nutrition research and dietetics. J Am Diet Assoc. 2002; 102(8):1105–18.
14. Brustad M, Parr C, Melhus M, Lund E. Childhood diet in relation to Sami and Norwegian ethnicity in northern and mid-Norway–the SAMINOR study. Public Health Nutr. 2008;11(02):168–75.
15. Nicolaou M, Doak CM, van Dam RM, Brug J, Stronks K, Seidell JC. Cultural and social influences on food consumption in Dutch residents of Turkish and Moroccan origin: a qualitative study. J Nutr Educ Behav. 2009;41(4): 232–41.
16. Lawton J, Ahmad N, Hanna L, Douglas M, Bains H, Hallowell N. 'We should change ourselves, but we can't': accounts of food and eating practices amongst British Pakistanis and Indians with type 2 diabetes. Ethn Health. 2008;13(4):305–19.
17. Andersen E, Høstmark AT, Holme I, Anderssen SA. Intervention effects on physical activity and insulin levels in men of Pakistani origin living in Oslo: a randomised controlled trial. Immigr Minor Health. 2013;15(1):101–10.
18. Kay T. Daughters of Islam family influences on Muslim young Women's participation in sport. International Review for the Sociology of Sport. 2006; 41(3–4):357–73.
19. Méjean C, Traissac P, Eymard-Duvernay S, Delpeuch F, Maire B. Influence of acculturation among Tunisian migrants in France and their past/present exposure to the home country on diet and physical activity. Public Health Nutr. 2009;12(06):832–41.
20. Pollard TM, Guell C. Assessing physical activity in Muslim women of south Asian origin. J Phys Act Health. 2012;9(7):970.
21. Kumanyika SK, Obarzanek E, Stettler N, Bell R, Field AE, Fortmann SP, et al. Population-based prevention of obesity: the need for comprehensive promotion of healthful eating, physical activity, and energy balance: a scientific statement from American Heart Association Council on epidemiology and prevention, interdisciplinary Committee for Prevention. Circulation. 2008;118(4):428–64.
22. Butland B, Jebb S, Kopelman P, McPherson K, Thomas S, Mardell J, et al. Foresight. Tackling obesities: future choices. Project report. Foresight. Tackling obesities: future choices. In: Project report; 2007. https://www.gov.uk/government/publications/reducing-obesity-future-choices.
23. Delavari M, Farrelly A, Renzaho A, Mellor D, Swinburn B. Experiences of migration and the determinants of obesity among recent Iranian immigrants in Victoria, Australia. Ethn Health. 2013;18(1):66–82.
24. Carey G, Malbon E, Carey N, Joyce A, Crammond B, Carey A. Systems science and systems thinking for public health: a systematic review of the field. BMJ Open. 2015;30(5):12.
25. Homer J, Hirsch G. Opportunities and demands in public health systems. Am J Public Health. 2006;96(3):452–8.
26. Rutter H, Savona N, Glonti K, et al. The need for complex systems model of evidence for public health. Lancet. 2017; https://doi.org/10.1016/S0140-6736(17)31267-9.
27. Lakerveld J, Van Der Ploeg HP, Kroeze W, Ahrens W, Allais O, Andersen LF, et al. Towards the integration and development of a cross-European research network and infrastructure: the DEterminants of DIet and physical ACtivity (DEDIPAC) knowledge hub. Int J Behav Nutr Phys Act 2014;11(1):1.
28. Stok FM, Hoffmann S, Volkert D, Boeing H, Ensenauer R, Stelmach-Mardas M, et al. The DONE framework: Creating, evaluating and updating of an interdisciplinary, dynamic framework 2.0 of determinants of nutrition and eating. PLoS One 2017;2;12(2):e0171077. doi:https://doi.org/10.1371/journal.pone.0171077.
29. Condello G, Ling FC, Bianco A, Chastin S, Cardon G, Ciarapica D, et al. Using concept mapping in the development of the EU-PAD framework (EUropean physical activity determinants across the life course): a DEDIPAC-study. BMC Public Health. 2016;16(1):1145.
30. Chastin S, De Craemer M, Lien N, Bernaards C, Buck C, Oppert J, et al. The SOS-framework (Systems of Sedentary behaviours): an international transdisciplinary consensus framework for the study of determinants, research priorities and policy on sedentary behaviour across the life course: a DEDIPAC-study. Int J Behav Nutr Phys Act. 2016;13(1):83. https://doi.org/10.1186/s12966-016-0409-3.
31. Booth SL, Sallis JF, Ritenbaugh C, Hill JO, Birch LL, Frank LD, et al. Environmental and societal factors affect food choice and physical activity: rationale, influences, and leverage points. Nutr Rev. 2001;59:S21–36.
32. Trochim WM. An introduction to concept mapping for planning and evaluation. Evaluation and program planning. 1989;12(1):1–16.
33. Daley BJ. Using concept maps in qualitative research. Theory, Methodology, Technology. Proc. of the First Int. Conference on Concept mapping Pamplona, Spain: Concept Maps; 2004.
34. Wheeldon J, Faubert J. Framing experience: concept maps, mind maps, and data collection in qualitative research. Int J Qual Methods. 2009;8:3.
35. Leischow SJ, Milstein B. Systems thinking and modeling for public health practice. Am J Public Health. 2006;96(3):403–5.
36. Osei-Kwasi HA, Nicolaou M, Powell K, Terragni L, Maes L, Stronks K, et al. Systematic mapping review of the factors influencing dietary behaviour in ethnic minority groups living in Europe: a DEDIPAC study. Int J Behav Nutr Phys Act. 2016;13(1):1.
37. Langøien LJ, Terragni L, Rugseth G, Nicolaou M, Holdsworth M, Stronks K, Lien N, Roos G. Systematic mapping review of the factors influencing physical activity and sedentary behaviour in ethnic minority groups in Europe: a DEDIPAC study. Int J Behav Nutr Phys Act. 2017;14:99.
38. Kockturk-Runefors TA. Model for adaptation to a new food pattern: the case of immigrants. Appetite. 1991;16(2):163.
39. Holdsworth M, Nicolaou M, Osei-Kwasi HA, Langøien LJ, Powell K, Terragni L, et al. Developing a framework map of the major determinants of dietary behaviour and physical activity/sedentary behaviour in minority ethnic groups living in Europe. Edinburgh (UK): abstract book of the conference of International Society for Behavioral Nutrition and Physical Activity (https://eventmobi.com/api/events/7231/documents/download/596c6adb-ef0f-4695-be2c-8a1927877d2c.pdf/as/ISBNPA%202015%20Abstract%20Book.pdf); 2015. p107, S6.73.
40. Powell K, Wilcox J, Clonan A, Bissell P, Preston L, Peacock M, et al. The role of social networks in the development of overweight and obesity among adults: a scoping review. BMC Public Health. 2015;15(1):1.
41. International organisation for Migration. Migration flows to Europe- 2017 Quarterly overview. 2017. http://migration.iom.int/docs/Q1_2017_statistical_Overview.pdf. Accessed 10 July 2017.
42. Shove E, Pantzar M, Watson M. The dynamics of social practice: everyday life and how it changes. London: Sage Publications; 2012.
43. Delormier T, Frohlich KL, Potvin L. Food and eating as social practice–understanding eating patterns as social phenomena and implications for public health. Sociol Health Illn. 2009;31(2):215–28.
44. Razum O, Spallek J. Addressing health-related interventions to immigrants: migrant-specific or diversity-sensitive. Int J Public Health. 2014;59(6):893–5.
45. Fisher TL, Burnet DL, Huang ES, et al. Cultural leverage: interventions using culture to narrow racial disparities in health care. Med Care Res Rev. 2007; 64:243S–82S.
46. Neamah HH, Sebert Kuhlmann AK, Tabak RG. Effectiveness of program modification strategies of the diabetes prevention program: a systematic review. Diabetes Educ. 2016;42(2):153–65.
47. Diaz E, Ortiz Barreda G, Ben-Shlomo Y, et al. Interventions to improve immigrant health. A scoping review. Eur J Pub Health. 2017;27(3):433–9.
48. Harris J, Springett J, Booth A, et al. Can community-based peer support promote health literacy and reduce inequalities? A realist review. J Public Health Res. 2015;3(3)
49. Bartholomew LK, Parcel GS, Kok G. Intervention Mapping: A Process for Developing Theory and Evidence-Based Health Education Programs. 1998; 25(5):545–63.

10

The use of entertainment and communication technologies before sleep could affect sleep and weight status: a population-based study among children

Nomathemba Dube[1], Kaviul Khan[1,2], Sarah Loehr[1], Yen Chu[1,3] and Paul Veugelers[1*]

Abstract

Background: Short sleep duration and poor sleep quality have been demonstrated to be associated with childhood obesity. It has been suggested that electronic entertainment and communication devices (EECDs) including TVs, computers, tablets, video games and cell phones interfere with sleep in children and youth. The aim of this study was to assess the impact that the use of EECDs in the hour before bedtime has on sleep and weight status to inform sleep promotion interventions and programs to prevent childhood obesity.

Methods: A provincially representative sample of 2334 grade 5 children and their parents in Alberta, Canada was surveyed. Parents reported their child's bedtime and wake-up time along with how often their child snored, felt sleepy during the day, woke-up at night and woke-up in the morning feeling unrefreshed. Sleep duration, sleep quality and sleep efficiency were derived from these indicators. Parents also reported on the presence of EECDs in their child's bedroom, while children reported use of EECDs during the day and frequency of using each of these devices during the hour before sleep. The height and weight of children were measured. Multivariable mixed effect linear and logistic regression models were used to determine how sleep duration, sleep quality, sleep efficiency and weight status are influenced by (i) access to EECDs in children's bedrooms, (ii) use of EECDs during the hour before sleep, and (iii) calming activities specifically reading during the hour before sleep.

Results: Sleep duration was shorter by −10.8 min (cell phone), −10.2 min (computer) and −7.8 min (TV) for those with bedroom access to and used these EECDs during the hour before sleep compared to no access and no use. Good sleep quality was hindered by bedroom access to and use of all EECDs investigated during the hour before sleep, particularly among users of cell phones (OR = 0.64, 95% CI: 0.58–0.71) and computers (OR = 0.72, 95% CI: 0.65–0.80). Very good sleep efficiency was decreased by access to and frequent use of a TV (54%), cell phone (52%), tablet (51%) and video games (51%). Odds of obesity were doubled by bedroom access to and use of a TV and computer during the hour before sleep. Children who rarely read a printed book in the bedroom during the hour before sleep had a shorter sleep duration and poorer sleep quality and sleep efficiency compared to their peers. Having access to an EECD in the bedroom was associated with increased obesity despite frequently reading during the hour before sleep.

(Continued on next page)

* Correspondence: paul.veugelers@ualberta.ca
[1]Department of Public Health Sciences, Population Health Intervention Research Unit, School of Public Health, University of Alberta, 3-50 University Terrace, 8303 112 Street, Edmonton, AB T6G 2T4, Canada
Full list of author information is available at the end of the article

(Continued from previous page)

Conclusions: Our findings suggest that sleep duration, sleep quality, sleep efficiency and weight status are better among children who do not have EECDs in the bedroom and frequently read a book during the hour before sleep as opposed to those who use EECDs during this hour. Education of limits against EECD use by parents may improve sleep outcomes. These findings will inform health promotion messages and may give rise to national recommendations regarding EECD use.

Trial registration: ClinicalTrials.gov NCT01914185. Registered 31 July 2013 Retrospectively registered.

Keywords: Sleep duration, Total time in bed, Sleep quality sleep efficiency, Weight status, Elementary school children, Electronic devices

Background

The National Sleep Foundation recommends 9–11 h of sleep per night for children aged 6–13 years [1]. Obtaining the recommended amount of sleep is important for mental and physical health [2, 3]. Despite this, children nowadays are sleeping much less than children 20 years ago [4]. Between 1974 and 1986 alone, sleep duration in children was found to have decreased by one hour [4]. The rising use of electronic entertainment and communication devices (EECDs) by children have been shown to play a role in shorter sleep duration [5] as well as poor sleep quality [6] and sleep efficiency [7]. Between 1996 and 2009, children aged 8–18 years old were reported to use EECDs (TVs, computers, tablets, video games and cell phones) for as much as 8 ½ hours daily, seven days a week [8, 9]. The negative effects of long periods of EECD use on sleep are well established [7, 9–11] and so are the effects of sleep deprivation on body weight [10, 12–14], demonstrated by the activation of a hormonal response when sleep is insufficient, which increases appetite and food consumption leading to obesity [15–19]. In an era of deteriorating sleep habits and rising childhood obesity rates, understanding fully which practices affect both sleep duration and sleep quality is essential to public health decision makers.

While access to and use of EECDs in the bedroom have been shown to shorten sleep duration [9], it remains unclear whether it is merely the presence of EECDs in the bedroom, or whether it is their use immediately before bedtime that is detrimental to sleep. It is therefore important to investigate how the presence and use of EECDs in the bedroom affect sleep, and specifically, how sleep may be affected when these devices are used during the hour before bedtime. In the present study, we have investigated the effects of independent and interdependent presence and use of EECDs by grade 5 children in the bedroom during the hour before sleep on: i) sleep duration, ii) sleep quality iii) sleep efficiency and iv) weight status. Furthermore, since reading a printed book has been recommended as a calming activity to help the body wind down and shift into sleep mode [20], we also investigated how reading during the hour before sleep is associated with these four outcomes. Reading a printed book was of interest as opposed to a self-luminous eReader because calming effects of eReaders require further validation [21].

Methods

Study population

In 2012, 181 geographically representative elementary schools in Alberta, Canada were invited to participate in the Raising healthy Eating and Active Living Kids in Alberta (REAL Kids Alberta) survey. Of those invited, 143 (77.9%) schools agreed to participate. Packets containing a consent form and a home-based questionnaire [22], both to be completed by parents, were sent home with 4957 grade 5 children, who typically are either 10 or 11 years old. Of the packets sent home, 2732 were returned (55.1% return rate) with 50.1% (2483/4957) of children receiving parental consent. Of the children with parental consent, 94.0% (2334/2483) completed the school-based questionnaire and had heights and weights measured by evaluation assistants while the remaining 6.0% (149/2483) of children with parental consent were either absent on the day of the survey or declined to participate. More information about study tools is available at http://www.REALKidsAlberta.ca.

Outcomes of interest

Sleep duration and Total time in bed

Parents were asked to report their child's usual bedtime, additional time required to fall asleep after going to bed and wakeup time for weekdays and weekend days. Sleep duration was calculated by subtracting the child's bedtime and additional time required to fall asleep from wakeup time. Total time in bed (TTIB) was calculated by subtracting the child's bedtime from wakeup time. For each child, sleep duration across the whole week was calculated by multiplying the weekday sleep duration by five and the weekend sleep duration by two before obtaining the sum of both and dividing it by seven. The same was done for TTIB using weekday and weekend TTIB in bed.

Sleep quality and sleep efficiency

Parents were asked four questions about their child's sleep quality. They were asked whether their child (i) snored; (ii) woke up feeling unrefreshed; (iii) felt sleepy during the daytime; and (iv) woke up during the night after falling asleep. Response options were 'Never', 'Sometimes', 'Frequently' and 'Almost always'. These sleep quality questions were adapted from validated questions among adults and were used in our population. To obtain sleep efficiency, sleep duration was divided by TTIB, before multiplying the result by 100. Sleep efficiency, was categorized into good (90–94%) and very good (≥95%).

Weight status

Body Mass Index (BMI) of each student was calculated using her or his measured height and weight. Children were asked to remove their shoes before the measurements were taken. Height was measured to the nearest 0.1 cm on a portable stadiometer, and body weight was measured to the nearest 0.1 kg on calibrated digital scales. The resulting BMI was used to define weight status based on the age- and gender-specific cut-off points specified by the Extended International Obesity Task Force [23, 24].

Exposures of interest

Access to EECDs in the bedroom

Parents were asked to indicate, which EECDs (TV, computer, tablet, video game or cell phone) their child had access to in the bedroom. Responses included: 'Yes', 'No' and 'Sometimes', where 'Sometimes' was considered as 'Yes' in the analysis. Additionally, in the analysis, children were considered to have access to "at least one device" in their bedroom if parents responded 'Yes' or 'Sometimes' to having access to any one of the EECDs in the bedroom.

Bedroom use of EECDs during the hour before sleep

Children were asked how often they used each EECD in their bedroom during the hour before sleep. Response options were 'Never', 'About once per month', '1–2 times a week', '3–4 times a week' and '5 or more times per week'. Children whose responses were 'Never' or 'About once per month' were regarded as 'Never' using the EECDs during the hour before sleep, while children providing alternative responses were regarded as 'Used' EECDs during that hour.

Frequency of reading a book one hour before sleep

Children were asked how often they read in their bedroom during the hour before sleep. Response options were categorized as 'Rarely' and 'Frequently'.

Other covariates

Parents who completed the survey were asked about the gender of their child, their highest level of educational attainment (secondary or less, college, university or above) and household income levels in Canadian dollars (CA$) (≤CA$50,000; CA$50,001–CA$100,000; or ≥CA$100,000). Region of elementary school (metropolitan, city or rural) was determined using school postal codes. Children were asked how many hours per day they spend (i) using the computer, (ii) playing video games and (iii) watching TV outside of school hours. Response options were 'Less than 1 hour a day' regarded as 0.5 h; '1 – 2 hours a day' regarded as 1.5 h; '3 – 4 hours a day' regarded as 3.5 h; and 5 or more hours a day' regarded as 5.5 h. The total sum of hours each student spent on EECDs was calculated to represent total daily exposure to EECDs.

Statistical analysis

Sleep quality was derived by using exploratory factor analysis with varimax rotations. The resulting factor scores were grouped into tertiles, with the first representing good sleep quality and the second and third tertiles representing poor sleep quality [9]. For descriptive statistics, one-way analysis of variance (ANOVA) was used to test for differences in the means of sleep duration, a normally distributed continuous variable, and exposure variables. Associations between sleep quality, sleep efficiency and weight status with the exposures of interest were evaluated with Rao-Scott chi-square statistics [25, 26]. When one or more of the variable frequencies was five or less, the Fishers Exact test was used instead. To accommodate clustering of student observations within schools, the effect of EECD access and use during the hour before sleep was evaluated using mixed effect linear regression for sleep duration and TTIB and mixed effect logistic regression for sleep quality and sleep efficiency. For weight status, thinness weight categories (grade 1, grade 2 and grade 3) were combined into one category (underweight) and obese and morbid obese were also combined to form the obese weight category. Multinomial logistic regression was used to evaluate the association between weight status categories (normal, overweight and obese) and the exposure groups. All multivariable analyses were adjusted for gender, household income, parental education, and area of residence as potential confounders. For all regression analyses, total daily exposure to EECDs outside of school hours was adjusted for and a combined effect of total daily exposure to EECDs and exposure during the hour before sleep was computed using linear combinations of estimators. Statistical analyses were performed in STATA version 14 (StataCorp, College Station, Texas). A p value of less than 0.05

(two-sided test) was considered statistically significant. Study ethical approval was obtained from University of Alberta Health Research Ethics Board.

Results

Demographic characteristics of the 2334 children who participated in the survey are shown in Table 1. Sleep duration on weekdays ranged between 7.33 h and 12.58 h, whilst it ranged between 7.00 h and 13.25 h on the weekend. TTIB ranged between 7.50 h and 13.00 h on weekdays and 7.50 h and 14.00 h on the weekend. On average, TTIB were statistically significantly longer for girls than boys. Compared to their peers, longer sleep duration and TTIB were observed amongst children in schools located away from metropolitan areas, who

Table 1 Sleep duration and Total time in bed of grade 5 children by gender, highest level of parental education, school region, household income, weight status, total daily exposure to devices and days of the week, Alberta, 2012

Variables	Frequency	(%)	Sleep duration (Hours)	*p-value*	Total Time in Bed (Hours)	*p-value*
Gender						
Girls	1235	(53.2)	9.85 (±0.56)	*0.05*	10.22 (±0.56)	*0.01*
Boys	1071	(46.8)	9.82 (±0.58)		10.16 (±0.59)	
Highest level of parental education						
No school/Elementary school	63	(3.0)	9.83 (±0.58)	0.65	10.19 (±0.58)	0.29
Secondary/college	1391	(59.0)	9.86 (±0.54)		10.21 (±0.54)	
University	792	(38.0)	9.83 (±0.58)		10.17 (±0.59)	
Region of elementary school						
Metropolitan	612	(49.0)	9.78 (±0.59)	*<0.001*	10.11 (±0.60)	*<0.001*
City	781	(16.3)	9.90 (±0.57)		10.21 (±0.54)	
Rural/town	941	(34.7)	9.88 (±0.54)		10.24 (±0.58)	
Household income						
< $50,000 (Low)	385	(19.7)	9.71 (±0.58)	*<0.001*	10.08 (±0.57)	*<0.001*
$50,001 - $100,000 (Middle)	614	(26.6)	9.84 (±0.55)		10.21 (±0.55)	
> $100,000 (High)	684	(28.2)	9.90 (±0.55)		10.22 (±0.56)	
Don't know/Prefer not to answer*	575	(25.5)	9.91 (±0.57)		10.22 (±0.59)	
Weight category						
Thinness grade 3	20	(0.9)	10.06 (±0.63)	*** < 0.001*	10.38 (±0.63)	*<0.001*
Thinness grade 2	49	(2.1)	9.91 (±0.71)		10.27 (±0.71)	
Thinness grade 1	233	(10.1)	9.98 (±0.51)		10.30 (±0.51)	
Normal	1503	(65.0)	9.88 (±0.57)		10.21 (±0.61)	
Overweight	399	(17.3)	9.75 (±0.60)		10.08 (±0.57)	
Obese	48	(2.1)	9.69 (±0.57)		10.01 (±0.01)	
Morbid Obese	3	(0.1)	9.80 (±0.14)		10.20 (±0.59)	
Total daily exposure to devices (hours)						
< 2	438	(18.8)	9.97(±0.55)	*<0.001*	10.29 (±0.56)	*<0.001*
2.0	1045	(44.1)	9.89 (±0.52)		10.22 (±0.53)	
3.5	48	(2.2)	9.71(±0.54)		10.04 (±0.51)	
4.0	264	(12.1)	9.82 (±0.62)		10.14 (±0.61)	
5.0	201	(9.5)	9.72 (±0.54)		10.07 (±0.66)	
5.5	318	(13.3)	9.78 (±0.60)		10.12 (±0.61)	
Days of the week						
Week days	2276	(97.5)	9.78 (±0.64)	*<0.001*	10.12 (±0.63)	*<0.001*
Weekend days	2.263	(97.0)	9.99 (±0.72)		10.37 (±0.79)	

*Household income category "Don't know/Prefer not to answer" excluded from p trend calculations.

***p* values generated using an aggregate of 'thinness grade 1', thinness grade 2' and thinness grade 3' and 'obese and morbid obese' categories

p value <0.05 was considered statistically significant

were from high-income families, who were of normal weight or less and were exposed to EECDs for less than two hours a day, ($p_{trend} > 0.001$) (Table 1).

Good sleep quality was more likely to be observed among children whose parents had a university education ($p_{trend} < 0.001$) and who were from high-income families ($p_{trend} < 0.001$) (Table 2). Average very good sleep efficiency was 97.6% ± 1.2% (range: 95.0% – 99.3%).

Sleep duration and TTIB were statistically significantly shorter for those with access to a TV, computer, video game and cell phone in the bedroom compared to those without (Table 3). Frequently reading a book in the bedroom with no access to EECDs was associated with longer sleep duration, longer TTIB (Table 3), the highest sleep quality and better sleep efficiency (Table 4) compared to other reading categories.

Furthermore, an increase in the proportion of children with good sleep quality (additional 2.1%) was observed amongst those who both frequently read during the hour before sleep and had no EECDs accessible in the bedroom (Data not shown).

Table 2 Sleep quality and sleep efficiency of grade 5 children by gender, highest level of parental education, school region, household income, weight status and total daily exposure to devices, Alberta, 2012

Variables	Frequency	(%)	Good sleep quality (%)	*p-value*	Very good sleep efficiency (%)	*p-value*
Gender						
Girls	1235	(53.2)	32.5	0.08	94.2	0.96
Boys	1071	(46.8)	37.1		94.2	
Highest level of parental education						
No school/Elementary school	63	(3.0)	30.3	*<0.001*	92.2	0.18
Secondary/college	1391	(59.0)	32.6		94.4	
University	792	(38.0)	39.8		95.2	
Region of elementary school						
Metropolitan	612	(49.0)	36.5	0.30	94.7	0.63
City	781	(16.3)	32.9		94.1	
Rural/town	941	(34.7)	33.7		93.5	
Household income						
< $50,000 (Low)	385	(19.7)	22.9	*<0.001*	94.0	0.60
$50,001 - $100,000 (Middle)	614	(26.6)	32.7		94.4	
> $100,000 (High)	684	(28.2)	35.1		94.2	
Don't know/Prefer not to answer*	575	(25.5)	38.4		94.7	
Weight category**						
Thinness grade 3	20	(0.9)	21.5	***0.10	100.0	***0.53
Thinness grade 2	49	(2.1)	38.0		89.6	
Thinness grade 1	233	(10.1)	35.9		94.5	
Normal	1503	(65.0)	36.2		94.9	
Overweight	399	(17.3)	29.8		92.8	
Obese	48	(2.1)	22.5		94.3	
Morbid Obese	3	(0.1)	26.6		100.0	
Total daily exposure to devices (hours)						
< 2	438	(18.8)	37.4	0.07	96.4	0.06
2.0	1045	(44.1)	36.8		94.5	
3.5	48	(2.2)	33.9		89.5	
4.0	264	(12.1)	32.7		93.8	
5.0	201	(9.5)	28.4		92.5	
5.5	318	(13.3)	30.4		92.5	

*Household income category "Don't know/Prefer not to answer" excluded from p trend calculations
**Missing weight category excluded
****p* values generated using an aggregate of 'thinness grade 1', thinness grade 2' and thinness grade 3' and 'obese and morbid obese' categories
p value <0.05 was considered statistically significant

Table 3 Sleep duration and Total time in bed of grade 5 children and electronic and entertainment communication device bedroom access and use during the hour before sleep

	%	Sleep duration (Hours)	*p-value*	Total Time in Bed (%)	*p-value*
TV					
No access and no use	53.7	9.87 (±0.56)	*<0.001*	10.19 (±0.56)	*<0.001*
Access but never used	14.2	9.80 (±0.59)		10.12 (±0.61)	
Access and used	20.1	9.75 (±0.60)		10.09 (±0.60)	
[a]No access and used	12.0	9.90 (±0.54)		10.23 (±0.54)	
Computer					
No access and no use	54.5	9.89 (±0.56)	*<0.001*	10.21 (±0.57)	*<0.001*
Access but never used	13.8	9.77 (±0.59)		10.10 (±0.60)	
Access and used	12.3	9.70 (±0.63)		10.02 (±0.64)	
[a]No access and used	19.4	9.84 (±0.54)		10.17 (±0.54)	
Tablet					
No access and no use	52.3	9.86 (±0.57)	0.50	10.18 (±0.58)	0.52
Access but never used	10.2	9.83 (±0.65)		10.15 (±0.65)	
Access and used	16.3	9.83 (±0.56)		10.17 (±0.56)	
[a]No access and used	21.2	9.83 (±0.55)		10.15 (±0.56)	
Video Games					
No access and no use	60.9	9.87 (±0.55)	*<0.001*	10.19 (±0.56)	*0.002*
Access but never used	15.9	9.78 (±0.58)		10.11 (±0.58)	
Access and used	10.3	9.78 (±0.65)		10.12 (±0.65)	
[a]No access and used	12.9	9.85 (±0.62)		10.19 (±0.60)	
Cell Phone					
No access and no use	59.0	9.89 (±0.57)	*<0.001*	10.21 (±0.58)	*<0.001*
Access but never used	23.1	9.78 (±0.53)		10.11 (±0.53)	
Access and used	11.8	9.73 (±0.57)		10.06 (±0.57)	
[a]No access and used	6.1	9.87 (±0.69)		10.19 (±0.69)	
At least one device					
No access and no use	12.2	9.93 (±0.56)	*<0.001*	10.27 (±0.57)	*<0.001*
Access but never used	17.8	9.82 (±0.58)		10.15 (±0.60)	
Access and used	56.4	9.80 (±0.57)		10.13 (±0.58)	
[a]No access and used	13.6	9.96 (±0.53)		10.26 (±0.54)	
Reading					
No access and frequent reading	19.9	9.97 (±0.53)	*<0.001*	10.28 (±0.54)	*<0.001*
Access but frequent reading	52.9	9.83 (±0.58)		10.16 (±0.59)	
Access and rarely reading	21.2	9.74 (±0.56)		10.08 (±0.56)	
No access and rarely reading	6.0	9.89 (±0.60)		10.19 (±0.60)	

[a]Response category considered illogical: No access to EECD in the bedroom and is used in the bedroom during the hour before sleep
p value <0.05 was considered statistically significant

When compared to normal weight children, a larger proportion of obese children had access to EECDs in the bedroom and used them during the hour before sleep, except for the tablet, which was used by a large proportion of normal weight children. However, a statistically significant difference in proportion of weight status was only observed with the TV (Table 5).

Effects of EECD access and use on sleep duration and Total time in bed

After adjusting for covariates, children with access to EECDs in the bedroom and reportedly used them during the hour before sleep reported shorter sleep duration of −10.8 min for a cell phone (β = −0.18 h; 95% CI = −0.26, −0.09), −10.2 min for a computer

Table 4 Sleep quality and sleep efficiency of grade 5 children and electronic and entertainment communication device bedroom access and use during the hour before sleep

	%	Good sleep quality (%)	*p-value*	Very good sleep efficiency (%)	*p-value*
TV					
No access and no use	53.7	36.3	0.67	94.5	*0.01*
Access but never used	14.2	35.9		96.4	
Access and used	20.1	32.1		90.8	
[a]No access and used	12.0	32.4		94.7	
Computer					
No access and no use	54.5	36.4	0.17	94.5	0.71
Access but never used	13.8	31.5		93.1	
Access and used	12.3	30.1		93.1	
[a]No access and used	19.4	36.2		93.5	
Tablet					
No access and no use	52.3	36.2	0.67	94.3	0.64
Access but never used	10.2	32.7		93.7	
Access and used	16.3	35.0		92.5	
[a]No access and used	21.2	33.5		94.3	
Video Games					
No access and no use	60.9	36.3	0.77	95.1	*0.01*
Access but never used	15.9	31.6		94.6	
Access and used	10.3	34.2		91.9	
[a]No access and used	12.9	35.0		90.6	
Cell Phone					
No access and no use	59.0	36.6	0.10	95.1	*0.03*
Access but never used	23.1	33.2		93.1	
Access and used	11.8	28.9		90.6	
[a]No access and used	6.1	38.8		94.6	
At least one device					
No access and no use	12.2	35.5	0.29	94.9	0.06
Access but never used	17.8	36.9		95.7	
Access and used	56.4	33.1		92.8	
[a]No access and used	13.6	39.1		96.0	
Reading					
No access and frequent reading	19.9	38.4	*<0.001*	96.3	*0.01*
Access but frequent reading	52.9	37.5		94.5	
Access and rarely reading	21.2	25.9		91.0	
No access and rarely reading	6.0	34.1		92.7	

[a]Response category considered illogical: No access to EECD in the bedroom and is used in the bedroom during the hour before sleep
p value <0.05 was considered statistically significant

(β = −0.17 h; 95% CI = −0.26, −0.08) and −7.8 min for a TV (β = −0.13 h; 95% CI = −0.20, −0.06) compared to the reference (Table 6). These findings coincided with a reduced TTIB of −7.8 min for a cell phone (β = −0.13 h; 95% CI = −0.22, −0.05), −9.0 min for a computer (β = −0.15 h; 95% CI = −0.23, −0.06) and −4.2 min for TV (β = −0.07 h; 95% CI = −0.14, −0.00) among children with access to EECDs in the bedroom and reportedly used them during the hour before sleep. Interestingly, when a child had access to a cell phone in the bedroom, their sleep duration decreased (−7.8 min) as well as their TTIB (−5.4 min) (Table 6). Access to and frequent use of tablets and video games

Table 5 Weight status characteristics of grade 5 children and electronic and entertainment communication device bedroom access and use during the hour before sleep

	%	[a]Underweight (13.4%) %	Normal (66.7%) %	Overweight (17.7%) %	[b]Obese (2.3%) %	*p-value*
TV						
No access and no use	53.7	61.7	54.0	49.7	28.6	*<0.001*
Access but never used	14.2	8.5	14.2	16.5	22.5	
Access and used	20.1	15.3	19.9	24.6	38.8	
[c]No access and used	12.0	14.6	11.9	9.2	10.2	
Computer						
No access and no use	54.5	55.5	57.1	57.0	43.8	0.23
Access but never used	13.8	12.3	13.8	12.7	16.7	
Access and used	12.3	10.3	10.2	12.1	22.9	
[c]No access and used	19.4	21.9	18.9	18.2	16.7	
Tablet						
No access and no use	52.3	50.7	50.7	54.4	50.0	0.82
Access but never used	10.2	9.3	9.9	8.8	8.7	
Access and used	16.3	16.4	17.7	13.6	15.2	
[c]No access and used	21.2	23.6	21.7	23.2	26.1	
Video Games						
No access and no use	60.9	64.1	60.3	62.6	52.1	0.17
Access but never used	15.9	12.1	15.9	16.3	27.1	
Access and used	10.3	9.3	10.4	10.3	14.6	
[c]No access and used	12.9	14.5	13.4	10.8	6.3	
Cell Phone						
No access and no use	59.0	56.7	61.1	55.6	53.1	0.39
Access but never used	23.1	25.9	21.5	26.6	24.5	
Access and used	11.8	10.2	11.9	12.3	14.3	
[c]No access and used	6.1	7.2	5.6	5.5	8.2	
At least one device						
No access and no use	12.2	12.8	12.3	12.1	6.0	0.56
Access but never used	17.8	17.2	17.9	17.7	8.0	
Access and used	56.4	54.7	56.3	57.7	72.0	
[c]No access and used	13.6	15.2	13.5	12.7	14.0	
Reading						
No access and frequent reading	19.9	21.6	20.1	16.8	14.0	0.66
Access but frequent reading	52.9	49.7	53.1	52.2	56.0	
Access and rarely reading	21.2	22.3	21.0	23.3	24.0	
No access and rarely reading	6.0	6.4	5.8	7.8	6.0	

[a]Thinness grade 1, Thinness grade 2 and Thinness grade 3 weight categories combined
[b]Obese and Morbid obese weight categories combined
[c]Response category considered illogical: No access to EECD in the bedroom and is used in the bedroom during the hour before sleep
p value <0.05 was considered statistically significant

in the bedroom during the hour before sleep had no statistically significant effect on sleep duration and TTIB.

Among children who frequently read during the hour before sleep, those with an EECD present in the bedroom had a shorter sleep duration of −9.0 min ($\beta = -0.15$ h; 95% CI = −0.23, −0.08) and a shorter TTIB of −6.6 min ($\beta = -0.11$ h; 95% CI = −0.18, −0.05) compared to those without an EECD in the bedroom. Rarely reading with an EECD present in the bedroom shortened sleep duration (−12.6 min) and TTIB (−9.6 min) further (Table 6).

Daily exposure to EECDs was associated with a decrease in sleep duration of between −2.1 and −2.2 min

Table 6 Effect of electronic entertainment and communication device use during the day and access and use in the bedroom during the hour before sleep on Sleep duration and Total time in bed in grade 5 children

	Sleep duration		Total time in bed	
	Unadjusted coefficient (95% CI)	[a]Adjusted coefficient (95% CI)	Unadjusted coefficient (95% CI)	[a]Adjusted coefficient (95% CI)
TV				
No access and no use	[b]Ref	Ref	Ref	Ref
Access but never used	−0.07 (−0.16, 0.02)	*−0.09 (−0.18, −0.01)*	−0.07 (−0.16, 0.02)	−0.07 (−0.15, 0.02)
Access and frequently used	*−0.10 (−0.17, −0.03)*	*−0.13 (−0.20, −0.06)*	*−0.08 (−0.15, −0.00)*	*−0.07 (−0.14, −0.00)*
Computer				
No access and no use	Ref	Ref	Ref	Ref
Access but never used	−0.05 (−0.17, 0.06)	−0.12 (−0.22, 0.02)	−0.10 (−0.20, 0.00)	−0.09 (−0.19, 0.01)
Access and frequently used	*−0.14 (−0.24, −0.05)*	*−0.17 (−0.26, −0.08)*	*−0.12 (−0.22, −0.02)*	*−0.15 (−0.23, −0.06)*
Tablet				
No access and no use	Ref	Ref	Ref	Ref
Access but never used	−0.03 (−0.15, 0.08)	−0.08 (−0.19, 0.03)	−0.05 (−0.13, 0.03)	−0.04 (−0.11, 0.03)
Access and frequently used	−0.05 (−0.15, 0.05)	−0.09 (−0.18, 0.01)	−0.05 (−0.15, 0.05)	−0.01 (−0.11, 0.07)
Video Games				
No access and no use	Ref	Ref	Ref	Ref
Access but never used	−0.06 (−0.14, 0.02)	*−0.08 (−0.16, −0.01)*	−0.02 (−0.13, 0.09)	−0.04 (−0.14, 0.07)
Access and frequently used	−0.07 (−0.18, 0.03)	−0.08 (−0.17, 0.02)	−0.03 (−0.13, 0.06)	−0.03 (−0.13, 0.06)
Cell Phone				
No access and no use	Ref	Ref	Ref	Ref
Access but never used	*−0.12 (−0.18, −0.05)*	*−0.13 (−0.20, −0.07)*	*−0.12 (−0.18, −0.05)*	*−0.09 (−0.15, −0.03)*
Access and frequently used	*−0.16 (−0.24, −0.08)*	*−0.18 (−0.26, −0.09)*	*−0.16 (−0.24, −0.08)*	*−0.13 (−0.22, −0.05)*
At least one device				
No access and no use	Ref	Ref	Ref	Ref
Access but never used	−0.08 (−0.20, 0.04)	−0.11 (−0.24, 0.03)	−0.08 (−0.20, 0.05)	−0.07 (−0.21, 0.06)
Access and frequently used	*−0.11 (−0.20, −0.02)*	*−0.13 (−0.23, −0.03)*	*−0.11 (−0.20, −0.02)*	*−0.10 (−0.20, −0.01)*
Reading				
No access and frequent reading	Ref	Ref	Ref	Ref
Access but frequent reading	*−0.12 (−0.19, −0.05)*	*−0.15 (−0.23, −0.08)*	*−0.11 (−0.18, −0.05)*	*−0.11 (−0.18, −0.05)*
Access and rarely reading	*−0.19 (−0.27, −0.11)*	*−0.21 (−0.30, −0.13)*	*−0.17 (−0.25, −0.09)*	*−0.16 (−0.24, −0.07)*
No access and rarely reading	−0.04 (−0.17, 0.08)	−0.07 (−0.19, 0.06)	−0.06 (−0.18, 0.06)	−0.05 (−0.18, 0.07)

[a]Adjusted for gender of the child, household income, region of elementary school, highest level of parental education and total daily exposure to electronic entertainment and communication devices
[b]Reference category

for all EECDs. A similar association was observed among children who used EECDs during the day and read during the hour before sleep (Data not shown).

Effects of EECD access and use on sleep quality

After adjusting for covariates, access to a computer, tablet, video games or cell phone in the bedroom, whether used or not during the hour before sleep (compared to the reference) decreased the odds of good sleep quality (Table 7). Having a TV in the bedroom affected good sleep quality when it was frequently used during the hour before sleep (OR = 0.86, 95% CI: 0.80, 0.94) (Table 7). Cell phone access and its frequent use during the hour before sleep had the greatest impact on good sleep quality, decreasing it by 36% (OR = 0.64, 95% CI: 0.58, 0.71) (Table 7).

Having access to any EECD and rarely reading during the hour before sleep (compared to no access and frequently reading) decrease good sleep quality by 43% (OR = 0.57, 95% CI: 0.52, 0.63) (Table 7). Among children with access to EECDs in the bedroom, those who rarely read (compared to those who frequently read) had a 34% decrease in good sleep quality (OR = 0.66, 95% CI: 0.61, 0.71) (Data not shown).

Table 7 Effect of electronic entertainment and communication device use during the day and access and use in the bedroom during the hour before sleep on sleep quality and sleep efficiency in grade 5 children

	Good sleep quality		Very good sleep efficiency (≥95%)	
	Unadjusted OR (95% CI)	[a]Adjusted OR (95% CI)	Unadjusted OR (95% CI)	[a]Adjusted OR (95% CI)
TV				
No access and no use	[b]Ref	Ref	Ref	Ref
Access but never used	*1.09 (1.01, 1.19)*	1.01 (0.93, 1.11)	*1.93 (1.56, 2.39)*	*1.45 (1.13, 1.85)*
Access and frequently used	*0.90 (0.84, 0.97)*	*0.86 (0.80, 0.94)*	*0.58 (0.50, 0.66)*	*0.46 (0.39, 0.56)*
Computer				
No access and no use	Ref	Ref	Ref	Ref
Access but never used	*0.82 (0.75, 0.90)*	*0.73 (0.67, 0.80)*	*0.77 (0.65, 0.91)*	*0.83 (0.69, 0.98)*
Access and frequently used	*0.83 (0.75, 0.91)*	*0.72 (0.65, 0.80)*	1.19 (0.98, 1.44)	0.96 (0.79, 1.18)
Tablet				
No access and no use	Ref	Ref	Ref	Ref
Access but never used	*0.84 (0.76, 0.93)*	*0.79 (0.71, 0.87)*	0.97 (0.81, 1.15)	*0.58 (0.48, 0.71)*
Access and frequently used	*0.87 (0.81, 0.95)*	*0.82 (0.76, 0.89)*	*0.55 (0.46, 0.65)*	*0.49 (0.42, 0.58)*
Video Games				
No access and no use	Ref	Ref	Ref	Ref
Access but never used	*0.86 (0.79, 0.93)*	*0.80 (0.74, 0.87)*	*0.74 (0.61, 0.89)*	0.91 (0.76, 1.10)
Access and frequently used	0.99 (0.90, 1.09)	*0.87 (0.79, 0.97)*	*0.55 (0.48, 0.64)*	*0.49 (0.41, 0.59)*
Cell Phone				
No access and no use	Ref	Ref	Ref	Ref
Access but never used	*0.84 (0.78, 0.90)*	*0.73 (0.69, 0.80)*	*0.84 (0.78, 0.90)*	*0.56 (0.49, 0.65)*
Access and frequently used	*0.67 (0.61, 0.74)*	*0.64 (0.58, 0.71)*	*0.67 (0.61, 0.74)*	*0.48 (0.41, 0.57)*
At least one device				
No access and no use	Ref	Ref	Ref	Ref
Access but never used	1.10 (0.99, 1.22)	0.97 (0.87, 1.08)	*1.29 (1.01 1.65)*	1.06 (0.82, 1.37)
Access and frequently used	0.96 (0.88, 1.05)	*0.87 (0.79, 0.95)*	*0.59 (0.48, 0.72)*	*0.52 (0.42, 0.63)*
Reading				
No access and frequent reading	Ref	Ref	Ref	Ref
Access but frequent reading	0.99 (0.92, 1.06)	*0.87 (0.81, 0.94)*	*0.62 (0.52, 0.75)*	*0.66 (0.55, 0.80)*
Access and rarely reading	*0.61 (0.56, 0.67)*	*0.57 (0.52, 0.63)*	*0.36 (0.29, 0.43)*	*0.33 (0.27, 0.40)*
No access and rarely reading	0.95 (0.83, 1.08)	*0.86 (0.76, 0.99)*	*0.57 (0.44, 0.76)*	0.77 (0.58, 1.03)

[a]Adjusted for gender of the child, household income, region of elementary school, highest level of parental education and total daily exposure to electronic entertainment and communication devices
[b]Reference category

Total daily exposure to EECDs was consistently associated with lower good sleep quality of between 8% and 9% for all EECDs investigated. Exposure to EECDs during the day also decreased good sleep quality among children who frequently read during the hour before sleep (Data not shown).

Effects of EECD access and use on sleep efficiency

Although frequently using the TV during the hour before sleep significantly decreased very good sleep efficiency by 54% (OR = 0.46, 95% CI: 0.39, 0.56), it was notable that, the odds of very good sleep efficiency were increased by 45% among children with access to a TV in the bedroom, though not used during the hour before sleep (OR = 1.45, 95% CI: 1.13, 1.85) (Table 7). The effect of having access to a tablet or cell phone in the bedroom, whether used or not during the hour before sleep, affected very good sleep efficiency to a similar extent (Table 7). Never using a computer during the hour before sleep, although accessible in the bedroom, decreased very good sleep efficiency by 17% (OR = 0.83, 95% CI: 0.69, 0.98) (Table 7).

Compared to having no access to EECDs and frequently reading during the hour before sleep, access to EECDs in the bedroom, whether one frequently read during the hour before sleep (OR = 0.66, 95% CI: 0.55, 0.80) or not (OR = 0.33, 95% CI: 0.27, 0.40), was associated with a 34% and 67% decrease in very good sleep efficiency respectively. Among children with access to EECDs in the bedroom, those who rarely read (compared to those who frequently read) had a 50% decrease in very good sleep efficiency (OR = 0.50, 95% CI: 0.33, 0.57) (Data not shown). Among those who rarely read, having no access to EECDs in the bedroom doubled the odds of having very good sleep efficiency (OR = 2.04, 95% CI: 1.57, 2.65) when compared to having access (Data not shown).

Effects of EECD access and use on weight status

After adjusting for covariates, when compared to the reference, access to a TV and a computer, when frequently used during the hour before sleep increased the odds of being overweight by more than 20% and doubled the odds of being obese (Table 8). When accessible in the bedroom, a cell phone was associated with an increase in odds of being overweight (OR = 1.44, 95% CI: 1.32, 1.58) and obese (OR = 1.56, 95% CI: 1.24, 1.98), despite it never being used during the hour before sleep. Similarly, access to a TV and video games in the bedroom greatly increased the odds of obesity although reportedly not used during the hour before sleep (Table 8). Overall,

Table 8 Effect of electronic entertainment and communication device use during the day and access and use in the bedroom during the hour before sleep on weight status in grade 5 children

	Overweight vs. Normal		Obese vs. Normal	
	Unadjusted OR (95% CI)	[a]Adjusted OR (95% CI)	Unadjusted OR (95% CI)	[a]Adjusted OR (95% CI)
TV				
No access and no use	[b]Ref	Ref	Ref	Ref
Access but never used	*1.20 (1.08, 1.32)*	*1.15 (1.04, 1.28)*	*2.42 (1.86, 3.14)*	*2.28 (1.74, 2.98)*
Access and frequently used	*1.22 (1.11, 1.33)*	*1.21 (1.10, 1.33)*	*2.90 (2.31, 3.64)*	*2.56 (2.02, 3.24)*
Computer				
No access and no use	Ref	Ref	Ref	Ref
Access but never used	1.01 (0.91, 1.13)	0.99 (0.89, 1.11)	1.08 (0.80, 1.46)	1.17 (0.86, 1.59)
Access and frequently used	*1.37 (1.23, 1.53)*	*1.34 (1.20, 1.50)*	*2.28 (1.77, 2.94)*	*2.79 (2.15, 3.63)*
Tablet				
No access and no use	Ref	Ref	Ref	Ref
Access but never used	*0.81 (0.71, 0.91)*	*0.76 (0.66, 0.86)*	0.73 (0.49, 1.07)	0.84 (0.57, 1.25)
Access and frequently used	*0.72 (0.65, 0.80)*	*0.75 (0.67, 0.84)*	1.12 (0.86, 1.46)	1.19 (0.91, 1.57)
Video Games				
No access and no use	Ref	Ref	Ref	Ref
Access but never used	1.03 (0.94, 1.14)	0.99 (0.89, 1.09)	*1.77 (1.40, 2.23)*	*1.61 (1.27, 2.05)*
Access and frequently used	1.02 (0.90, 1.14)	*0.80 (0.70, 0.91)*	1.32 (0.98, 1.78)	1.10 (0.80, 1.50)
Cell Phone				
No access and no use	Ref	Ref	Ref	Ref
Access but never used	*1.41 (1.29, 1.53)*	*1.44 (1.32, 1.58)*	*1.45 (1.15, 1.82)*	*1.56 (1.24, 1.98)*
Access and frequently used	*1.20 (1.08, 1.34)*	*1.28 (1.14, 1.43)*	1.25 (0.93, 1.68)	1.31 (0.96, 1.78)
At least one device				
No access and no use	Ref	Ref	Ref	Ref
Access but never used	0.99 (0.86, 1.12)	0.92 (0.80, 1.05)	*0.55 (0.34, 0.90)*	*0.54 (0.33, 0.88)*
Access and frequently used	*1.13 (1.01, 1.27)*	1.06 (0.94, 1.19)	*2.04 (1.44, 2.89)*	*1.82 (1.28, 2.59)*
Reading				
No access and frequent reading	Ref	Ref	Ref	Ref
Access but frequent reading	*1.22 (1.22, 1.34)*	*1.18 (1.07, 1.31)*	*1.42 (1.09, 1.86)*	*1.35 (1.03, 1.77)*
Access and rarely reading	*1.41 (1.26, 1.58)*	*1.19 (1.06, 1.34)*	*1.43 (1.05, 1.96)*	1.09 (0.79, 1.51)
No access and rarely reading	*1.64 (1.40, 1.92)*	*1.42 (1.20, 1.68)*	1.38 (0.86, 2.19)	1.11 (0.69, 1.79)

[a]Adjusted for gender of the child, household income, region of elementary school, highest level of parental education and total daily exposure to electronic entertainment and communication devices
[b]Reference category

access to at least one device in the bedroom, and frequently using it was associated with an 82% increase in odds of obesity (OR = 1.82, 95% CI: 1.28, 2.59) (Table 8).

Amongst those with no bedroom EECD access, rarely reading during the hour before sleep (compared to frequently reading) increased the odds of being overweight by 42% (OR = 1.42, 95% CI: 1.20, 1.68) (Table 8). In addition, frequently reading with access to EECDs in the bedroom (compared to without) increased the odds of obesity by 35% (Table 8).

Total daily exposure to EECDs was statistically significantly associated with an increase in weight status ranging from 4% to 7% increase in the odds of being overweight and 24% to 28% increase in odds of being obese for all EECDs (Data not shown).

Discussion

In the present study, we found that for most EECDs, both their presence in the bedroom and their frequent use during the hour before sleep was negatively associated with sleep duration, good sleep quality and very good sleep efficiency and positively associated with weight status. As expected, the magnitude at which sleep and weight status was affected depended on the EECD in question, however, the TV, computer and cell phone were identified as common culprits. Rarely reading during the hour before sleep was associated with a decrease in sleep duration, sleep quality and sleep efficiency and an increase in the chance of being overweight. Having access to EECDs in the bedroom was associated with an increase in being obese even if children read frequently during the hour before sleep. Exposure to EECDs during the day also contributed to their effect on sleep and weight status when they were used in the bedroom during the hour before sleep.

Our findings support the American Academy of Pediatrics recommendation to remove EECDs from the bedroom to improve sleep amongst children [27]. The observed negative effect on sleep and weight status that the presence of EECDs and their use during the hour before sleep have, suggests that an interdependent relationship exists between EECD presence and use in the bedroom during the hour before sleep. This finding begs for restrictions to EECD use during the hour before sleep as well as their accessibility in the bedroom. Some may argue that the decrease in sleep duration associated with the use of EECDs an hour before sleep is modest. On the contrary, as little as 15 min difference in sleep duration has been shown to have clinical significance on mental, behavioral and daytime functioning [28]. Where multiple EECDs are used, this threshold of 15 min will be exceeded as demonstrated in a similar study [9]. Our findings also show an association of sleep and weight status with total exposure to EECDs during the day. Parents should therefore be encouraged to implement EECD limits on use during the daytime in addition to restrictions to bedroom accessibility and use during the hour before sleep. This should begin while their children are young so as to develop habits that can be continued through to the teenage and adult years.

The negative impact of EECDs when used in the bedroom during the hour before sleep may be related to the bright light emitted from many of these devices [16]. The backlight of many EECDs currently being manufactured emits diodes rich in blue light. Exposure to blue light close to bedtime suppresses the release of the sleep-facilitating hormone; melatonin, thereby delaying sleep onset, shortening total sleep duration and affecting good sleep quality [29, 30]. Exposure time needed to significantly suppress melatonin production may however, differ between products depending on their built-in ability to decrease brightness as well as filter out blue light [21]. In an experimental trial involving tablets, researchers found that after exposure to light from self-luminous Apple iPad® tablets for one hour, the tablets' built-in lighting did not suppress melatonin production significantly, and therefore, did not delay sleep onset. However, after a two-hour exposure to the same tablets, melatonin production was significantly suppressed, delaying sleep onset [21]. The effect of tablets on sleep latency observed in this trial is consistent with the effect of tablets on sleep duration and weight status observed in our study. We suspect that the duration of exposure (1 h or less) amongst children who used tablets before sleep was insufficient to significantly suppress melatonin production and to have a meaningful effect on sleep duration.

A number of cross-sectional studies have shown that EECDs affect sleep and weight status when accessible in the bedroom even if they are reportedly not used [31–34]. Similarly, in our study, a large number of EECDs investigated negatively affected sleep and weight status when accessible in the bedroom even if children reported these were not used during the hour before sleep. A possible reason for this maybe that the presence of EECDs in the bedroom is a mediator for use [35]. Therefore, we speculate that reporting bias regarding actual use of EECDs during the hour before sleep may exist which explains why sleep (duration, quality, and efficiency) as well as weight status was negatively affected when EECDs were accessible in the bedroom, though reportedly never used during the hour before sleep. These children may have used these devices but reported otherwise due to fear of their parents finding out. The positive effect that TV access in the bedroom had on very good sleep efficiency among students who never used it during the hour before sleep is notable. This is inconsistent with the effect that other screens investigated here have shown. Chaput et al. (2014) recently found that the presence of one screen in the bedroom does not lower sleep efficiency. Although number of screens in the bedroom was not investigated here, the presence of only the TV in the bedroom that was never used decreased any sleep interruptions and therefore increased very good sleep efficiency. As opposed to a TV, having access to a computer, tablet, video games and a cell phone though never used an hour before sleep negatively affected very good sleep efficiency. Cell phone access in the bedroom, even when not in use, has previously been shown to impact negatively on sleep by giving off alerts for incoming calls or messages [36]. By the same token, tablets may give off alerts even when not in use while computers and video games may continually flicker and make sounds that disturb sleep, particularly when left in stand-by mode.

The increase in weight status associated with the interdependent presence and use of EECDs during the hour before sleep is consistent with our previous study which reported that both presence of EECDs in the bedroom and their use at night were associated with lower diet quality, less physical activity and increased odds of being overweight or obese in a different sample of grade 5 students [9]. As expected, the use of EECDs at night displaces sleep thereby shortening sleep duration. Typically, short sleep duration impacts weight status by decreasing the production of leptin, an appetite-suppressing hormone, and increasing that of ghrelin, an appetite-stimulating hormone causing those using EECDs closer to bedtime to eat more [37, 38].

The potential for negative long-term impacts of EECD use at night, may indicate an urgency to address the use of EECDs before sleep. Nuutinen et al. (2013) reported that children who watched TV and used a computer in their bedroom had significantly shorter sleep duration and later bedtimes than their counterparts. Shorter sleep duration persisted 18 months later [31], suggesting long-term negative effects of EECD use in the bedroom. In fact, the World Health Organization has classified exposure to bright light after dark as a carcinogen after observations of increased incidence of cancers amongst night-shift workers [39–41]. Prolonged exposure to bright light after dark, such as what occurs among chronic night-users of EECDs, causes chronic suppression of melatonin.

In place of engaging in stimulating interactive activities with bright lights, we found that frequently reading a book during the hour before sleep without EECD access in the bedroom, is key to a longer sleep duration, good sleep quality, very good sleep efficiency, and normal weight status. A recent study showed that reading a printed book under reflected light has a significant positive impact on restorative sleep, morning alertness and the circadian cycle compared to reading a book from a light-emitting eReader [29]. Based on our results and other supporting literature [29, 30], we recommend that children should not have access EECDs in their bedroom, and should refrain from using EECDs during the hour before sleep. Instead, parents should encourage children to read a book, preferably printed and with dim lighting, during the hour before sleep. Parental rules to control chronic EECD use have been found to be effective [42], and may be applied in our population.

Our findings need to be interpreted within confines of a number of limitations. Firstly, as a cross sectional study, temporality, hence, causality cannot be determined. The relationship of the exposures (EECDs access and use) and the outcomes (sleep duration, sleep quality, sleep efficiency and weight status) may be bidirectional [43]. Secondly, all sleep measures are self-reported and based mainly on parental reports. Parental reports regarding sleep problems have been shown to disagree widely with reports from children, and are therefore prone to error [44]. Reports of children as young as 6 years old have been shown to be valid and add valuable information regarding medical history, behavior and health care [45]. Nonetheless, a more objective measure of sleep, such as that from actigraphy, may improve the validity of study findings. Thirdly, the sample, comprising exclusively of grade 5 elementary school children, is not representative of the general population limiting generalizability; however, this does not discredit any associations found. Lastly, the outcomes studied may have been associated with additional factors such as how long the children were exposed to EECDs during the hour before sleep. Such factors not investigated here could have resulted in residual confounding. Further experimental studies should be conducted to explore how EECD content, type of video games or various uses of cell phones (e.g. calling versus social media) affects sleep and weight status. Additionally, experimental studies on how best to prevent EECD use during the hour before sleep in an era of booming technology and promote reading a printed book instead are required. Despite these limitations, our study has several strengths. As a school-based survey, the response rate and resulting large sample size increased our study power. This is the first study, to our knowledge, to specifically focus on the use of a wide range of EECDs and distinguish between mere bedroom access and actual use within a specified time period before sleep, and how this impacts sleep and weight status. Finally, our study assessed the impact of reading a book on sleep duration, good sleep quality, very good sleep efficiency and weight status comparing and contrasting this with the use of various EECDs which adds to its novelty.

Conclusions

In conclusion, we have demonstrated that there may indeed be unappreciated effects of access to EECDs in the bedroom on sleep (duration, quality and efficiency) and weight status, more so, when EECDs are reportedly used during the hour before sleep. Our findings highlight the importance of ensuring that parents not only remove all EECDs from their children's bedroom but also discourage their use during the hour before sleep. Alternatively, children should be encouraged to read a book during the hour before sleep as this may improve sleep duration, sleep quality and sleep efficiency and decrease prevalence of overweight and obesity.

Abbreviations

BMI: Body Mass Index; CA$: Canadian dollars; EECD(s): Electronic entertainment and communication device(s); OR: Odds ratio; REAL Kids: Raising healthy Eating and Active Living Kids; TTIB: Total time in bed; TV(s): Television(s)

Acknowledgements

We would like to thank the reviewers who gave valuable feedback regarding this publication. We are grateful to all grade 5 children, parents, and schools for their participation in the study. We also thank the evaluation assistants and school health facilitators for their contribution during data collection. All interpretations and opinions in the current study are those of the authors. Part of the results from this research have been presented at the 15th Annual meeting of the International Society of Behavioral Nutrition and Physical Activity, Cape Town, South Africa, 8 – 11 June 2016.

Funding

The REAL Kids Alberta survey was funded through Alberta Health. The present analysis was funded through the Collaborative Research and Innovation Opportunities (CRIO) Team program from Alberta Innovates-Health Solutions. ND received a postdoctoral stipend through this CRIO program and through the Women and Children's Health Research Institute. PJV holds a Canada Research Chair in Population Health, an Alberta Research Chair in Nutrition and Disease Prevention, and an Alberta Innovates Health Scholarship. All interpretations and opinions in the present study are those of the authors.

Authors' contributions

Conceived and designed the study: ND MK PV. Analyzed the data: NM, MK. Wrote the paper: ND MK SL YC PV. All authors read and approved the final manuscript.

Competing interests

The authors declare that they have no competing interests.

Author details

[1]Department of Public Health Sciences, Population Health Intervention Research Unit, School of Public Health, University of Alberta, 3-50 University Terrace, 8303 112 Street, Edmonton, AB T6G 2T4, Canada. [2]Dalla Lana School of Public Health, University of Toronto, Toronto, ON, Canada. [3]Centre for Clinical Epidemiology and Evaluation, University of British Columbia, Vancouver, BC, Canada.

References

1. Foundation NS. How much sleep do we really need? 2016; https://sleepfoundation.org/how-sleep-works/how-much-sleep-do-we-really-need. Accessed 8 May 2016.
2. Corkum P, Tannock R, Moldofsky H. Sleep disturbances in children with attention-deficit/hyperactivity disorder. J Am Acad Child Adolesc Psychiatry. 1998;37(6):637–46.
3. Khan MKA, Chu YL, Kirk SFL, Veugelers PJ. Are sleep duration and sleep quality associated with diet quality, physical activity, and body weight status? A population-based study of Canadian children. Can J Public Health. 2015;106(5):E277–82.
4. Iglowstein I, Jenni OG, Molinari L, Largo RH. Sleep duration from infancy to adolescence: reference values and generational trends. Pediatrics. 2003; 111(2):302–7.
5. Hale L, Guan S. Screen time and sleep among school-aged children and adolescents: a systematic literature review. Sleep Med Rev. 2015;21:50–8.
6. Arora T, Broglia E, Thomas GN, Taheri S. Associations between specific technologies and adolescent sleep quantity, sleep quality, and parasomnias. Sleep Med. 2014;15(2):240–7.
7. Dworak M, Schierl T, Bruns T, Struder HK. Impact of singular excessive computer game and television exposure on sleep patterns and memory performance of school-aged children. Pediatrics. 2007;120(5):978–85.
8. Rideout V. Generation M2: Media in the Lives of 8- to 18-year-olds. Menlo Park, CA: Kaiser Family Foundation; 2010.
9. Chahal H, Fung C, Kuhle S, Veugelers PJ. Availability and night-time use of electronic entertainment and communication devices are associated with short sleep duration and obesity among Canadian children. Pediatr Obes. 2013;8(1):42–51.
10. Arora T, Hosseini-Araghi M, Bishop J, Yao GL, Thomas GN, Taheri S. The complexity of obesity in U.K. adolescents: relationships with quantity and type of technology, sleep duration and quality, academic performance and aspiration. Pediatr Obes. 2013;8(5):358–66.
11. Falbe J, Davison KK, Franckle RL, et al. Sleep duration, restfulness, and screens in the sleep environment. Pediatrics. 2015;135(2):e367–75.
12. Chen X, Beydoun MA, Wang Y. Is sleep duration associated with childhood obesity? A systematic review and meta-analysis. Obesity. 2008;16(2):265–74.
13. Nielsen LS, Danielsen KV, Sorensen TI. Short sleep duration as a possible cause of obesity: critical analysis of the epidemiological evidence. Obes Rev. 2011;12(2):78–92.
14. Wolfson AR, Carskadon MA. Understanding adolescents' sleep patterns and school performance: a critical appraisal. Sleep Med Rev. 2003;7(6): 491–506.
15. Vgontzas AN, Bixler EO, Chrousos GP. Metabolic disturbances in obesity versus sleep apnoea: the importance of visceral obesity and insulin resistance. J Intern Med. 2003;254(1):32–44.
16. Fossum IN, Nordnes LT, Storemark SS, Bjorvatn B, Pallesen S. The association between use of electronic media in bed before going to sleep and insomnia symptoms, daytime sleepiness, morningness, and chronotype. Behav Sleep Med. 2014;12(5):343–57.
17. Kuehni CE, Strippoli MP, Chauliac ES, Silverman M. Snoring in preschool children: prevalence, severity and risk factors. Eur Respir J. 2008;31(2):326–33.
18. Li S, Jin X, Yan C, Wu S, Jiang F, Shen X. Habitual snoring in school-aged children: environmental and biological predictors. Respir Res. 2010;11:144.
19. Spilsbury JC, Storfer-Isser A, Drotar D, et al. Sleep behavior in an urban US sample of school-aged children. Arch Pediatr Adolesc Med. 2004;158(10):988–94.
20. National Sleep Foundation. Health sleep tips. 2015; https://sleepfoundation.org/sleep-tools-tips/healthy-sleep-tips. Accessed 18 June 2015.
21. Wood B, Rea MS, Plitnick B, Figueiro MG. Light level and duration of exposure determine the impact of self-luminous tablets on melatonin suppression. Appl Ergon. 2013;44(2):237–40.
22. Fraught E. REAL Kids Alberta. 2015; http://www.realkidsalberta.ca. Accessed 25 May 2015.
23. Cole TJ, Lobstein T. Extended international (IOTF) body mass index cut-offs for thinness, overweight and obesity. Pediatr Obes. 2012;7(4):284–94.
24. de Onis M, Lobstein T. Defining obesity risk status in the general childhood population: which cut-offs should we use? Int J Pediatr Obes. 2010;5(6):458–60.
25. Rao JNK, Scott AJ. The analysis of categorical data from complex sample surveys: chi-squared tests for goodness of fit and independence in two-way tables. J Am Stat Assoc. 1981;76(374):10.
26. Rao JNK, Scott AJ. On chi-squared tests for multiway contingency tables with cell proportions estimated from survey data. Ann Stat. 1984;12(1):46–60.

27. American Academy of Pediatrics Council on Communications and Media. Children, adolescents, and the media. Pediatrics. 2013;132(1):958–61.
28. Chan NY, Zhang J, Yu MW, et al. Impact of a modest delay in school start time in Hong Kong school adolescents. Sleep Med. 2017;30:164–70.
29. Chang AM, Aeschbach D, Duffy JF, Czeisler CA. Evening use of light-emitting eReaders negatively affects sleep, circadian timing, and next-morning alertness. Proc Natl Acad Sci U S A. 2015;112(4):1232–7.
30. Van Gelder RN. A tablet that shifts the clock. Proc Natl Acad Sci U S A. 2015; 112(4):946–7.
31. Nuutinen T, Ray C, Roos E. Do computer use, TV viewing, and the presence of the media in the bedroom predict school-aged children's sleep habits in a longitudinal study? BMC Public Health. 2013;13:684.
32. Borghese MM, Tremblay MS, Katzmarzyk PT, et al. Mediating role of television time, diet patterns, physical activity and sleep duration in the association between television in the bedroom and adiposity in 10 year-old children. Int J Behav Nutr Phys Act. 2015;12:60.
33. Garmy P, Nyberg P, Jakobsson U. Sleep and television and computer habits of Swedish school-age children. J Sch Nurs. 2012;28(6):469–76.
34. Van den Bulck J. Television viewing, computer game playing, and internet use and self-reported time to bed and time out of bed in secondary-school children. Sleep. 2004;27(1):101–4.
35. Cameron AJ, van Stralen MM, Brug J, et al. Television in the bedroom and increased body weight: potential explanations for their relationship among European schoolchildren. Pediatr Obes. 2013;8(2):130–41.
36. National Sleep Foundation. 2014 sleep in America® poll sleep in the modern family: summary of findings. 2014; http://sleepfoundation.org/sites/default/files/2014-NSF-Sleep-in-America-poll-summary-of-findings—FINAL-Updated-3-26-14-.pdf. Accessed 23 June 2015.
37. Spiegel K, Tasali E, Penev P, Van Cauter E. Brief communication: sleep curtailment in healthy young men is associated with decreased leptin levels, elevated ghrelin levels, and increased hunger and appetite. Ann Intern Med. 2004;141(11):846–50.
38. Spiegel K, Leproult R, L'Hermite-Baleriaux M, Copinschi G, Penev PD, Van Cauter E. Leptin levels are dependent on sleep duration: relationships with sympathovagal balance, carbohydrate regulation, cortisol, and thyrotropin. J Clin Endocrinol Metab. 2004;89(11):5762–71.
39. Erren TC. Shift work, cancer and "white-box" epidemiology: association and causation. Epidemiol Perspect Innov. 2010;7:11.
40. Straif K, Baan R, Grosse Y, et al. Carcinogenicity of shift-work, painting, and fire-fighting. Lancet Oncol. 2007;8(12):1065–6.
41. Costa G, Haus E, Stevens R. Shift work and cancer - considerations on rationale, mechanisms, and epidemiology. Scand J Work Environ Health. 2010;36(2):163–79.
42. Pieters D, De Valck E, Vandekerckhove M, et al. Effects of pre-sleep media use on sleep/wake patterns and daytime functioning among adolescents: the moderating role of parental control. Behav Sleep Med. 2014;12(6):427–43.
43. Magee CA, Lee JK, Vella SA. Bidirectional relationships between sleep duration and screen time in early childhood. JAMA Pediatr. 2014;168(5):465–70.
44. Fatima Y, Doi SA, O'Callaghan M, Williams G, Najman JM, Mamun AA. Parent and adolescent reports in assessing adolescent sleep problems: results from a large population study. Acta Paediatr. 2016;105(9):e433–9.
45. Riley AW. Evidence that school-age children can self-report on their health. Ambul Pediatr. 2004;4(4 Suppl):371–6.

11

Perceptions of overweight by primary carers (mothers/grandmothers) of under five and elementary school-aged children in Bandung, Indonesia: a qualitative study

Cut Novianti Rachmi[1*], Cynthia Louise Hunter[2,3], Mu Li[3] and Louise Alison Baur[1,3]

Abstract

Background: The prevalence of childhood overweight has increased in the past two decades in Indonesia. Even though prevalence is escalating, there is a lack of qualitative evidence to assist in the design and implementation of strategies to tackle this issue. This study aimed to explore the view of primary carers (mothers and grandmothers) from different socio-economic-status groups, on childhood overweight in the Greater Bandung Area, Indonesia.

Methods: We conducted 12 focus groups discussions with a total of 94 carers of under-five and 7–12 years children, from June to October 2016. We used the grounded theory approach in our analysis.

Results: Three main categories emerged: the concept of overweight, factors contributing to overweight, and awareness and feelings towards overweight children. Most carers from all SES groups defined overweight subjectively, while a few from the low SES group defined it objectively. Most carers from low and high SES groups agreed with the concept "chubbier is healthier". All carers had some knowledge of the main factors that contribute to childhood overweight: dietary factors, activity levels and sedentary behavior, and hereditary factors. Carers from all SES groups described similar characteristics of overweight; carers from low and intermediate SES groups had mixed feelings while all high SES carers have negative feelings about overweight children, mostly related to stigma. However, carers who identified their own children as being overweight expressed sensitivity about this weight status, especially their physical abilities. Almost all carers knew their children's current weight while less than two thirds knew their children's height.

Conclusions: There are several policy implications. Firstly, health-related knowledge of the primary carers is of great importance and needs augmenting. To increase that knowledge, there is a role for front-line health practitioners (doctors/midwives/nurses) to be more active in educating the community. Secondly, simpler and more effective ways to disseminate healthy lifestyle messages to carers is required. Thirdly, by placing more emphasis on carers monitoring their children's growth may encourage carers to take steps to keep their children in the healthy weight and height ranges. Fourthly, the Department of Education may need to improve the quality and quantity of physical activity in schools.

Keywords: Overweight, Children, Perceptions, Mothers, Indonesia, Qualitative

* Correspondence: Crac8243@uni.sydney.edu.au; cutnovianti@gmail.com
[1]Discipline of Child & Adolescent Health, The Children's Hospital at Westmead, University of Sydney Clinical School, Locked Bag 4001, Westmead, NSW 2145, Australia
Full list of author information is available at the end of the article

Background

Overweight/ obesity in both children and adults, while initially an issue mainly in western countries, is now a major emerging health problem in countries undergoing economic transition – including Indonesia [1, 2]. Indonesia, the world's fourth most populous country, has been dealing with the problem of children's undernutrition, including stunting and underweight for decades, as a consequence of which many nutrition policies and programs were focused on addressing these issues [3]. Overweight, on the other hand, has only been recognised as an Indonesian health problem for little more than a decade [2, 3].

The prevalence of childhood overweight in Indonesia has significantly increased in the last 20 years, with higher prevalence rates found among boys in general and boys and girls living in urban areas [2]. To our knowledge, qualitative evidence about overweight in Indonesia is scarce, with the available evidence mainly focused on mothers with overweight children, [4] and none considering the views of people from different socio-economic groups.

Parents, particularly mothers, hold an important role in child feeding, role modelling for healthy eating and active living, and the prevention of overweight [5–11]. Many potential strategies in tackling overweight will involve working with families, especially the primary carers of young children. These strategies will benefit from an understanding of the knowledge, attitudes, and behaviours of the primary carers. Thus, this study aimed to explore the perceptions of Indonesian mothers and grandmothers from different socio-economic groups towards child overweight/ obesity and related issues. In the Indonesian language, people refer to overweight/ obesity with the same word, *kegemukan*, except those in the health sector/ academics. Hereafter, we will refer to overweight/ obesity as overweight.

Methods

Study design and location

We undertook a qualitative study in Bandung, West Java, Indonesia. West Java Province consists of 27 cities/regencies and we selected three cities/regencies (Bandung City, Bandung Regency, and Bandung Barat Regency) based on high population numbers and mixed ethnic groups, to explore the situation in Indonesia [12]. Every district in each city/regency was numbered and we chose the selected areas based on the last digit from a table of random numbers. These three areas have different Human Development Index scores (high, medium, and low); these were used as a measure of different levels of socioeconomic status [12]. The locations of the selected areas (Cisarua, Margahayu, and Sukasari districts) represent the low, intermediate, and high socio-economic status areas, respectively.

The rationale for selecting areas of different SES was to obtain a diversity of views of mothers/grandmothers towards children's growth, development and overweight and to observe whether SES is a contributing factor to overweight. Hereafter, we will refer to mothers/grandmothers as carers.

Participants and recruitment process

Twelve focus group discussions (FGDs) were conducted, six with carers of under five children and six with carers of elementary-school-aged children (7–12 years),[1] from June to October 2016 (Fig. 1). Inclusion criteria were carers of children who hold or share the primary role in decision-making for the care of the child or were responsible, in part or in whole, for child feeding and eating, including food shopping and budgeting.

To recruit participants from low and intermediate SES areas, we contacted Community Health Centres (*Puskesmas*) in the chosen areas to reach carers of under five children. We collaborated with local midwives and health *kader* (mothers who are trained and work for the *Puskesmas* and Community Health Posts [*Posyandu*] for a small incentive). These *kader* have knowledge of the people living in the communities [13]. We provided a verbal explanation of the project, and disseminated the participant information statement to invite participation. To recruit carers of 7–12 years children, we asked for assistance from class coordinators in public elementary schools (a mother from each grade in elementary school who acts as the information source for fellow mothers). We also placed project information including contact details in students' communication books (book that teachers use to communicate with mothers of individual children).

Recruitment of participants from high SES groups was by invitation to local private schools and paediatricians' offices. In Indonesia, children from socially advantaged families do not go to *Puskesmas*, but to private medical practices or specialists, and they attend private schools. We used the same approach in each school (i.e. contacting the class coordinator), and asked the nurse in the paediatrician's office to assist us in providing information about and contact details for the study to the carers.

Interested carers then directly contacted the research team who gave further explanation about the discussion process and took details. Carers who gave verbal consent to participate were later approached to set the date and time for the FGD.

Research team, data collection and approach to analysis

The field research team consisted of the first author (CNR) and two research assistants (DMP and TMF). They

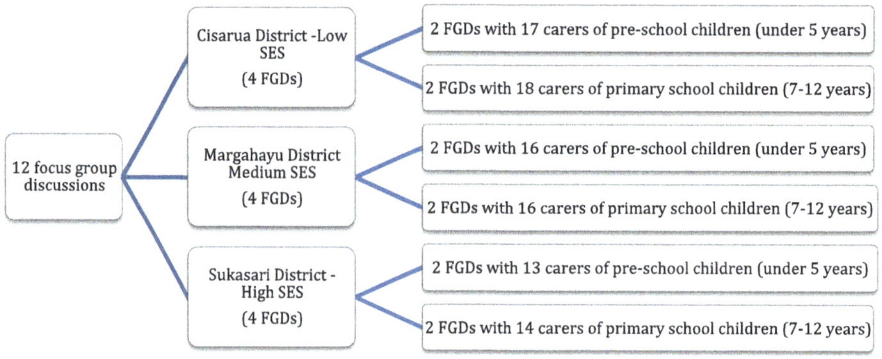

Fig. 1 Numbers and participants of focus group discussions in Bandung, Indonesia. SES: socio economic status; Low SES: FGDs 5, 6, 7, and 8; Intermediate SES: FGDs 3, 4, 7, and 8; High SES: FGDs 1, 2, 11, and 12

underwent a three-day training program in qualitative research, concentrating on FGDs, with CLH in Bandung. Question guidelines were developed in English and finalised during the training. Afterwards, the guidelines were translated into the Indonesian and Sundanese languages and a pilot FGD was conducted to test the questions guidelines (Table 1). This process included a discussion of potential issues and possible resolutions that might be encountered during the FGDs.

CNR acted as a moderator in all of the FGDs, with two research assistants (DMP and TMF) observing and managing the recordings and time keeping. Prior to each FGD, the study team explained the FGD process to the participants and asked them to fill in the basic demographic information form and provide written informed consent. Participants were offered the language of their choice to be used during the FGDs, either Indonesian or Sundanese (the language of West Java), in which all three moderators were fluent. Each FGD began with a 30-min ice-breaker, to build rapport between participants and researchers. We highlighted how much everyone's opinion was valued and encouraged the participants to speak freely. Similarly, and to ensure confidentiality, we did not videotape the discussion. To ensure consistency of the discussion the moderator used the same guideline, including a set of prompt questions. All discussions were digitally recorded, and lasted 50–90 min. Group size ranged from 6 to 9 people. Participants each received 11 USD for participation.

Transcription and translation started immediately after the first FGD, giving the team some time to reflect on the discussion results. Transcription was done only in Indonesian by DMP and TMF and checked by CNR to confirm that the transcripts were verbatim to the recordings. The research assistants then translated the transcripts into English; both Indonesian and English transcripts were checked by CLH and CNR to ensure the quality of the translation. Sundanese or Indonesian terms that have no exact English translation were kept and explained in English inside parentheses next to those terms.

We used the grounded theory approach in our analysis [14–16]. All transcripts were analysed using NVivo for Mac version 11.0.0 [17]. The research assistants were not involved in the analysis phase. The analysis was conducted following the steps: 1) CNR and CLH read all transcripts several times to familiarise themselves with the data. 2) CNR undertook the open coding and compared the coding within and between transcripts. 3) CNR and CLH identified categories and sub-categories of ideas/concepts. 4) Once the final version of categories and subcategories was agreed upon, a final combination of subcategories took place. 5) CNR and CLH identified similarities and differences between and within the different SES groups. 6) The quotations that best represented each category and subcategory were identified. As part of the analysis, CNR quantified comments throughout the transcripts looking at responses from individual carers. Quotations representing each SES grouping were selected from multiple FGD groups. 7) All authors (CNR, CLH, ML, and LAB) agreed upon the final version of the categories and subcategories. LAB and ML, experts in childhood obesity and childhood nutrition, were significantly involved in the design phase of the research and writing up of the manuscript.

Credibility and trustworthiness

Credibility and trustworthiness were addressed in several ways. One researcher (CNR) was the moderator of all 12 FGDs and could, therefore, describe the situation and convey the opinions stated directly (words) or indirectly (intonation of voice or facial expressions) consistently. We reduced interpretive bias by involving another analyst (CLH) who was not present during the data collection. CNR also conducted triangulation with the two research assistants and used the notes made during the

Table 1 Questions used in focus group discussions in Greater Bandung Area, Indonesia

No	Questions (English)	Indonesian	Sundanese
1	There is quite a lot of talk around these days about being obese or being overweight in both adults and in children and babies - can you tell me what you think this means? When I say overweight/obesity, what is the first thing that comes in your mind? In your opinion, which celebrities have the ideal body?	*Akhir-akhir ini banyak pembicaraan tentang terlalu gemuk pada anak dan dewasa, termasuk bayi, menurut ibu, apa arti terlalu gemuk? Ketika saya mengatakan terlalu gemuk, apa hal pertama yang ibu pikirkan? Menurut ibu, artis yang berat badannnya ideal siapa?*	*Jaman ayeuna seuer pisan pacariosan tentang bayi, barudak sareng dewasa anu parawakanna ageung teuing, menurut ibu, kumaha artina ari parawakanna ageung teuing teh? Upami abdi nyarios parawakan anu ageung teuing, naon hal pertama anu ibu pikirkeun? Menurut ibu, saha artis anu parawakanna ideal?*
2	In your opinion, when can you say a baby/ child is overweight/obese? Prompts: e.g. they have multiple chins, they wear clothes several sizes bigger than their age, they have trouble learning how to walk/ run, they eat adult size portion of food	*Menurut ibu, kapan seorang bayi/anak bisa dibilang terlalu gemuk?* *Bantuan:* • *Mukanya (dagu berlipat)* • *Ukuran baju* • *Terlambat belajar berjalan/lari (bayi)* • *Makan banyak seperti orang dewasa*	*Menurut ibu, iraha bayi/barudak teh disebat parawakanna ageung teuing?* *Bantuan:* • *Rarayna (dagu berlipat)* • *Ukuran bajuna* • *Telat diajar jalan/lumpat(bayi)* • *Tuangna siga jalmi dewasa*
3	What do you think of the saying 'chubbier is healthier'? What do you think about the relationship between body weight and health?	*Apa pendapat ibu tentang ungkapan "lebih gemuk lebih sehat"? Bagaimana pendapat ibu tentang hubungan berat badan dengan kesehatan?*	*Kumaha pendapat ibu tentang paribasa "langkung ageung langkung sehat"? Kumaha pendapat ibu tentang hubungan abot badan sareng kasihatan?*
4	What factors do you think contribute/ influence to a baby/ child's weight? Prompts: Is it dietary? Mention the following only if they are not mentioned: genetic, family eating patterns, physical activity, screen time (length of time spends in front of a screen – TV, computers, iPad, video games, reading, phone/games, playing cards, board games, etc), sleep, other activities (soccer, kite flying, hide and seek, hop scotch, jump rope, other outside activities: buying something at store)? In your knowledge, what do your children usually have as snacks? Prompts: • Soda • Instant noodles How do you feel about your children's snacks choices?	*Menurut ibu, hal apa saja yang mempengaruhi berat badan bayi/anak?* *Bantuan: Apakah makanan?* *Sebut hal berikut hanya bila hal-hal ini tidak disinggung: turunan/ bawaan (genetik), pola makan keluarga, kegiatan fisik, waktu layar (waktu yang dihabiskan di depan layar - TV, komputer, iPad, permainan video, membaca, telefon/ permainan, bermain kartu, permainan lainnya), tidur, kegiatan lainnya (main bola, layangan, petak umpet, engkle, lompat tali, kegiatan lain di luar rumah: belanja ke warung)?* *Sepengetahuan ibu, apa yang dimakan anak ibu sebagai cemilan?* *Bantuan:* • *Soda* • *Mie instan* *Bagaimana perasaan ibu tentang pilihan cemilan anak ibu?*	*Menurut ibu, naon wae anu ngaruh kana berat badan bayi/anak?* *Bantuan: Apakah makanan?* *Sebut hal berikut hanya bila hal-hal ini tidak disinggung: turunan/ bawaan (genetik), pola makan keluarga, kegiatan fisik, waktu layar (waktu yang dihabiskan di depan layar - TV, komputer, iPad, permainan video, membaca, telefon/ permainan, bermain kartu, permainan lainnya), tidur, kegiatan lainnya (main bola, layangan, petak umpet, engkle, lompat tali, kegiatan lain di luar rumah: belanja ke warung)?* *Sapengetahuan ibu, naon wae cemilan anu dituang ku anak ibu?* *Bantuan:* • *Soda* • *Mie instan* *Kumaha perasaan ibu tentang pilihan cemilan anak ibu?*
5	How much do you expect your baby to weigh at birth? About how much do you think a healthy baby should weigh by 6 months and by age 12 months?	*Menurut ibu berapa berat badan bayi yang diharapkan saat lahir? Menurut ibu berapa seharusnya berat badan bayi saat usia 6 bulan dan 1 tahun?*	*Menurut ibu, sabaraha abot bayi anu diharapkeun pas lahir? Menurut ibu, sabaraha kedahna abot bayi pas usia 6 sasih sareng sataun?*
6	Can you tell me how much your child weighs and his/her height now?	*Apakah ibu tahu berapa berat badan dan tinggi badan anak ibu sekarang?*	*Kinten-kintena ibu terang teu sabaraha abot sareng tinggi anak ibu ayeuna?*
7	Are you satisfied with your child's growth up to this point? If there is anything you would like to change about your child's weight, what would it be?	*Apakah ibu puas dengan pertumbuhan anak ibu sampai saat ini? Kalau ada hal yang ingin diubah mengenai berat badan anak ibu, kira-kira hal apa?*	*Apa ibu puas sareng pertumbuhan anak ibu dugika ayeuna? Upaya aya hal anu bade diubah soal berat badan anak ibu, naon anu bade diubah?*
8	Who do you think plays an important role in influencing your child's weight in the house? Prompts: • Who is responsible in determining the kind of food the child consume? • Who feed the child?	*Ibu, kalau di rumah siapa yang berperan dalam pertumbuhan anak ibu?* *Bantuan:* • *Siapa yang menentukan jenis makanan anak?* • *Siapa yang memberikan makanan anak?*	*Ibu, upami di bumi saha anu berperan dina pertumbuhan anak ibu?* *Bantuan:* • *Saha anu nangtoskeun jenis makanan anak?* • *Saha anu masihan makanan anak?*
9	Have you ever had any discussions regarding your baby/ child's growth? If yes, what is the discussion about? Prompts: For example if you think he/ she is the tallest/ biggest one in the class/ neighbourhood? With who do you usually have the discussion with? Prompts: • Husband	*Apakah ibu pernah berdiskusi tentang pertumbuhan anak ibu?* *Mengenai apa?* *Bantuan: Misalnya apakah menurut ibu anak ibu yang paling tinggi/ besar di kelas/ lingkungan.* *Dengan siapa?* *Bantuan:* • *Suami* • *Mertua*	*Apa ibu pernah diskusi tentang pertumbuhan anak ibu?* *Diskusina tentang apa?* *Bantuan: Misalnya apa menurut ibu anak ibu nu pang tinggi/ besarna di kelas/ lingkunganna.* *Sareng saha?* *Bantuan:* • *Suami* • *Mertua* • *Kader*

Table 1 Questions used in focus group discussions in Greater Bandung Area, Indonesia *(Continued)*

	• In laws • Posyandu (health post) *kader* • *Doctor* • *Neighbours*	• *Kader posyandu* • *Dokter* • *Tetangga*	• *Dokter* • *Tatanggi*
10	What do you think when you see children who appear overweight/obese? Can you elaborate more on that?	*Apa yang ibu pikirkan ketika melihat anak yang menurut ibu terlalu gemuk? Tolong jelaskan!*	*Naon anu ibu pikirkeun upami ningali anak anu menurut ibu parawakanna ageung teuing? Tiasa dijelaskeun bu.!*

FGDs to ensure the nuances captured during the discussions were agreed upon by three facilitators.

Results

Characteristics of participants

A total of 94 carers gave their consent and participated in the FGDs. We had similar numbers of carers in the under 5 years and elementary groups. Most carers from the low and intermediate SES groups had graduated either from elementary or middle and high school, but none from university. In contrast, most carers from the high SES groups were university graduates with only a few having middle and high school qualifications alone. We had more mothers compared to grandmothers in all three SES groups (Table 2). We had carers from 11 different ethnicities; however, we did not find that ethnicity played a part in the differences in the discussions.

Emerging categories

Emerging categories are shown in Table 3. There were several marked differences between the three SES groups involved. Although we expected differences would arise from carers of children under 5 years old and carers of elementary school children within the same SES group, such differences were not found.

Concepts of overweight

This broad category portrays carers' opinions around the concepts of overweight in children, "chubbier is healthier" and the ideal adult body, including their expectations of normal weight ranges at certain ages. Relevant excerpts from the transcripts are presented in Table 4.

How carers define overweight

Most (23 out of 27) carers in the high SES category defined overweight subjectively, for example through visual interpretation of body size. The researchers did not provide any particular definition of overweight nor differentiate between overweight and obesity at the beginning of our discussions, since most Indonesians use the same word, *kegemukan*. One carer stated that in her opinion the two terms are the same. Few (4/27) high SES carers defined it in a more objective way (i.e. based on specific measurements).

In contrast, although the same subjective pattern was seen in the low SES groups (32/35), three carers defined overweight objectively, based on Kartu Menuju Sehat (KMS – Health Card). KMS is a card used since the 1970s in Indonesia (Additional file 1). In 2010, the Indonesian Ministry of Health released a regulation to use this card for children aged under 5. The purpose of the KMS is to monitor children's growth, to record children's immunisation history, health services usage, and a tool to educate the community [18].

All carers (32/32) from the intermediate SES groups defined overweight in a subjective way. A few (3/32) described overweight differently.

Normal birthweight range

Carers from different SES groups had similar expectations for a baby's birthweight. Carers from high SES groups expected their children to be heavier at age 6 months and 1 year, compared to the other two groups.

"chubbier is healthier"

One third (12/35) of carers from the low SES groups agreed and two thirds (23/35) disagreed with the term "chubbier is healthier". They mentioned the concept of healthy overweight as an overweight baby/child who is still very active and is developmentally normal.

All carers (32/32) from the intermediate SES groups were against the concept of "chubbier is healthier". They specifically differentiated between cuteness and health status in overweight children. However, they also included the concept of healthy overweight.

One fourth (7/27) of the high SES carers agreed with "chubbier is healthier", while the rest (20/27) disagreed, highlighting past experiences of dealing with the overweight status of their children.

Ideal body

Carers from all three SES groups referred to Indonesian media celebrities they considered had ideal bodies. The ideal body was described as tall, slim, skinny, or model-like in women and a well-muscled body in men. However, it was difficult to name child celebrities they felt had an ideal body.

Table 2 Characteristics of participants from 12 focus group discussions in Greater Bandung Area, Indonesia

	Low SES (groups 5, 6, 7, 8)	Intermediate SES (groups 3, 4, 9, 10)	High SES (groups 1, 2, 11, 12)
Number of participants			
Total	35	32	27
Under five	17 (48.6%)	16 (50.0%)	13 (48.1%)
Elementary	18 (51.4%)	16 (50.0%)	14 (51.9%)
Education			
Elementary or less	16 (45.7%)	11 (34.4%)	0
Middle & High School	16 (45.7%)	19 (59.4%)	3 (11.1%)
Diploma	3 (8.6%)	2 (6.2%)	6 (22.2%)
University or higher	0	0	18 (66.7%)
Distribution of participants			
Mothers	31	23 (71.9%)	25 (92.6%)
Grandmothers	4	9 (28.1%)	2 (7.4%)
Number of children at home			
Two or less	24 (68.6%)	16 (50.0%)	17 (63.0%)
More than two	11 (31.4%)	16 (50.0%)	10 (37.0%)
Ethnicities	5 (Sunda, Jawa, Padang, Batak, Bali)	5 (Sunda, Jawa, Betawi, Minahasa, Aceh)	7 (Sunda, Jawa, Riau, Dayak, Batak, Betawi, Bugis)

SES socio economic status

Factors contributing to overweight

This category represents carers' views on what they considered were the three main factors contributing to overweight: dietary factors, physical activity and sedentary behaviours, and heredity (Table 5).

Table 3 Category and subcategories on the perception of overweight in carers in Greater Bandung Area, Indonesia

Category	Subcategory
1. Concept of overweight	1.1 How carers define overweight
	1.2 Normal weight range
	1.3 Chubbier is healthier
	1.4 Ideal body shape
2. Factors contributing to overweight	2.1 Dietary factors
	2.2 Activity levels and sedentary behaviour in children
	2.3 Heredity
3. Awareness and feelings towards overweight in children	3.1 Characteristics of overweight
	3.2 Food portion size in overweight children
	3.3 Eating frequency in overweight children
	3.4 Feelings about overweight children
	3.5 Sensitivity in carers of own overweight children
	3.6 Children's current weight and height

Dietary factors

Carers from all SES groups stated that there was a range of dietary factors contributing to overweight such as excessive sugar consumption, unhealthy snacks, certain types of food, big portions, frequent eating, and parental eating/snacking habits.

Intermediate and high SES groups commented upon vitamin supplements, milk, cooking oil, and mealtimes (especially dinner). Diets high in carbohydrate (rice or noodles) were also a factor.

Rice is Indonesia's staple food. All SES groups considered rice as a "must have", everyday food. One mother (high SES group) admitted that it is part of their identity as an Indonesian.

It seems that what the family will cook/eat depended heavily on what the children requested, because if the carers did not fulfill the children's wishes the children's behaviour may become difficult, for example by being cranky or do not want to eat anything through out the day. Most carers (25/32) from intermediate SES groups admitted that their children were heavily influenced by TV food commercials.

Low and intermediate SES carers in particular mentioned that the ideal menu should consist of *empat sehat lima sempurna* (Four Healthy, Five Perfect – an Indonesian ideal meal incorporating carbohydrates, proteins, vegetables, fruits, and milk). This concept, introduced by the Indonesian government in 1952, is now considered dated because it only gives information about variety of food without considering quantity [19]. In 1995 the government

Table 4 Quotes on concept of overweight according to carers from Bandung, Indonesia

	Low SES (FGD 5, 6, 7, 8)	Intermediate SES (FGD 3, 4, 7, 8)	High SES (FGD 1, 2, 11, 12)
How carers define overweight	• P1: Too much fat. • P3: Big body. • P4: Posture not appropriate with height and age range. • P8: Weight exceeds normal range based on age, based on the chart in KMS-Kartu Menuju Sehat (Health Card)	• P2: Excessive fat. • P5: Body weighs more than it should be. • P7: Around here it means you are healthy. • P6: In here it means you are happy.	• P1: Weight and height not balanced/ proportional. • P4: (Someone who has a) big body. • P8: Excessive weight. • P7: Obesity is the same with overweight. • P8: Weight is more than standard; I know there's a way to measure it.
Normal weight range	• Birth: 2.5–3.5 kg • 6 months: 5–9 kg • 1 year: 9–12 kg	• Birth: 2.8–3.5 kg • 6 months: 6–8 kg • 1 year: 7–11 kg	• Birth: 2.5–3.5 kg • 6 months: 8–10 kg • 1 year: 8–13 kg
Chubbier is healthier	• P5: I personally don't know what measurements would count as obese, what obesity is. But according to my knowledge... I agree with "the chubbier, the healthier". Being chubby is healthy. That's what I think. • P4: But, if it's me, Doc, I want to have a fat child. Who doesn't want a fat child, right? Fat and healthy, they're so nice to look at. • 1P2: If you mean a healthy fat, well... then that is okay, maybe. But... if it's unhealthy fat, it means they have too much. • P5: Cholesterols. • P7: I want a child who is fat and healthy.. it would be better.. uh, I want it to be that way.	• P4: I think it's cute, but definitely not healthier. • P8: (They have) lots of diseases. • P3: If they're too fat, they are often sick and that's not good. • P1: Well, there are fat people who are healthy and unhealthy. • P7: I think I agree with chubbier is healthier, if it's in toddlers. And also in babies, I think	• P3: Umm... When she was 6 months old, the doctor said she was obese. So yeah, she was fat, chubby. At the beginning I thought she was cute. But when the doctor said she was obese, it frightened me. • P2: My child often got an asthma attack when she was fat. • P6: It's (chubbier is healthier) not true. • P7: The child can be big, but actually, the child is not healthy.
Ideal body shape	• P6: Luna Maya (famous model and movie star in Indonesia). • P7: Krisdayanti (famous singer in Indonesia), she still has a nice body even though she has children. • P8: Ideally, approximately 40 kg. • P3: Being ideal is about having nice height, too. P2:Steven William (half Indonesian, half English movie star). • P6: Like a model, hahaha.		

introduced new guidelines *Pedoman Umum Gizi Seimbang* (PUGS - Balanced Nutrition Guidelines) that contain information on both food variety and portion size along with the importance of exercise and water consumption [19, 20]. None of the carers mentioned PUGS.

Activity levels and sedentary behaviours in children

All elementary schools in Indonesia have a mandatory 2 h physical education class per week. This was considered not enough by all low and intermediate SES carers, who said children should engage in more physical activity. Carers stated that boys spent their time in PE class by playing soccer and girls by having aerobic activities. They also mentioned the 2 h includes time to change clothes and sometimes time to walk to the nearby sports field (low and intermediate SES), leaving only 45–60 min for playing sports. All children in the low SES groups went to public schools (free of any charge), while children in intermediate SES groups went to public schools or Islamic schools (madrasah; some fee payment required but not as expensive as private schools). Public kindergartens start at 7.30 am and end at 9.30 am, 1st-3rd grades of elementary schools start at 7.00 am and end at 10.00 am, while 4th–6th grades start at 7.00 am and end at 12.00 pm. Children from low and intermediate SES groups spent their time after school playing outside although they also had screen time (watching TV at night). These families usually had "physical activity time" once a week such as hiking the mountains, running, and family sports time. In many low and intermediate SES areas in Indonesia children must spend time (from 5 pm–6.30 pm) in Quran recitation class every day at the mosque.

In contrast, children from high SES groups spent most of their after school time indoors at home. In addition to the school physical education class, there were extracurricular activities such as dancing, martial arts, and soccer. Eight (8/27) carers thought that, ideally, children should have more (maybe around 3 h) physical activities outside school every day because the activities at school are not enough. Half (13/27) of the carers stated children do not need extra activity outside school because they are moving around the house anyway - they have bigger houses. All children in these groups went to private schools. Classes in private schools start at 7 am and finish at 11.30 am for kindergarten, 1.30 pm for 1st and 2nd grade of elementary school, and 3.30 pm for 3rd-6th graders. Most children had other extracurricular activities e.g. piano class, math class, swimming class. These arrangements resulted in children arriving home at 6 pm or even 6.30 pm, when they usually had dinner, watched TV or played with their tablets and then went to sleep.

Table 5 Quotes on factors contributing to weight according to carers from Bandung, Indonesia

	Low SES	Intermediate SES	High SES
Dietary factors	• P1: It's mainly caused by one's dietary habit that is too... where one does not have appropriate portions. Also, frequent eating can cause obesity. • P4: It could be that, Ma'am, aa, obesity comes from eating too many sugary foods, excessive sugar consumption. Or it could be from the snacks, Ma'am; they're not very healthy. • P7: Even if he has eaten two packs of noodles, if he has not eaten rice, he'll consider it as if he hasn't eaten yet.	• P2: They eat too much P5: It has to be empat sehat lima sempurna (Four Healthy, Five Perfect – an Indonesian ideal meal incorporating carbohydrates, proteins, vegetables, fruits, and milk). • P2: Like when you sleep right after you eat, lack of exercise, eating snacks… these things make you bigger. • P9: Aa, they eat a bowl of noodle and a plateful of rice. M: So, noodles and rice. How often do they eat that, Ma'am? P9: Aa, sometimes they eat those twice a day. P5: Noodle can also cause obesity. • P7: Initially, A (name) drank too many sugary drinks like... something like Teh Gelas (sugary drinks brand). So he became obese.	• P1: We are Indonesians, we have to eat rice. • P7: She has a big appetite, drinks a lot of milk, and her father is also fat. Could that be a factor? • P2: I rarely consume noodles now, when I do, I only put half of the MSG. Hahaha. • P6: So you add salt to it? • P2: Aa, nope, I add eggs and mix them with butter, so it has the right amount of saltiness from the butter. • P6: But that's where the fat come from (the butter). • P4: It can be the quantity of the milk.P5: It can be how much the children drink the milk. • P3: Maybe it's because they drink a lot of milk. • P4: For example, he drinks brand A, although he only drinks a little, but the composition is different. Maybe one of the compositions stimulates the appetite.
Activity levels and sedentary behaviours in children	• P1: After they eat, they're just sitting down, watching TV. So that, aa, there is no chance for them to burn the calories. That might have caused (the person to be). • P7: Fat. • P2: He is out somewhere to play (right after he came home from school). Changes his uniform, then goes straight outside to play. • P3: After school my daughter usually have her lunch, then….. Then after lunch, that's in... in the afternoon, aa, she is joining Qur'an (Moslem's holy book) recitation. • P7: Maybe, being fat is caused by lack of...maybe lack of activities? • P8: They fly kites. • P5: They just run around. • P8: They ride bicycles, Doc. • P7: Right, bicycles.	• P6: Lifestyle. M: What kind of lifestyle? P6: One that lacks exercise. • P8: My child can't stand staying at home, so he plays outside. • M: What do you think about the physical education class at school? • P6: It's not long enough. • P4: Right, it's not enough. • P3: They mostly play outside, of course.P5: Yeah, outdoors. • P8: He reads Qur'an in the evening. • P5: He reads the Qur'an, ma'am. • P3: My child reads the Qur'an in the evening and afterwards he plays for a while M: Outside or inside the house? • P3: He plays outside.	• P4: Video games. • P5: This (imitates someone playing video games) isn't being active. • All: Hahaha • P4: Because, the children can, umm, even if they don't go outside, they can do the activities at home.P3: They can play around the house, moving here and there, right? P4: Yes. They can go up and down. P5: On the stairs, right? • P2: For my son of course it's inside. • P3: Heeh, he arrived in the afternoon, and then go straight to his math course. And then it's Maghrib (praying times-6 pm) when he came home; he only spends some time outside the house on Saturdays and Sundays, and that doesn't happen a lot either. • P2: Yeah, same here. Even on Saturdays and Sundays he doesn't spend much time outside.
Heredity	• P1: Those who have inherited it from.... • P6: From the parents. • P3: Being large is in my family's blood • P8: But he inherits it from his father. His father is also fat. • P2: That's when an excessive diet is not balanced by exercise, which was mentioned earlier. Heredity is a factor that can play into this, too, right? Like genes? Right? • P9: People in the village always think like this, it's normal if the children are fat because the father is also fat, just like that.	• P8: There's the heredity factor. • P3: Yes, it's inherited. • P5: That's why the children become fat. • P7: If the parents were fat, the children would also be fat. • P1: Heredity. • P2: It can be inherited. • P4: Fatness can be inherited.	• P2: It's inherited. I am one of the big families. Yeah, my husband and I, we're big and tall people. • P7: Several diseases are heredity like cancer, asthma, but not overweight. • P8: The shape and size of the body is probably not affected by heredity. • P6: It might be both. Maybe, the fat people already has a heredity factor and then… • P5: It's worsened by wrong dietary habit. • P6: The heredity, maybe, heredity factor? • P4: Do you mean genetic factor? • P6: So, their bones are naturally big. • P5: Yes, since they were little, it's already big.

Heredity

Carers from low and intermediate SES groups had a similar understanding of heredity i.e. overweight is simply what has been going on in their family for several generations. Carers from high SES groups elaborated further on the concept of heredity based on their personal observation of their children/nephews. A few (5/27) from high SES groups thought that heredity is *not* a factor that contributes to overweight.

Awareness and feelings towards overweight in children

Relevant excerpts for this category are available in Table 6.

Characteristics of overweight

All SES groups mentioned similar characteristics: physical appearance ("bulging belly", head circumference, "stomach folds", plump cheeks, "hulk like", "big butt", no neck), size of their clothes, difficulty in movements, tiring easily, panting breath, and having a lower IQ level. Intermediate and high SES carers added that overweight children get sick more often compared to their healthy weight counterparts.

Food portions in overweight children

All carers stated that overweight children eat bigger portions compared to healthy weight children, admitting that sometimes their children eat the same portion of food as their parents. One mother (low SES group) stated that as one of her efforts to reduce her child's weight, she gave her smaller portions, different from the recommended serving size on the box of instant food.

Eating frequency in overweight children

Carers from the low SES groups were aware that their overweight children eat more than three times a day. One carer stated that her obese child eats regularly three times a day at home, but every time he visits a relative or a neighbour, he accepts their invitation to eat. It is customary in Indonesia to offer people (children or adults) food whenever they visit. It is considered polite and respectful for the host to do so, and the guest should accept, in order to show respect.

Carers in the intermediate and high SES groups also raised the issue of snacks, as their children would eat three or four times a day and snack in between.

Feelings about overweight children

Carers from low SES groups had mixed feelings about overweight babies/children, one fourth (9/35) having positive feelings such as happiness and an eagerness to pinch the child to express their feelings. Pinching children on their cheeks to express their feelings is common in Indonesia, for example when people think the child is cute. However, more carers (26/35) had negative feelings such as fear that their children will become overweight, feeling sorry for the overweight child because they might be bullied at school or because of their inability to participate in some of the schools' physical activities, or feeling that overweight children are "just lazy".

Similar to carers from the low SES groups, carers from the intermediate SES groups also had mixed feelings about overweight babies/children. Several (6/32) expressed positive feelings but most (26/32) portrayed negative feelings.

All carers from the high SES groups shared the same negative feelings towards overweight children. Carers from all SES groups shared their concern about overweight-related health problems such as heart disease, diabetes, difficulty in breathing, cholesterol problems, or high blood pressure.

Sensitivity in carers of overweight children

All carers who mentioned that their children were overweight expressed similar sensitive attitudes when it came to their own children, irrespective of SES. For example, they placed more attention on their children's capabilities in physical activities rather than their weight status.

Children's current weight and height

Most carers of the low and intermediate SES groups knew their children's current weight (29/35 and 25/32, respectively), but only some (21/35 and 15/32, respectively) knew their children's height. These families had their children's height and weight measured regularly at the *Posyandu* until they were 5 years old. From the carers' facial expressions and the way they stated their experience of going to *Posyandu* to have the child measured, it is indicative that carers from low and intermediate SES groups may consider this as just an obligation to tick the checklist instead of an opportunity to monitor their children's development. In public elementary schools, weight and height are measured once a year.

All high SES group carers agreed that their indicator of health is their children's weight, with 22/27 knowing their children's current weight, while only a little more than half (15/27) knew their height. Five carers (5/13) admitted they were only concerned about the children's weight and not height; one even stated she never paid attention to her children's heights. One mother stated that the only opinion that matters for her was her trusted doctor's. Under 5 children are weighed during visits to the paediatrician whereas 7–12 year old children are weighed every 2 months at (private) school. Even with this scheme, many carers did not pay much attention to their children's current weight or height.

One third (35/94) of all carers from all SES groups were satisfied with their children's growth; (including all carers who stated that their children were healthy weight/overweight), while 59/94 carers were not satisfied. Carers admitted that they compared their children's weight or height to that of their peers at school, in the playground or other public places. One mother from the intermediate SES groups stated that she compared her son's height with his friends because she thinks that he is short and felt relieved when she saw that his peers were mostly 'as short as he is'.

Table 6 Quotes on awareness and feelings towards overweight in children according to carers from Bandung, Indonesia

	Low SES	Intermediate SES	High SES
Characteristics of overweight	• P5: If it's in babies, Ma'am, from here (pointing at her arms), we can see it from their arms. So, in Sundanese, gegeretan (Sundanese term- babies with fat folds; it looks as if their flesh have been sliced). • P7: The size should be the plus one; otherwise it must be sewn. Hahaha • P3: ... for example after they walk for a little while, they go hah hah hah (laboured breathing noises). • P5: Sundanese people said that the way they walk is ngajegag (walking with the leg open, like frog legs), right?	• P8: Uh... the belly is bloated and it looks like the person is pregnant. • P2: When you bring them out to walk, they get tired easily. • P6: They run for a little bit and they are like (makes panting noises). • P7: They are slow; they walk slowly. • P5: So, for example, when the baby is 4 months old, the other child can lie flat on the stomach, but the fat baby can't do it.	• P4: For example, babies his age are supposed to be in the standing and started to walking stage (but the fat baby cannot do that just yet). P6: Yeah, it's like, the children seem to experience difficulties to move. It looks difficult for them to walk. I see that a lot, and I use to think, "That is overweight". • P5: It's probably because she has tough bones, bigger bones and however much weight she loses she will never be as thin as other kids. The problem is, currently she moves slower than her younger sibling and she has breathing problems, too • P7: If the person is overweight, he's prone to diseases and becomes sick easily.
Food portion size in overweight children	• P9: So when I gave her the food, I gave her less, I don't follow the serving size guidelines from the box. • P1: For normal children, it's just the standard serving...for the overweight children, they will have as much as adults.	• P3: My son (elementary school) eats the same portion as mine. • P7: Like earlier this morning, before I came here, we have breakfast with fried rice. Well, after fried rice, he asked more, he asked for noodles. I gave him one pack of noodle, and he ate it until there's nothing left. • P4: In a day? Well, actually, he eats three times a day, but the portion is more than me. For me, for example, I eat one full plate. My child can eat up to three full portion.	• P6: She only eats zuppa soup as main meal.P2: How many bowls?P6: Only three bowls. • P5: Because we think the children are still on the growth period (so we let the children eat a lot). • P7: Parents are also afraid if the children get sick, because there are so many diseases right now. • P6: So sometimes they make their children eat a lot to prevent them from getting sick.
Eating frequency in overweight children	• P4: My niece, 5th grade, 58 kg, she eats at 6 pm, then she eats again at 8 pm. Mostly, she eats meatballs, she rarely eats any vegetables. • P2: A child should eat three meals a day right? This one eats more than three times and she eats noodles, sometimes two packages aren't enough for her, only four is. • P9: My (obese) child eats regularly, three times at home, but even when he has eaten and our neighbour offers him something to eat, he will eat it. When he comes to his aunt's house and she offers him food, he will eat it.	• P7: He's always eating. He never stops eating. • P5: He eats four times a day, and he also eats snacks like bread, cakes, sweets. • P2: He eats…he eats at noon. The others only eat in the morning and after Isya (the last Moslem's prayer time in a day, in Indonesia, it's at about seven o'clock p.m). When the others eat after Isya, my son also joins them. After that, he watches TV until 11 o'clock. Sometimes, at ten o'clock, he eats again. That means he doesn't make a move (after his last meal), then he directly goes to sleep.	• P5: Yeah, people do that you know. My son, my eldest one weighs almost 70 k. He eats one meal at 10 am, and then another one at 12. In the afternoon, when he finally gets home, he eats another meal. He just wanders around the kitchen looking for food, and suddenly he has a plate full of rice. • P4: For my child, if he eats regularly like three times a day, his weight is stable. Three meals: morning, noon, and afternoon around six pm. Stable, but once there are snacks. Oh, his weight goes skyrocketing.
Feelings about overweight children	• P5: Who doesn't want a fat child? • P7: They are cute. I want to pinch them. • P2: I feel gereget (kind of loving something cute mixed with desire to pinch, in Sundanese), Ma'am. • P8: Happy to see a fat child, but pity him as well • P6: Because it's a pity. It's difficult. Yes, the fat children have difficulties to move. They become uh, they're lazy, they sleep a lot. • P7: Out of fear of becoming like A (name), so we limit our child's diet... • P9: Horrified.	• P7: When they're little, it's kind of cute (to be fat). • P3: Yes, cute, like on TV. • P6: It scares me. • P1: If the child is too fat, sometimes I feel pity for him/her, just like the one on TV. • P8: I feel sorry for him, Doctor.	• P8: When we look at the fat children, we'll think they are cute…But actually it's a pity, fat children are having difficulties to move. • P6: I'm afraid my child will become that fat. • P2: The problem is that they are vulnerable to diseases, I'm afraid of that. Underweight children are vulnerable to diseases, but so are the big ones, hahaha.
Sensitivity in carers of own overweight children	• P6: This doesn't happen to my child, he is fat but healthy. • P9: Well, when he runs around, he doesn't get tired easily.	• P8: I don't think a fat person gets tired easily because mine is fat (and he does not get tired easily).	• P5: My child, who is fat, is actually very active and can run quickly. • P8: When he's racing with his thinner friends, he runs faster. • P4: Fat people are not always slower.

Table 6 Quotes on awareness and feelings towards overweight in children according to carers from Bandung, Indonesia *(Continued)*

Children's current weight and height	• P2: I just want it [my child's weight] to be just normal, ascending in a straight line [on the KMS- Kartu Menuju Sehat (Health Card)].	• P3: I have too many under 5 children, everytime I go to Posyandu (community health post) to weigh them; I bring 3 or 4 children. • P4: I thought that my child was the only short one, but it turns out that there are a lot of kids who are as short as he is.	• P7: Importantly, it must be according to the chart, or the doctor's opinion. If the doctor says okay, I'll be thankful. • P6: I'm aware that I am short, so my children won't be tall.

Discussion

This is the first study in Indonesia that investigates the knowledge, attitudes and beliefs surrounding childhood overweight of mothers/grandmothers from different SES groups. We identified 3 categories and 13 subcategories as stated in Table 3. However, due to word limitations, we can only discuss several subcategories: normal weight range, ideal body shape, characteristics of overweight, activity levels and sedentary behaviour, heredity, how carers define overweight, children's current weight and height, and chubbier is healthier.

All three SES groups had similar expectations about an appropriate weight at birth, 6 and 12 months. This might have resulted from the participation of mothers in the *Posyandu,* [21] community counselling usually done in *Puskesmas,* or consultations with health practitioner or paediatricians. All participants had similar ideas about the ideal adult body type, demonstrating the influence of the media in their lives. It is very likely children of parent participants watched television with their parents and were influenced by what is considered the ideal adult body type. Thus, children who absorbed large amounts of screen time could relate to the ideal for adults but not have a connection with the young child's bodyweight because there is no such ideal for children either in the media or in everyday reality. Linking this to inadequate PE in school curricula seems to suggest that a child's ideal body type is not considered as important. All carers had similar opinions about the characteristics of overweight children: overweight children had bigger portion sizes and ate more frequently compared to their healthy weight counterparts. How carers characterised overweight is similar to studies in the United Kingdom [22] and the United States [23] where parents were found to rely on visual appearance, exercise capability in relation to peers, and clothing sizes.

The carers recognised that dietary factors, activity levels and sedentary behaviours, and heredity all contributed to the development of overweight. Most carers agreed that the 2-h physical education (PE) class at school is not enough, especially as this includes changing clothes and getting to the sportsfield. One qualitative study with US school principals, PE teachers and students highlighted the need for improvement in the in-school physical activity; one student referred to PE class as a "dumping ground", where children were sent when other "subject matter" teachers were not available [24]. Another US study, using pedometers to count steps, showed that typical PE classes only account for 8–11% of the total steps made throughout the day [25]. A 3-year intervention study of primary school children in Sweden showed that to successfully reduce weight gain, children needed to be physically active for more than 40 min in each physical education setting every day [26]. Carers seemed less worried about physical education at school because children from low and intermediate SES groups spend most of their after school hours playing outside the house, which add to their physical activity hours; while the high SES children engaged more in extracurricular activities.

Many carers assigned heredity or genetic predisposition as the 'expected and accepted' cause of childhood overweight, a finding also documented in Australia [27] and the United States [23, 28, 29].

Most carers knew the current weight of their children but less than 60% of these carers knew about their children's height. Most carers defined overweight subjectively from physical appearance. This finding is in keeping with studies from Germany, [30] the United Kingdom, [22] the United States, [23, 31] and in Vietnam [32]. While some carers knew how to define overweight objectively, this knowledge is not very useful when they do not know their child's current weight or height. Knowing how to measure overweight and then knowing a child's weight and height status may be important first steps in recognising whether children are underweight, of a healthy weight or overweight [22, 31–33].

Some carers agreed with the 'chubbier is healthier' concept that is also found in other cultures. For example in Turkey (plump kids are healthy), [34] Vietnam (chubbiness is good), [32] the United States ("baby fat" is cute and healthy [31]; a bigger infant is a better infant [28]) and the United Kingdom (a big baby is a healthy baby) [35]. The concept of overweight symbolising family wellbeing is also found in China [36].

Carers from the high SES groups expressed their opinions freely and in a more confident manner compared to the other two groups. This is probably related to their educational background, with more carers from the high SES groups being university graduates, compared to none from the other groups. Within the low SES groups, we found that the women from villages with an active midwife (in terms of educating the carers) were involved more actively in the discussion. This may highlight the significant role played by front line staff in the health system, e.g. midwives and general practitioners. Two studies in Indonesia support this issue, stating that the availability and higher participation in *Posyandu* in Indonesia have significantly improved children's nutrition status and had a protective effect on the development of overweight in children [21, 37].

One aspect to highlight in our study is the interaction between participants within each focus group, an advantage of conducting FGDs [38]. Some carers supported each other and some questioned another's opinion, bringing many insights to the topic and richness to our data. Comparison between the three SES groups revealed more similarities in low and intermediate SES groups in the way they perceived childhood overweight and related topics. We also found that in a few subcategories (how carers define overweight; chubbier is healthier), carers from low SES groups shared similar knowledge with their counterparts from the higher SES groups. For some issues, the low SES carers even showed better knowledge compared to their counterparts from higher SES, for example in the knowledge to define overweight objectively and knowledge about the current weight and height of their children.

A strength of this study is that it is the first in Indonesia to investigate the perceptions of overweight in carers from three different SES groups. Secondly, in contrast to the other Indonesian study where only mothers of overweight children were involved, our study recruited carers with children of diverse weight status, providing a variety of perspectives. Thirdly, we had the same number of groups in each status category, allowing us to compare the results between the three groups involved. Fourthly, we successfully attracted participation from carers of low SES groups, even though low SES participants are considered by some to be difficult to recruit [31]. One of our study's limitations is that because the number of mother participants outweighed the number of grandmother participants, comparison of these two groups' perspectives was unavailable. Although our qualitative research findings may lack generalisability, we believe our findings are supportive of findings from other countries while producing new replicable findings that will represent carers' views if done in other regions of Indonesia.

Conclusions

This study sought to explore the perceptions of carers towards childhood overweight. Although there were similarities in the way carers from different SES groups perceived overweight, the differences were of great interest. In discussion of health-related issues, there were differences on the perceptions of overweight not only between different SES groups but also within the same SES groups.

Recommendations

Irrespective of these differences, one of the policy implications around the perception of carers is the importance of educating mothers and other primary carers of children around healthier lifestyles. This study highlights the need for improvement within Indonesia in the dissemination of current policies such as PUGS and the use of KMS, for example through the media (newspaper and television). The use of the KMS card needs to be implemented with all levels of health practitioners, making it the national reference in Indonesia to regularly monitor children's growth. Consideration should be given to routine anthropometric measurements, currently undertaken in private elementary schools, being implemented in every school, thus providing feedback to parents about their children's weight and height status. There is room for review and revision of the quality and quantity of physical education class in elementary schools. The Department of Education may need to increase the times for children's physical activities during school hours, e.g. during recess or before and after school physical activities. Future research should aim to explore the food choices made by carers and the involvement of other people in the household (father, grandparents) in making diet-related decisions.

Endnotes

[1]We included carers of under five and elementary school children because of the practicalities in recruiting these mothers through Community Health Centers, private practices and schools. Carers of 5 and 6-year-olds (kindergarten age) are much harder to recruit because kindergarten is not mandatory in Indonesia.

Acknowledgements
CNR would like to thank Lembaga Pengelola Dana Pendidikan (LPDP), the Republic of Indonesia for her PhD scholarship.

Funding
This study was funded by the Children's Hospital at Westmead (CHW), Australia. CHW did not have any role in the design of the study and collection, analysis, and interpretation of data and in writing the manuscript.

Authors' contributions
All authors contributed equally in designing the study. CNR analysed and interpreted the data under the supervision of CLH, ML and LB. All authors contributed in writing the manuscript and have read, revised and approved the final draft of the manuscript.

Competing interests
The authors declare that they have no competing interest.

Author details
[1]Discipline of Child & Adolescent Health, The Children's Hospital at Westmead, University of Sydney Clinical School, Locked Bag 4001, Westmead, NSW 2145, Australia. [2]School of Social and Political Sciences, The University of Sydney, RC Mills Building (A26), Sydney, NSW 2006, Australia. [3]Sydney School of Public Health, The University of Sydney, Edward Ford Building (A27), Fisher Rd, Sydney, NSW 2006, Australia.

References

1. International Food Policy Research Institute. Global nutrition report 2015: actions and accountability to advance nutrition and sustainable development. Washington, DC: International Food Policy Research Institute; 2015.
2. Rachmi CN, Li M, Baur L. Overweight and obesity in Indonesia: prevalence and risk factors–a literature review. Public Health. 2017;
3. Shrimpton R, Rokx C. The double burden of malnutrition in Indonesia. Jakarta, Indonesia: World Bank Jakarta; 2013.
4. Rizona F, Susetyowati S, Lusmilasari L. Mother's feeding behaviours on overweight children. Int J Community Med Public Health. 2016;3:831–6.
5. Tucker P, Irwin JD, He M, Bouck LM, Pollett G. Preschoolers' dietary behaviours: parents' perspectives. Can J Diet Pract Res. 2006;67:67–71.
6. Towns N, D'Auria J. Parental perceptions of their child's overweight: an integrative review of the literature. J Pediatr Nurs. 2009;24:115–30.
7. Scaglioni S, Salvioni M, Galimberti C. Influence of parental attitudes in the development of children eating behaviour. Br J Nutr. 2008;99(Suppl 1):S22–5.
8. Oude Luttikhuis H, Baur L, Jansen H, Shrewsbury VA, O'Malley C, Stolk RP, Summerbell CD. Interventions for treating obesity in children. Cochrane Database Syst Rev. 2009. doi:10.1002/14651858.CD001872.pub2.
9. Golley RK, Hendrie GA, Slater A, Corsini N. Interventions that involve parents to improve children's weight-related nutrition intake and activity patterns - what nutrition and activity targets and behaviour change techniques are associated with intervention effectiveness? Obes Rev. 2011;12:114–30.
10. Niemeier BS, Hektner JM, Enger KB. Parent participation in weight-related health interventions for children and adolescents: a systematic review and meta-analysis. Prev Med. 2012;55:3–13.
11. Gibson EL, Kreichauf S, Wildgruber A, Vogele C, Summerbell CD, Nixon C, Moore H, Douthwaite W, Manios Y, ToyBox-Study G. A narrative review of psychological and educational strategies applied to young children's eating behaviours aimed at reducing obesity risk. Obes Rev. 2012;13(Suppl 1):85–95.
12. Indeks Pembangunan Manusia [https://jabar.bps.go.id/Subjek/view/id/26-subjekViewTab3|accordion-daftar-subjek1].
13. Operational Working Group Ministry of Health: Pedoman Umum Pengelolaan Posyandu. (Health Mo ed. pp. 6–7. Jakarta: Departemen Kesehatan Republik Indonesia; 2011:6–7.
14. Strauss A. Qualitative analysis for social scientists. Cambridge: Cambridge University Press; 1987.
15. Strauss A, Corbin J. Basics of qualitative research: grounded theory procedures and techniques. Newbury Park, CA: Sage; 1990.
16. Glaser B, Strauss A. The discovery of grounded theory: strategies for qualitative research. Chicago: Aldine; 1967.
17. NVivo qualitative data analysis Software. vol. Version 11: QSR International Pty Ltd.; 2014. http://www.qsrinternational.com/support/faqs/how-do-i-cite-nvivo-10-nvivo-9-or-nvivo-8-in-my-wo.
18. Kartu Menuju Sehat [http://www.depkes.go.id/resources/download/info-terkini/Kartu Menuju Sehat KMS.pdf].
19. Inilah Perbedaan '4 Sehat 5 Sempurna' Dengan 'Gizi Seimbang' [http://www.depkes.go.id/article/view/16051300001/inilah-perbedaan-4-sehat-5-sempurna-dengan-gizi-seimbang-.html].
20. Departemen Kesehatan RI. Direktorat Jenderal Bina Kesehatan Masyarakat DKR: Pedoman Umum Gizi Seimbang (PUGS) - panduan untuk petugas. Indonesia DKR ed. Jakarta, Indonesia: Depkes RI; 2003.
21. Anwar F, Khomsan A, Sukandar D, Riyadi H, Mudjajanto ES. High participation in the Posyandu nutrition program improved children nutritional status. Nutr Res Pract. 2010;4:208–14.
22. Jones AR, Parkinson KN, Drewett RF, Hyland RM, Pearce MS, Adamson AJ. Gateshead millennium study Core T: parental perceptions of weight status in children: the Gateshead millennium study. Int J Obes. 2011;35:953–62.
23. Goodell LS, Pierce MB, Bravo CM, Ferris AM. Parental perceptions of overweight during early childhood. Qual Health Res. 2008;18:1548–55.
24. Gamble A, Chatfield SL, Cormack ML Jr, Hallam JS. Not enough time in the day: a qualitative assessment of in-school physical activity policy as viewed by administrators, teachers, and students. J Sch Health. 2017;87:21–8.
25. Tudor-Locke C, Lee SM, Morgan CF, Beighle A, Pangrazi RP. Children's pedometer-determined physical activity during the segmented school day. Med Sci Sports Exerc. 2006;38:1732–8.
26. Sollerhed AC, Ejlertsson G. Physical benefits of expanded physical education in primary school: findings from a 3-year intervention study in Sweden. Scand J Med Sci Sports. 2008;18:102–7.
27. Jackson D, McDonald G, Mannix J, Faga P, Firtko A. Mothers' perceptions of overweight and obesity in their children. Aust J Adv Nurs. 2005;23:8–13.
28. Baughcum AE, Burklow KA, Deeks CM, Powers SW, Whitaker RC. Maternal feeding practices and childhood obesity: a focus group study of low-income mothers. Arch Pediatr Adolesc Med. 1998;152:1010–4.
29. Jain A, Sherman SN, Chamberlin LA, Carter Y, Powers SW, Whitaker RC. Why don't low-income mothers worry about their preschoolers being overweight? Pediatrics. 2001;107:1138–46.
30. Sikorski C, Riedel C, Luppa M, Schulze B, Werner P, Konig HH, Riedel-Heller SG. Perception of overweight and obesity from different angles: a qualitative study. Scand J Public Health. 2012;40:271–7.
31. Eli K, Howell K, Fisher PA, Nowicka P. "a little on the heavy side": a qualitative analysis of parents' and grandparents' perceptions of preschoolers' body weights. BMJ Open. 2014;4:e006609.
32. Do LM, Larsson V, Tran TK, Nguyen HT, Eriksson B, Ascher H. Vietnamese mother's conceptions of childhood overweight: findings from a qualitative study. Glob Health Action. 2016;9:30215.
33. He M, Evans A. Are parents aware that their children are overweight or obese? Do they care? Can Fam Physician. 2007;53:1493–9.
34. Esenay FI, Yigit R, Erdogan S. Turkish Mothers' perceptions of their Children's weight. J Spec Pediatric Nurs. 2010;15:144–53.
35. Southwell O, Fox JR. Maternal perceptions of overweight and obesity in children: a grounded theory study. Br J Health Psychol. 2011;16:626–41.
36. Li J, Lei J, Wen S, Zhou L. Sex disparity and perception of obesity/overweight by parents and grandparents. Paediatr Child Health. 2014;19:e113–6.
37. Andriani H, Liao CY, Kuo HW. Association of Maternal and Child Health Center (Posyandu) availability with child weight status in Indonesia: a National Study. Int J Environ Res Public Health. 2016;13
38. Green J, Thorogood N. Qualitative methods for Health Research. Second edition edn. Great Britain: SAGE Publications Ltd; 2009.

12

Comparison of an alternative schedule of extended care contacts to a self-directed control: a randomized trial of weight loss maintenance

Gareth R. Dutton[1*], Marissa A. Gowey[1], Fei Tan[2], Dali Zhou[2], Jamy Ard[3], Michael G. Perri[4] and Cora E. Lewis[1]

Abstract

Background: Behavioral interventions for obesity produce clinically meaningful weight loss, but weight regain following treatment is common. Extended care programs attenuate weight regain and improve weight loss maintenance. However, less is known about the most effective ways to deliver extended care, including contact schedules.

Methods: We compared the 12-month weight regain of an extended care program utilizing a non-conventional, clustered campaign treatment schedule and a self-directed program among individuals who previously achieved ≥5% weight reductions. Participants (N = 108; mean age = 51.6 years; mean weight = 92.6 kg; 52% African American; 95% female) who achieved ≥5% weight loss during an initial 16-week behavioral obesity treatment were randomized into a 2-arm, 12-month extended care trial. A clustered campaign condition included 12 group-based visits delivered in three, 4-week clusters. A self-directed condition included provision of the same printed intervention materials but no additional treatment visits. The study was conducted in a U.S. academic medical center from 2011 to 2015.

Results: Prior to randomization, participants lost an average of −7.55 ± 3.04 kg. Participants randomized to the 12-month clustered campaign program regained significantly less weight (0.35 ± 4.62 kg) than self-directed participants (2.40 ± 3.99 kg), which represented a significant between-group difference of 2.28 kg (p = 0.0154) after covariate adjustments. This corresponded to maintaining 87% and 64% of lost weight in the clustered campaign and self-directed conditions, respectively, which was a significant between-group difference of 29% maintenance of lost weight after covariate adjustments, p = 0.0396.

Conclusions: In this initial test of a clustered campaign treatment schedule, this novel approach effectively promoted 12-month maintenance of lost weight. Future trials should directly compare the clustered campaigns with conventional (e.g., monthly) extended care schedules.

Trial registration: Clinicaltrials.gov NCT02487121. Registered 06/26/2015 (retrospectively registered)

Keywords: Obesity, Behavioral treatment, Extended care, Weight loss maintenance, Weight regain, Adults

* Correspondence: gdutton@uabmc.edu
[1]Division of Preventive Medicine, Department of Medicine, University of Alabama at Birmingham, Birmingham, AL, USA
Full list of author information is available at the end of the article

Background

Behavioral weight management interventions typically produce initial reductions in body weight of 7–10%, which provides meaningful benefits for the prevention and management of various health conditions [1, 2]. Within the first year following treatment, however, individuals commonly regain 50–65% of their lost weight [3–5]. To attenuate this weight regain, extended care contacts are recommended for at least 1 year following initial treatment [1]. Indeed, extended care programs significantly reduce weight regain when compared to minimal or no additional contact [6–10]. By providing continued intervention contact focused on maintaining weight loss, participants are assisted in sustaining the self-management strategies necessary for long-term weight management [5, 7, 8].

Despite the documented benefits of maintenance programs, less is known about the best schedule for delivering these programs. Weight loss maintenance programs generally provide contacts on an evenly-spaced schedule, such as bi-weekly or monthly visits [1, 11, 12]. According to learning theory and theories of behavior change [13–15], this fixed-interval schedule is appropriate for the *initiation* of treatment and learning of new behaviors. This intensive contact schedule provides ongoing opportunities to learn and practice self-management skills while receiving support and corrective feedback from trained interventionists [5, 16].

However, as individuals transition to maintaining self-management behaviors in the extended care phase of behavioral obesity treatment, it is unclear whether the same schedule or intensity of contact is appropriate. In fact, operant learning, self-regulation, and relapse prevention theories [5, 6, 13–20], combined with preliminary research, suggest that an alternative schedule of treatment delivery may be useful for behavior *maintenance* [21, 22]. More specifically, a temporally-clustered campaign includes periods of frequent contact separated by extended periods without contact, which provides opportunities for intensive support and expert feedback over a shorter time period to further develop skills for weight maintenance behaviors; yet, it also allows for independent practice of self-management skills for extended periods.

Additionally, a clustered campaign schedule during the maintenance phase of treatment may protect against diminished reinforcement, boredom, and behavioral habituation that are common with conventional maintenance schedules [5, 16, 23–26]. Such clustered campaigns can be organized around different themes that may further reduce monotony, which is not typically used in the initial phase of behavioral obesity treatment when novel content is being introduced regularly. It also allows advanced knowledge acquisition and honing of advanced skills during maintenance. Variability in the schedule and content may counter the boredom that can occur during the sessions (e.g., participants get a 'break' from group participation for several weeks between campaigns that might in turn improve engagement when returning to group) as well as habituation with engaging in the same routine and behaviors between sessions. Despite the potential benefits, temporally-clustered sessions may increase the risk of attrition and less timely support due to extended periods without contact.

Contemporary weight loss programs, such as the Look AHEAD trial and Diabetes Prevention Program [27, 28], have incorporated "refresher groups" or "motivational campaigns" delivered on this temporally-clustered type of schedule during the maintenance phases of treatment. However, this alternative maintenance schedule was one part of a multi-component intervention that included continuation of evenly-distributed, fixed-interval contacts. Two other trials also used temporally-clustered extended care contacts to reduce weight regain [21, 29], although novel scheduling was one of several simultaneous treatment modifications, including different intensities of contact [29] and different behavioral prescriptions and goals [21].

Thus, the specific effect of temporally-clustered schedules for extended care remains unclear. To provide an initial test of this alternative extended care schedule in the absence of other treatment components, the purpose of this behavioral extended care trial was to compare 12-month outcomes of a clustered campaign maintenance delivery schedule to a self-directed comparison condition among individuals who previously achieved ≥5% weight reductions. It was hypothesized that an extended care program that included 12 maintenance visits delivered in three, 4-week clusters, would result in significantly better maintenance of lost weight than the comparison condition.

Methods

Participants

Participants were adults (≥21 years-old) who had taken part in a 16-week weight loss program and lost ≥5% of their initial body weight by month 4 of the program. Inclusion criteria for the initial, 16-week program included a body mass index (BMI; kg/m^2) between 28 and 45. Individuals were ineligible to participate in the initial program if they had lost >4.5 kg and/or taken a weight loss medication in the past 6 months, had a medical condition for which weight loss or physical activity would be inadvisable, planned to relocate from the area in the next 18 months, were unable or unwilling to attend sessions, or were unwilling to accept random assignment. Participants were recruited through local newspaper, television, flyer, and university-affiliated website and e-newsletter advertisements.

Procedures

Interested individuals contacted project staff to complete a pre-screening interview by telephone to determine preliminary eligibility. Based on the telephone screening, eligible individuals were scheduled to attend an orientation session and provide informed consent. This included brief, in-person screening to confirm eligibility (i.e., measurement of height and weight for BMI). Participant flow is summarized in Fig. 1. Participants providing consent returned for a baseline assessment visit and enrolled in an initial 16-week weight loss program.

This initial program included weekly, group-based sessions at an academic medical center with 15–20 participants. Groups were facilitated by a team of trained

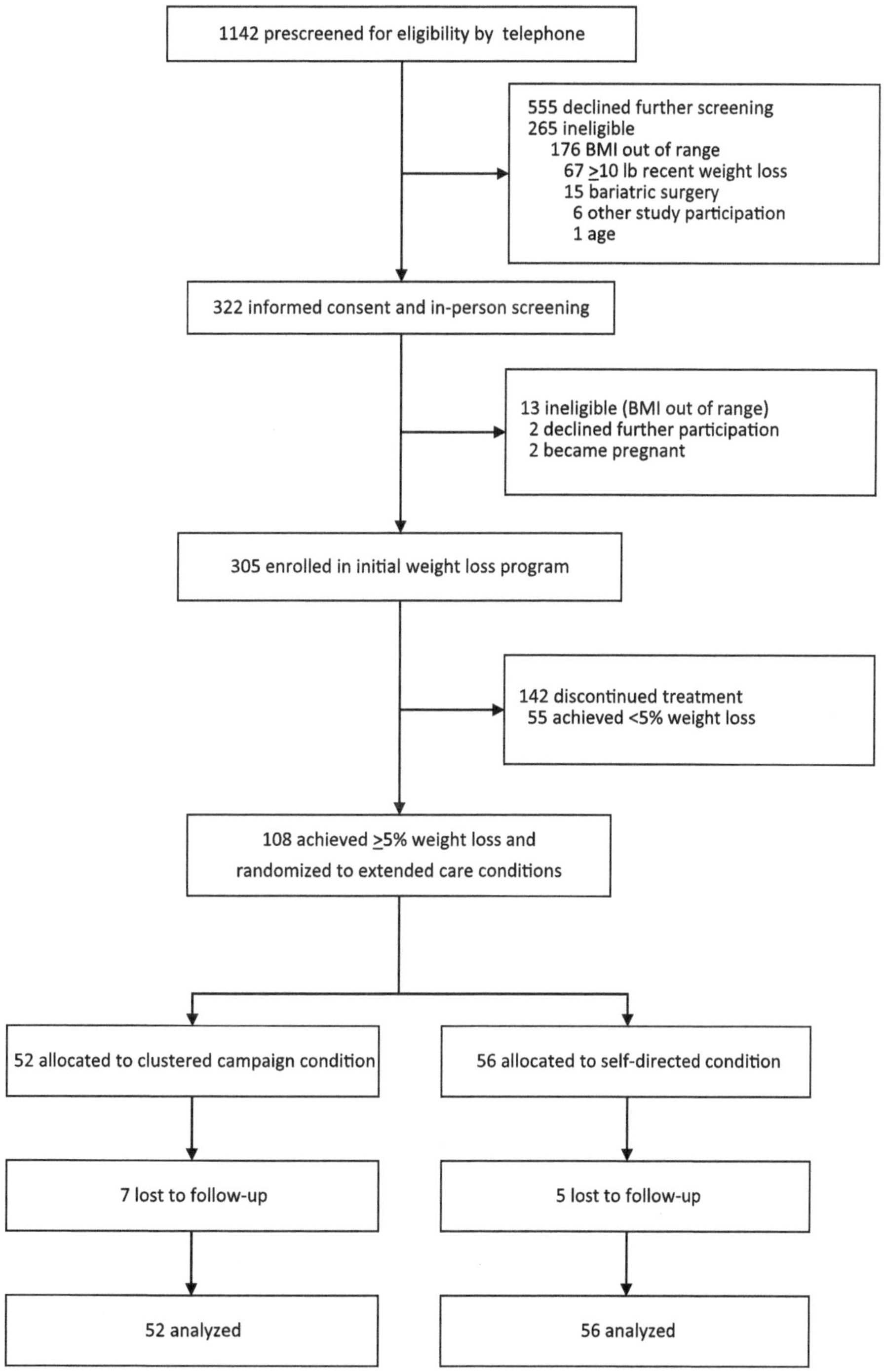

Fig. 1 CONSORT flow diagram

interventionists, including dieticians, exercise specialists, and clinical psychologists. Program content was modeled after the Diabetes Prevention Program (DPP) [28] and weight loss protocols by Perri and colleagues [7]. Participants were encouraged to work toward a 5% weight loss goal, and they were aware this criterion was required to continue into the maintenance trial. They were instructed to reduce caloric intake to 1200 kcal/day (for participants weighing <250 lb) or 1500 kcal/day (for participants weighing ≥250 lb) and encouraged to work toward a physical activity goal of at least 180 min/week. Participants received training in behavioral strategies designed to support weight loss, including goal-setting, problem-solving, and self-monitoring. Participants also received pedometers, food scales, and measuring cups/spoons to facilitate self-monitoring. Although the initial program provided intensive (i.e., weekly) contact and evidence-based content, treatment did not include an extensive behavioral run-in period, individual make-up sessions for missed groups, or other supplemental resources or strategies to maximize adherence and weight loss as provided in prior programs such as DPP and other weight loss trials.

Upon completion of the initial program, participants attended an assessment visit and those who achieved ≥5% weight loss were randomized in a parallel 1:1 ratio to one of two maintenance conditions for a 12-month extended care trial. At this visit, staff provided eligible participants with a numbered, sealed envelope, which indicated to which condition they were randomized. Randomization was prepared by PROC PLAN in SAS (Ver. 9.3), and a unique randomization number was generated for each participant. A permuted-block randomization scheme with block sizes of 4 was used to maintain assignment balance. Approval for this study was obtained from the IRB of the participating academic health center. Informed consent was obtained from all individual participants included in the study. This trial is registered with clinicaltrials.gov (NCT02487121).

Extended care interventions

Clustered campaign maintenance program

Consistent with other extended care programs [7, 30], the purpose was to maintain adherence, bolster motivation, and reinforce information previously discussed with a focus on the maintenance of healthy lifestyle behaviors. Sessions included some review of previously-learned concepts and skills as well as incorporation of novel material pertaining to diet, physical activity, and behavior/motivation. The main focus of the extended care sessions was on the maintenance (rather than initial adoption) of healthy lifestyle behaviors associated with continued weight loss and/or weight loss maintenance and the avoidance of returning to less healthy behaviors.

The unique feature of this maintenance program was the non-conventional schedule of delivery. Rather than an evenly-distributed, fixed-interval (e.g., monthly) schedule of contact, the program included 12 extended care group sessions divided into three intensive, 4-week campaigns. These occurred during months 7, 10, and 13 of the 16-month study (Table 1). Thus, the periodic episodes of frequent visits were separated by extended periods without contact. Session content of the three campaigns was organized to reflect themes, including overviews of dietary practices (sessions 1–4), physical activity (sessions 5–8), and behavioral and motivational strategies and relapse prevention (sessions 9–12). This schedule of several weekly meetings separated by extended periods with less frequent contact is consistent with the campaigns or refresher groups offered in the Look AHEAD trial during extended care [27].

During extended care, participants established weight goals mutually agreed upon by them and interventionists. Goals could include additional weight loss or weight maintenance, depending on individuals' progress, desired weight loss, and current BMI. Across all three campaigns, recommended behavioral goals for each participant included dietary and activity self-monitoring at least 3 days/week. In addition to self-monitoring goals, participants were encouraged to set campaign-specific dietary, physical activity, or behavioral/relapse prevention goals corresponding to specific session content (e.g., applying volumetric techniques to modify meals, identifying a new structured exercise to implement). Although general goals were provided to participants at each session, participants were encouraged to develop individualized action plans to tailor and implement each goal.

Because the trial included only participants losing ≥5% of baseline weight, fewer groups were required to deliver extended care treatment than during the initial weight reduction program. Therefore, extended care participants were consolidated into new treatment groups at randomization, which included a combination of familiar and new group

Table 1 Clustered campaign intervention schedule for weight loss maintenance

Month	1	2	3	4	5	6	7[a]	8	9	10[b]	11	12	13[c]	14	15	16
Treatment	X X	X X	X X	X X			X X			X X			X X			
Contacts	X X	X X	X X	X X			X X			X X			X X			
	Initial intervention (16 contacts in months 1-4)						Clustered campaign extended care intervention (12 contacts in months 5-16)									

X = Group-based treatment contact; [a] Dietary campaign; [b] Physical activity campaign; [c] Behavioral strategies campaign members. The same team of interventionists delivered the initial and extended care programs. To ensure fidelity to treatment delivery, all interventionists participated in initial training on the intervention protocol, which included structured facilitator guides and participant treatment materials. Although treatment fidelity was not formally assessed, all interventionists participated in ongoing weekly group supervision directed by the study PI, a licensed clinical psychologist with extensive experience in the delivery of behavioral weight management programs. Content of these group discussions indicated consistent protocol adherence.

Self-directed program

Participants in the self-directed program received printed intervention materials at the initiation of the 12-month extended care period. These materials were identical to those provided in the clustered campaign condition. Self-directed participants initially met with an interventionist to review the treatment materials and answer any questions about the extended care program. They were encouraged to continue using behavioral strategies for weight management including self-monitoring and independently work through the written materials provided. The self-directed control group did not receive further in-person contacts with interventionists during the 12-month follow-up. If participants initiated contact with interventionists by telephone or email during the extended care period, the interventionist provided brief feedback, responded to questions or concerns, and referred participants back to the intervention materials provided at randomization.

Measures

Demographics and medical history

At baseline, participants self-reported a variety of characteristics, including age, sex, race, educational attainment, income, and marital status.

Anthropometric measures

Height was measured at baseline to the nearest 0.1 cm using a wall-mounted stadiometer. Weight was measured to the nearest 0.1 kg using a calibrated digital scale at three time points, including baseline (i.e., pretreatment), month 4 (i.e., randomization), and month 16. The experimental sample included those participants who lost ≥5% body weight by month 4 and were randomized into the 12-month trial. The primary outcome was change in body weight during the 12-month randomized trial, which occurred between months 4 and 16. Secondary outcomes included the proportion of participants in each extended care condition that maintained ≥5% and ≥7% weight reductions at month 16. These values were selected because 5% weight loss is considered a clinically significant value for chronic disease risk reduction [1], greater weight loss (e.g., 7%) is associated with more pronounced health benefits [1, 31], and 7% weight loss is consistent with the goals of other lifestyle interventions such as Look AHEAD and the Diabetes Prevention Program [27, 28]. Height and weight were measured in a research clinic affiliated with the academic medical center by trained assessment staff with no involvement in initial or extended care treatment delivery.

Statistical analyses

A priori calculations indicated that $N = 96$ was required to provide statistical power of 80% to detect a between-group difference of 2.6 kg with a standard deviation of 4.5 kg at month 16. Accounting for 10% attrition, the required sample was 106, which was exceeded in this trial ($N = 108$). Based on previous trials [32, 33], it was conservatively estimated that one-third of participants would achieve ≥5% weight loss. Thus, to achieve 106 randomized participants, we estimated that 318 participants would need to be enrolled initially.

To summarize sample characteristics, descriptive statistics (sample mean, proportions and standard deviations) are provided. To analyze the effect of the clustered campaign maintenance program on the primary outcome of weight change over the extended care period (month 4 to month 16), two multiple regression models were fitted with response variables being weight change (kg) and weight regain (percent). In both models, the variables accounted for included age, marital status, race, education level, weight at randomization, and initial weight change (between months 0 and 4). To analyze the secondary outcome of the likelihood of maintaining a certain percentage of weight reduction at month 16, we dichotomized the weight loss percentage from month 0 to month 16 at ≥5% and ≥7% reductions from month 0. Logistic regression model was applied to each outcome. In addition to the treatment variable, we also accounted for baseline weight at month 0, age, marital status, race, and education. Odds ratio estimates and *p*-values were obtained.

As summarized in Fig. 1, 12 of 108 randomized participants were missing weight values at month 16 (i.e., 11% attrition). Attrition did not differ between conditions, $p = 0.45$. Due to these missing follow-up weight data and based on current recommendations for handling such data in weight loss trials [34], primary and secondary analyses were conducted based on multiple imputation in which we imputed the missing month 16 values 100 times to create 100 complete data sets, applied the desired analysis model to every imputed data set, and then pooled parameter estimates from the 100 data sets to form the final model results. Available variables used as predictors of missing data included treatment condition, race, marital status, education, age, income, height, initial weight (kg), and randomization weight (kg). Sensitivity analyses also were conducted with complete cases only, which yielded comparable results to those including multiple imputations. Thus, only the full sample intent-to-treat results with multiple imputation of missing data are presented here. Statistical analyses were implemented in R software [35] and SAS software, Version 9.4 of the SAS System for Windows.

Results

Participant characteristics

Recruitment, treatment delivery, and data collection were ongoing for this project from 11/01/11 to 3/31/15. Baseline (month 0) characteristics of the randomized sample are summarized in Table 2. The sample was comprised primarily of women (n = 103; 95.4%) and racial/ethnic minorities (n = 59; 54.6%). Of the 59 minority participants, most self-identified as African American (n = 56) followed by Asian (n = 1) and "other" racial group (n = 2).

Initial weight loss (months 0 to 4)

While 305 participants initially enrolled in the pre-randomization weight loss program, 108 (35.4% of original sample) completed the initial program and achieved the specified criterion of ≥5% weight loss. Therefore, 108 participants were randomized into the 12-month extended care trial (Fig. 1). All subsequent analyses are based on the randomized, extended care sample. Table 3 summarizes the pre-randomization weight change of these participants during the initial 16-week program, which represented significant within-group reductions in body weight (mean [SD], −7.45 [3.11] kg in the clustered campaign group and −7.64 [2.99] kg in the self-directed group).

Weight loss maintenance (months 4 to 16)

Participants randomized to receive the clustered campaign program regained less weight (unadjusted mean [SD], 0.35 [4.62] kg) compared to those in the self-directed condition (unadjusted mean [SD], 2.40 [3.99] kg) over the 12-month extended care period (Fig. 2). After adjustment for covariates in the multiple regression model, this represented a significant between-group difference in weight regain of 2.28 kg, P-value = 0.0154, favoring the clustered campaign program (Table 4). Similar results were obtained when the outcome was proportion of weight regain. These values equated to clustered campaign participants regaining 13% (unadjusted mean [SD], 13.11 [57.51] percent) of their initial weight loss, which compared favorably to the nearly 36%

Table 2 Baseline characteristics of randomized participants [a]

Characteristic [a]	Clustered Campaign Group (n = 52)	Self-directed Group (n = 56)	Total Randomized Sample (N = 108)
Age, years	52.13 (11.75)	51.18 (14.22)	51.64 (13.03)
Gender, No. (%)			
Male	1 (1.92)	4 (7.14)	5 (4.63)
Female	51 (98.08)	52 (92.86)	103 (95.37)
Race, No. (%)			
Non-Caucasian	28 (53.85)	31 (55.36)	59 (54.63)
Caucasian	24 (46.15)	25 (44.64)	49 (45.37)
Marital status, No. (%)			
Not Married	20 (38.46)	30 (53.57)	50 (46.30)
Married	32 (61.54)	26 (46.43)	58 (53.70)
Education, No. (%)			
Associates or lower degree	17 (32.69)	23 (41.07)	40 (37.04)
Bachelors or higher degree	35 (67.31)	33 (58.93)	68 (62.96)
Income, No. (%)			
≤ $40,000	13 (25.00)	19 (33.93)	32 (29.63)
$40,000 - $80,000	23 (44.23)	21 (37.50)	44 (40.74)
≥ $80,000	16 (30.77)	16 (28.57)	32 (29.63)
Body weight, kg	92.44 (13.77)	92.69 (12.86)	92.57 (13.24)
BMI, kg/m^2	34.93 (4.04)	35.26 (4.21)	35.10 (4.11)

Abbreviations: *BMI* body mass index

[a]Data are given as mean (SD) unless otherwise indicated. All values are at the start of the initial weight loss program (i.e., month 0)

Table 3 Changes in weight during the initial 4-month weight loss program (Months 0 to 4) [a]

Outcome	Clustered Campaign Group (*n* = 52)	Self-directed Group (*n* = 56)	Total Randomized Sample (*N* = 108)
Body weight, kg	−7.45 (3.11)	−7.64 (2.99)	−7.55 (3.04)
Body weight, %	−8.05 (3.01)	−8.22 (2.83)	−8.14 (2.91)
BMI, kg/m^2	−2.86 (1.17)	−3.03 (1.13)	−2.95 (1.15)

Abbreviations: *BMI* body mass index
[a]Data are given as mean (SD)

regain (unadjusted mean [SD], 35.55 [61.85] percent) observed for self-directed participants. After adjustment for relevant covariates, this represented a significant between-group difference of nearly 29% greater regain in the self-directed condition, *P*-value = 0.0396 (Table 5).

Secondary analyses compared the proportions of participants maintaining a reduced body weight that was at least 5% and 7% below initial (month 0) levels upon completion of the 12-month extended care program at month 16. A slightly greater proportion of clustered campaign participants (62.2%) maintained ≥5% weight reductions compared to self-directed participants (54.9%), although this was not significantly different, $p = 0.47$. However, the proportion achieving ≥7% reductions differed significantly between clustered campaign (51.1%) and self-directed (29.4%) conditions, $p = 0.03$. The adjusted likelihood of achieving ≥5% and ≥7% weight loss at the final follow-up was 1.45 and 2.79 times greater for clustered campaign participants as compared to self-directed participants, *p*'s = 0.3959 and 0.0283, respectively (Table 6).

Discussion

While previous trials have incorporated clustered campaign schedules into extended care programs to improve long-term weight management, this approach has been included along with other treatment components [27, 28] and/or additional alterations in delivery [21, 22, 29]. Thus, our understanding remains limited about the effect of using only a clustered campaign schedule to prevent weight regain, so the purpose of this study was to conduct an initial evaluation of such a schedule without other treatment components or adaptations (e.g., ongoing fixed-interval contacts, changes in dietary or behavioral targets). In the current sample of treatment-seeking, racially-diverse adults, a clustered campaign extended care program without major additional treatment components significantly improved maintenance of lost weight compared to a self-directed condition. The clustered campaign program resulted in the regain of only 13% of initial weight losses. Individuals in the self-directed condition regained nearly 29% more weight on average.

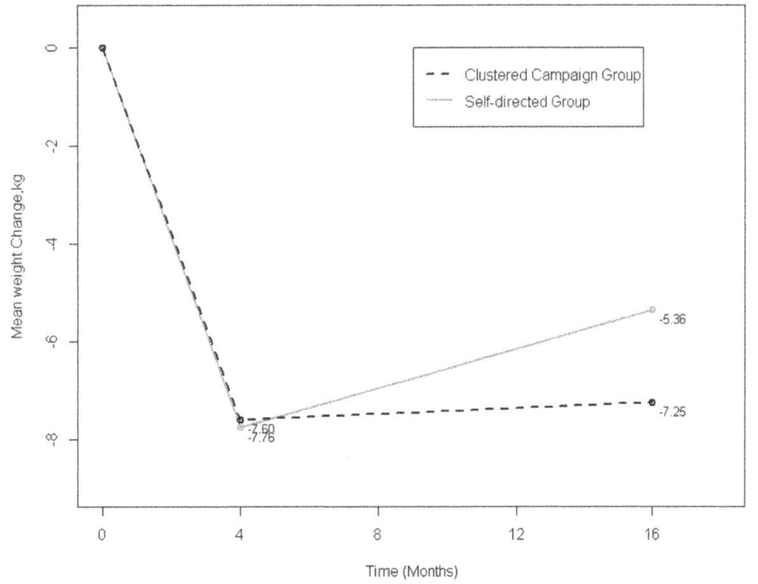

Fig. 2 Mean weight change by extended care condition. Randomization occurred at month 4. Reported mean weight change includes unadjusted, observed means for 96 randomized participants who completed the follow-up assessment at month 16. Multiple linear regression indicated significantly less weight regain in the clustered campaign group vs. the self-directed group between months 4 and 16 ($p = 0.0154$)

Table 4 Linear regression analysis of weight change (kg) during the 12-month extended care program (Months 4 to 16) [a]

Independent Variable [b]	Weight Change, kg		
	Parameter Est.	Std. Err	*P*-value
Treatment Condition	−2.28	0.92	0.0154
Randomization Weight	−0.02	0.04	0.6193
Initial Weight Change	0.26	0.15	0.0779
Age	<0.01	0.04	0.9197
Race	−0.73	1.08	0.5015
Marital Status	−1.33	0.94	0.1589
Education	−0.62	0.95	0.5124

[a]Analyses are based on multiple imputation of missing data
[b]For categorical independent variables, the comparison level versus reference level are as follows: Treatment Condition (Clustered Campaign vs. Self-directed), Race (Non-Caucasian vs. Caucasian), Marital Status (Not-married vs. Married), Education (Bachelors or higher degree vs. Associates or lower degree)

These findings are encouraging, since the first year following treatment represents a particularly high-risk period for weight regain. During this time, documented levels of weight regain are as high as 65%, which often precedes full weight regain within 3–5 years after treatment [4]. While comparisons to other weight loss maintenance trials are complicated by differences in aspects of treatment, populations, and settings investigated, the current effects appear consistent with outcomes achieved in conventional fixed-interval interventions [4, 6, 7, 30, 36]. Across a number of trials, fixed-interval sessions provided after the first 6 months of treatment resulted in the maintenance of approximately 66% of lost weight [4].

In the intensive lifestyle intervention of the Look AHEAD trial, which included periodic campaigns during maintenance in conjunction with other treatment components, weight losses were 8.5%, 6.3%, and 4.7% at 12-, 24-, and 48-months post-randomization, respectively [37]. Direct comparisons between Look AHEAD and the current trial are complicated by differing study designs (i.e., randomization occurring at baseline versus after initial weight reduction), different lengths of follow-up, and different target populations (i.e., adults with type 2 diabetes in Look AHEAD). However, the current 7–8 kg weight loss observed at month 4 and the maintenance of >7 kg weight loss observed at month 16 (i.e., 12 months post-randomization) are generally consistent with the first 2 years of follow-up in Look AHEAD.

Table 5 Linear regression analysis of percentage weight regain during the 12-month extended care program (Months 4 to 16) [a]

Independent Variable [b]	Weight Change, %		
	Parameter Est.	Std. Err	*P*-value
Treatment Condition	0.29	0.14	0.0396
Randomization Weight	<0.01	0.01	0.4582
Initial Weight Change	−0.06	0.02	0.0170
Age	<0.01	0.01	0.9578
Race	0.04	0.17	0.8106
Marital Status	0.21	0.14	0.1409
Education	0.10	0.14	0.4830

[a]Analyses are based on multiple imputation of missing data
[b]For categorical independent variables, the comparison level versus reference level are as follows: Treatment Condition (Clustered Campaign vs. Self-directed), Race (Non-Caucasian vs. Caucasian), Marital Status (Not-married vs. Married), Education (Bachelors or higher degree vs. Associates or lower degree)

Table 6 Likelihood of achieving ≥ 5% and ≥ 7% weight loss maintenance at month 16 in the clustered campaign versus self-directed condition[a]

Weight Loss	Odds Ratio Estimate[b]	95% Confidence Interval	*P*-value
≥5%	1.45	0.62–3.41	0.3959
≥7%	2.79	1.12–6.98	0.0283

[a]Analyses are based on multiple imputation of missing data
[b]Odds ratio estimates and *P*-values for treatment effect (Clustered campaign vs. Self-directed) were obtained from logistic regressions. Variables accounted for in each logistic model included: baseline weight at month 0, age, race, marital status and education. None of these variables was significant

The other trial most similar to the current one involved delivery of six, 8-week units of sessions that were separated by 4 weeks without contact [21]. While this novel timing of contacts seemed beneficial for weight loss maintenance in particular [21, 22], this alternative intervention included a number of other modifications that potentially impacted outcomes, including variety in the behavioral prescriptions, foci, and homework assignments of each unit as well as the use of structured financial incentives/contracts in one unit. Together, findings from the current trial and those observed by Jeffery, Levy, and colleagues [21, 22] support the potential value of a clustered campaign schedule of contacts to promote the maintenance of lost weight and highlight the need for additional research to more fully examine this approach.

Strengths and limitations

The study design and protocol adhered to a structured, intensive, evidence-based program consistent with current treatment guidelines [1]. Randomizing participants to maintenance and comparator conditions after completion of an initial program and achievement of a pre-specified weight loss criterion is consistent with current methodological recommendations [38] and other trials of weight loss maintenance [6, 7, 36]. In contrast, some trials randomize all participants at the beginning of treatment, which is appropriate for understanding overall, long-term weight change rather than weight loss maintenance in particular [38]. Each design has strengths and limitations, and randomizing a subset of the original sample may limit generalizability of findings to the broader population of individuals seeking weight loss treatment. In the current study, for example, only

35% of initially enrolled participants lost ≥5% to become eligible for randomization. In addition, only 53% of the original (pre-randomization) sample completed the initial, 4-month weight loss program. Although this protocol included evidence-based levels of contact during initial treatment, it provided minimal additional resources, make-up sessions, or other efforts to bolster attendance or adherence for those who were not initially responding to treatment. In addition, there was limited pre-screening of individuals and relatively modest exclusion criteria for enrollment, which contrasts with extensive screening procedures and behavioral run-in periods common to other weight loss trials (e.g., DPP, Look AHEAD).

The racially-balanced sample was a strength, as well as the high retention rate (89%) at follow-up. However, as 95% of participants were women, findings may not generalize to men. Furthermore, there were a high proportion of African American women, a group demonstrating more modest weight loss during the first few months of lifestyle interventions [39–41]. The current treatment response (i.e., 35% achieved pre-specified criterion of success) is lower than the 61% of participants who achieved a > 4-kg loss in the similarly-designed Weight Loss Maintenance (WLM) trial [36]. Compared to the WLM trial, however, the current trial included a higher proportion of African American women (51% vs. 32%), a shorter duration of initial treatment (16 vs. 20 weekly sessions), and a slightly different weight loss criterion (5% vs. 4 kg) [40].

Although the clustered campaigns may promote novelty and offer an alternative approach to a conventional fixed-interval schedule, the experimental treatment schedule is most accurately conceptualized as a modified, fixed-interval schedule. This schedule did not include unpredictable, variable contacts, and other schedules of contact may prove superior to the one examined here [13–15]. Also, the self-directed control condition does not provide a direct comparison of the clustered campaign to a conventional, fixed-interval schedule that is comparable in treatment intensity. Given the limited literature on differing contact schedules for extended care programs, this was designed as an initial test of a clustered campaign maintenance schedule isolated from the effects of other treatment components. Importantly, this initial test included a randomized design, which offers a more rigorous approach than a quasi-experimental or single-group study design. Thus, the current findings are a novel, methodologically-sound addition to the literature that offers a promising approach to promote weight loss maintenance that requires replication and further exploration. Furthermore, other behavioral and/or psychological changes that were not measured may have occurred during treatment and could potentially mediate or moderate the effects observed for weight loss. Finally, while the duration of extended care is consistent with other maintenance trials [4, 7, 9, 30, 42], it is unknown what would occur with the maintenance of lost weight beyond the 12-month extended care period.

Future research

This trial provides a promising first step in understanding the effects of an alternative schedule of contacts for extended care weight management programs. Future research directly comparing clustered campaign and fixed-interval schedules is needed to determine whether alternative extended care schedules minimize weight regain relative to conventional schedules of continued contact. Moreover, the examination of potential moderators and/or mediators of treatment effects are needed to understand why certain maintenance schedules may be advantageous. Alternative methods of delivering clustered campaign extended care treatment should be considered, including other schedules of contact and modalities of delivering treatment. The success with the clustered campaign approach for maintenance of weight loss in the current study raises the question of whether this approach may also be worthwhile for initial weight management treatment. Similarly, it may be useful to explore this approach for the maintenance of other behavioral changes prone to relapse that adhere to similar structured programs (e.g., smoking cessation).

Conclusions

In summary, these findings demonstrated that individuals who participated in an extended care intervention with a novel, clustered campaign delivery approach had better weight maintenance following an intensive lifestyle intervention than those who participated in a self-directed maintenance condition. Thus, extended care interventions for sustained weight loss may be efficaciously delivered via clustered campaign schedules or other alternative treatment schedules. Further research is needed to test these novel delivery methods against more conventional extended care delivery approaches to determine whether they have added weight maintenance or cost benefits.

Acknowledgements
Not applicable.

Funding
This work was supported by K23DK081607 and T32DK062710 from the National Institute of Diabetes and Digestive and Kidney Diseases (NIDDK).

Authors' contributions
GRD led the conceptualization and implementation of the study and led the interpretation of findings and writing of the manuscript. MAG contributed to initial drafting of the manuscript and interpretation of findings. FT and DZ led statistical analyses. JA, MGP, and CEL contributed to the design, conduct, and evaluation of the intervention. All authors contributed to the drafting of the manuscript and interpretation of study findings. All authors read and approved the final manuscript.

Competing interests

The authors declare that they have no competing interests.

Author details

[1]Division of Preventive Medicine, Department of Medicine, University of Alabama at Birmingham, Birmingham, AL, USA. [2]Department of Mathematical Sciences, Indiana University-Purdue University Indianapolis, Indianapolis, IN, USA. [3]Department of Epidemiology and Prevention, Wake Forest University School of Medicine, Winston Salem, NC, USA. [4]Department of Clinical and Health Psychology, University of Florida, Gainesville, FL, USA.

References

1. Jensen MD, Ryan DH, Apovian CM, Ard JD, Comuzzie AG, Donato KA, Hu FB, Hubbard VS, Jakicic JM, Kushner RF, et al. 2013 AHA/ACC/TOS guideline for the management of overweight and obesity in adults: a report of the American College of Cardiology/American Heart Association task force on practice guidelines and the Obesity Society. J Am Coll Cardiol. 2014;63(25 Pt B):2985–3023.
2. Butryn ML, Webb V, Wadden TA. Behavioral treatment of obesity. Psychiatr Clin North Am. 2011;34(4):841–59.
3. Institute of Medicine (IOM). Weighing the options: Criteria for evaluating weight management programs. Washington, DC: National Academy Press; 1995.
4. Perri MG, Corsica JA. Improving the maintenance of weight lost in behavioral treatment of obesity. In: Wadden TA, Stunkard AJ, editors. Handbook of Obesity Treatment. New York: Guilford; 2002. p. 357–79.
5. Dutton GR, Perri MG. Delivery, Evaluation, and Future Directions for Cognitive Behavioral Treatments of Obesity. In: Wadden TA, Stunkard AJ, editors. The Oxford Handbook of Cognitive and Behavioral Therapies. New York: Oxford University Press; 2015. p. 419–37.
6. Wing RR, Tate DF, Gorin AA, Raynor HA, Fava JL. A self-regulation program for maintenance of weight loss. N Engl J Med. 2006;355(15):1563–71.
7. Perri MG, Limacher MC, Durning PE, Janicke DM, Lutes LD, Bobroff LB, Dale MS, Daniels MJ, Radcliff TA, Martin AD. Extended-care programs for weight management in rural communities: the treatment of obesity in underserved rural settings (TOURS) randomized trial. Arch Intern Med. 2008;168(21):2347–54.
8. Perri MG, McAdoo WG, McAllister DA, Lauer JB, Jordan RC, Yancey DZ, Nezu AM. Effects of peer support and therapist contact on long-term weight loss. J Consult Clin Psychol. 1987;55(4):615–7.
9. Perri MG, Nezu AM, McKelvey WF, Shermer RL, Renjilian DA, Viegener BJ. Relapse prevention training and problem-solving therapy in the long-term management of obesity. J Consult Clin Psychol. 2001;69(4):722–6.
10. Perri MG, Sears SF Jr, Clark JE. Strategies for improving maintenance of weight loss. Toward a continuous care model of obesity management. Diabetes Care. 1993;16(1):200–9.
11. Middleton KM, Patidar SM, Perri MG. The impact of extended care on the long-term maintenance of weight loss: a systematic review and meta-analysis. Obes Rev. 2012;13(6):509–17.
12. Dombrowski SU, Knittle K, Avenell A, Araujo-Soares V, Sniehotta FF. Long term maintenance of weight loss with non-surgical interventions in obese adults: systematic review and meta-analyses of randomised controlled trials. BMJ. 2014;348:g2646.
13. Voils CI, King HA, Maciejewski ML, Allen KD, Yancy WS Jr, Shaffer JA. Approaches for informing optimal dose of behavioral interventions. Ann Behav Med. 2014;48(3):392–401.
14. Ferster C, Nurnberger J, Levitt E. The control of eating. J Mathetics. 1962;1: 87–109.
15. Stuart R. Behavioral control of overeating. Behav Res Ther. 1967;5:357–65.
16. Wadden TA, Foster GD. Behavioral treatment of obesity. Med Clin North Am. 2000;84(2):441–61. vii
17. Kanfer F, Goldstein A: Helping people change: a textbook of methods. 1975.
18. Brownell KD, Marlatt GA, Lichtenstein E, Wilson GT. Understanding and preventing relapse. Am Psychol. 1986;41(7):765–82.
19. DiMatteo MR. Variations in patients' adherence to medical recommendations: a quantitative review of 50 years of research. Med Care. 2004;42(3):200–9.
20. Cramer JA, Scheyer RD, Mattson RH. Compliance declines between clinic visits. Arch Intern Med. 1990;150(7):1509–10.
21. Jeffery RW, Levy RL, Langer SL, Welsh EM, Flood AP, Jaeb MA, Laqua PS, Hotop AM, Finch EA. A comparison of maintenance-tailored therapy (MTT) and standard behavior therapy (SBT) for the treatment of obesity. Prev Med. 2009;49(5):384–9.
22. Levy RL, Jeffery RW, Langer SL, Graham DJ, Welsh EM, Flood AP, Jaeb MA, Laqua PS, Finch EA, Hotop AM, et al. Maintenance-tailored therapy vs. standard behavior therapy for 30-month maintenance of weight loss. Prev Med. 2010;51(6):457–9.
23. Fisher EB, Jeffery RW, Absetz P, Oldenburg B. Sustaining behavior change in health promotion, diabetes prevention and management, and weight loss. Ann Behav Med. 2008;35(Suppl):s96.
24. Jeffery RW, Kelly KM, Rothman AJ, Sherwood NE, Boutelle KN. The weight loss experience: a descriptive analysis. Ann Behav Med. 2004;27(2):100–6.
25. Wadden TA, Butryn ML, Byrne KJ. Efficacy of lifestyle modification for long-term weight control. Obes Res. 2004;12(Suppl):151S–62S.
26. Wing RR, Jeffery RW. Prescribed "breaks" as a means to disrupt weight control efforts. Obes Res. 2003;11(2):287–91.
27. Look Ahead Research Group, Wadden TA, West DS, Delahanty L, Jakicic J, Rejeski J, Williamson D, Berkowitz RI, Kelley DE, Tomchee C, et al. The look AHEAD study: a description of the lifestyle intervention and the evidence supporting it. Obesity. 2006;14(5):737–52.
28. Diabetes Prevention Program Research G. The diabetes prevention program (DPP): description of lifestyle intervention. Diabetes Care. 2002;25(12):2165–71.
29. Perri MG, Limacher MC, von Castel-Roberts K, Daniels MJ, Durning PE, Janicke DM, Bobroff LB, Radcliff TA, Milsom VA, Kim C, et al. Comparative effectiveness of three doses of weight-loss counseling: two-year findings from the rural LITE trial. Obesity. 2014;22(11):2293–300.
30. West DS, Gorin AA, Subak LL, Foster G, Bragg C, Hecht J, Schembri M, Wing RR, Program to Reduce Incontinence by D, Exercise Research G. A motivation-focused weight loss maintenance program is an effective alternative to a skill-based approach. Int J Obes. 2011;35(2):259–69.
31. Wing RR, Koeske R, Epstein LH, Nowalk MP, Gooding W, Becker D. Long-term effects of modest weight loss in type II diabetic patients. Arch Intern Med. 1987;147(10):1749–53.
32. Jeffery RW, Sherwood NE, Brelje K, Pronk NP, Boyle R, Boucher JL, Hase K. Mail and phone interventions for weight loss in a managed-care setting: weigh-to-be one-year outcomes. Int J Obes Relat Metab Disord. 2003;27(12):1584–92.
33. Wylie-Rosett J, Swencionis C, Ginsberg M, Cimino C, Wassertheil-Smoller S, Caban A, Segal-Isaacson CJ, Martin T, Lewis J. Computerized weight loss intervention optimizes staff time: the clinical and cost results of a controlled clinical trial conducted in a managed care setting. J Am Diet Assoc. 2001; 101(10):1155–62. quiz 1163-1154
34. Elobeid MA, Padilla MA, McVie T, Thomas O, Brock DW, Musser B, Lu K, Coffey CS, Desmond RA, St-Onge MP, et al. Missing data in randomized clinical trials for weight loss: scope of the problem, state of the field, and performance of statistical methods. PLoS One. 2009;4(8):e6624.
35. R: A Language and Environment for Statistical Computing [http://www.R-project.org].
36. Svetkey LP, Stevens VJ, Brantley PJ, Appel LJ, Hollis JF, Loria CM, Vollmer WM, Gullion CM, Funk K, Smith P, et al. Comparison of strategies for sustaining weight loss: the weight loss maintenance randomized controlled trial. JAMA. 2008;299(10):1139–48.
37. The Look Ahead Research Group. Long term effects of a lifestyle intervention on weight and cardiovascular risk factors in individuals with type 2 diabetes: four year results of the look AHEAD trial. Arch Intern Med. 2010;170(17):1566–75.
38. MacLean PS, Wing RR, Davidson T, Epstein L, Goodpaster B, Hall KD, Levin BE, Perri MG, Rolls BJ, Rosenbaum M, et al. NIH working group report: innovative research to improve maintenance of weight loss. Obesity. 2015; 23(1):7–15.
39. Rickel KA, Milsom VA, Ross KM, Hoover VJ, Peterson ND, Perri MG. Differential response of African American and Caucasian women to extended-care programs for obesity management. Ethn Dis. 2011;21(2):170–5.
40. Hollis JF, Gullion CM, Stevens VJ, Brantley PJ, Appel LJ, Ard JD, Champagne CM, Dalcin A, Erlinger TP, Funk K, et al. Weight loss during the intensive intervention phase of the weight-loss maintenance trial. Am J Prev Med. 2008;35(2):118–26.
41. West DS, Elaine Prewitt T, Bursac Z, Felix HC. Weight loss of black, white, and Hispanic men and women in the diabetes prevention program. Obesity. 2008;16(6):1413–20.
42. Harvey-Berino J, Pintauro S, Buzzell P, Gold EC. Effect of internet support on the long-term maintenance of weight loss. Obes Res. 2004;12(2):320–9.

13

Food parenting practices for 5 to 12 year old children: a concept map analysis of parenting and nutrition experts input

Teresia M. O'Connor[1*], Louise C. Mâsse[2], Andrew W. Tu[3], Allison W. Watts[4], Sheryl O. Hughes[1], Mark R. Beauchamp[5], Tom Baranowski[1], Truc Pham[1], Jerica M. Berge[6], Barbara Fiese[7], Rebecca Golley[8], Melanie Hingle[9], Stef P. J. Kremers[10], Kyung E. Rhee[11], Helen Skouteris[12] and Amber Vaughn[13]

Abstract

Background: Parents are an important influence on children's dietary intake and eating behaviors. However, the lack of a conceptual framework and inconsistent assessment of food parenting practices limits our understanding of which food parenting practices are most influential on children. The aim of this study was to develop a food parenting practice conceptual framework using systematic approaches of literature reviews and expert input.

Method: A previously completed systematic review of food parenting practice instruments and a qualitative study of parents informed the development of a food parenting practice item bank consisting of 3632 food parenting practice items. The original item bank was further reduced to 110 key food parenting concepts using binning and winnowing techniques. A panel of 32 experts in parenting and nutrition were invited to sort the food parenting practice concepts into categories that reflected their perceptions of a food parenting practice conceptual framework. Multi-dimensional scaling produced a point map of the sorted concepts and hierarchical cluster analysis identified potential solutions. Subjective modifications were used to identify two potential solutions, with additional feedback from the expert panel requested.

Results: The experts came from 8 countries and 25 participated in the sorting and 23 provided additional feedback. A parsimonious and a comprehensive concept map were developed based on the clustering of the food parenting practice constructs. The parsimonious concept map contained 7 constructs, while the comprehensive concept map contained 17 constructs and was informed by a previously published content map for food parenting practices. Most of the experts (52%) preferred the comprehensive concept map, while 35% preferred to present both solutions.

Conclusion: The comprehensive food parenting practice conceptual map will provide the basis for developing a calibrated Item Response Modeling (IRM) item bank that can be used with computerized adaptive testing. Such an item bank will allow for more consistency in measuring food parenting practices across studies to better assess the impact of food parenting practices on child outcomes and the effect of interventions that target parents as agents of change.

Keywords: Food, Nutrition, Child, Parenting, Parenting practices, Family, Concept mapping, Measurement

* Correspondence: teresiao@bcm.edu
[1]USDA/ARS Children's Nutrition Research Center, Baylor College of Medicine, 1100 Bates St, Houston, TX, USA
Full list of author information is available at the end of the article

Background

Most children's eating patterns and behaviors are shaped by family influences and ultimately can have an important impact on their weight status [1–3]. Research designed to better understand how parents influence their children's eating has grown over the past two decades and has resulted in over 75 published articles related to the development of unique food parenting instruments [4]. Most of this work has focused on food parenting practices, or the specific goal-directed parent actions designed to influence children's eating behaviors or dietary intake [5]. With this growing number of available instruments, there is little consensus on how to measure food parenting practices, including which instrument to use and how food parenting constructs relate to or correlate with each other. This significantly limits our ability to evaluate the relationships between various food parenting constructs and children's intake or weight status; or compare findings across studies [6, 7].

Proposed ways to advance or improve the measurement of food parenting practices on children's eating behaviors and dietary intake include using direct or video observational methods [8] or employing digital technologies or simulations [6]. However, many large descriptive cross-sectional or prospective studies, or interventions will not be able to utilize such assessments due to the associated costs or burden on participants. Enhancing the ways in which behavioral and public health scientists can reliably and validly assess food parenting practices in a standard way via self-report is vital to advancing the field. One method for improving and standardizing the measurement of latent constructs measured by self-report is Item Response Modeling (IRM) of an item bank, supplemented with computerized adaptive testing [6, 9, 10]. In this approach, a bank of items that assesses the latent construct is developed and calibrated by IRM analysis. Computer adaptive testing of the calibrated item bank allows researchers to select all or a subset of the calibrated items to use, while maintaining the ability to compare the resulting score for the latent construct across studies. For a complex idea with multiple constructs, such as those that correspond to food parenting practices, a conceptual framework is needed to inform how the food parenting practice constructs are operationalized. While a content map for food parenting practices has recently been proposed [11], there is no tested consensus for how specific food parenting practice concepts or corresponding items fit within each construct of the proposed framework. To inform this process, this study aimed to develop a food parenting practice conceptual framework for parents with children 5–12 years old based on an existing systematically derived item bank of food parenting practices [4] using i) an online card sort task conducted by an international sample of experts of food parenting and feeding, followed by ii) a concept mapping analysis of the resulting grouping of food parenting concepts into constructs and a larger framework. The long-term goal of this project is to develop a calibrated IRM item bank that can be used with computerized adaptive testing and can be utilized by other researchers in the food parenting field internationally.

Method

Identification of expert panel

Scientific experts were recruited to help develop the conceptual framework. Experts were defined as researchers who have either a) developed nutrition-based, family interventions aimed at treating or preventing childhood obesity and/or modifying dietary behaviors; or b) studied the role of parenting and nutrition in the etiology of childhood obesity. A list of experts was created by reviewing: 1) the membership list of the International Society of Behavioral Nutrition and Physical Activity (ISBNPA); 2) the list of attendees to the 2012 pre-ISBNPA workshop focused on improving measures of physical activity and food parenting practices; 3) recent publications on food parenting practices through searches on PubMed, ERIC, PsycINFO, and ScienceDirect; and 4) asking our network of researchers for additional suggestions. In total 32 experts were identified and 25 experts from 8 countries (Australia, Canada, Finland, Japan, Mexico, Netherlands, UK, and USA) agreed to participate (78% response rate). All experts were offered an honorarium ($150) for their participation. The sorting task included participation of 28 experts, the 25 outside experts and three primary members of the research team (*TB, TMO, and SOH*) who did not conduct the statistical analysis. The protocol was approved by the Institutional Review Boards at the University of British Columbia and Baylor College of Medicine.

Identification, reduction and sorting of food parenting practices

An overview of the methods of this study can be found in Fig. 1. Previous work by our group [4] systematically identified published food parenting instruments and supplemented the published items with additional items reported by parents to populate a food parenting practice item bank. Briefly, published articles containing at least one scale on parenting or caregiver behaviors related to 2 to 16 year old children's eating, nutrition, or food intake were extracted from 1) articles identified from two recent systematic reviews; [12, 13] 2) an additional systematic review of articles published between January 2009 and March 2013 in PubMed, ERIC, PsycINFO, and ScienceDirect; [4] and 3) reviewing and back-tracing the reference of articles from steps 1 and 2. The broader age range for

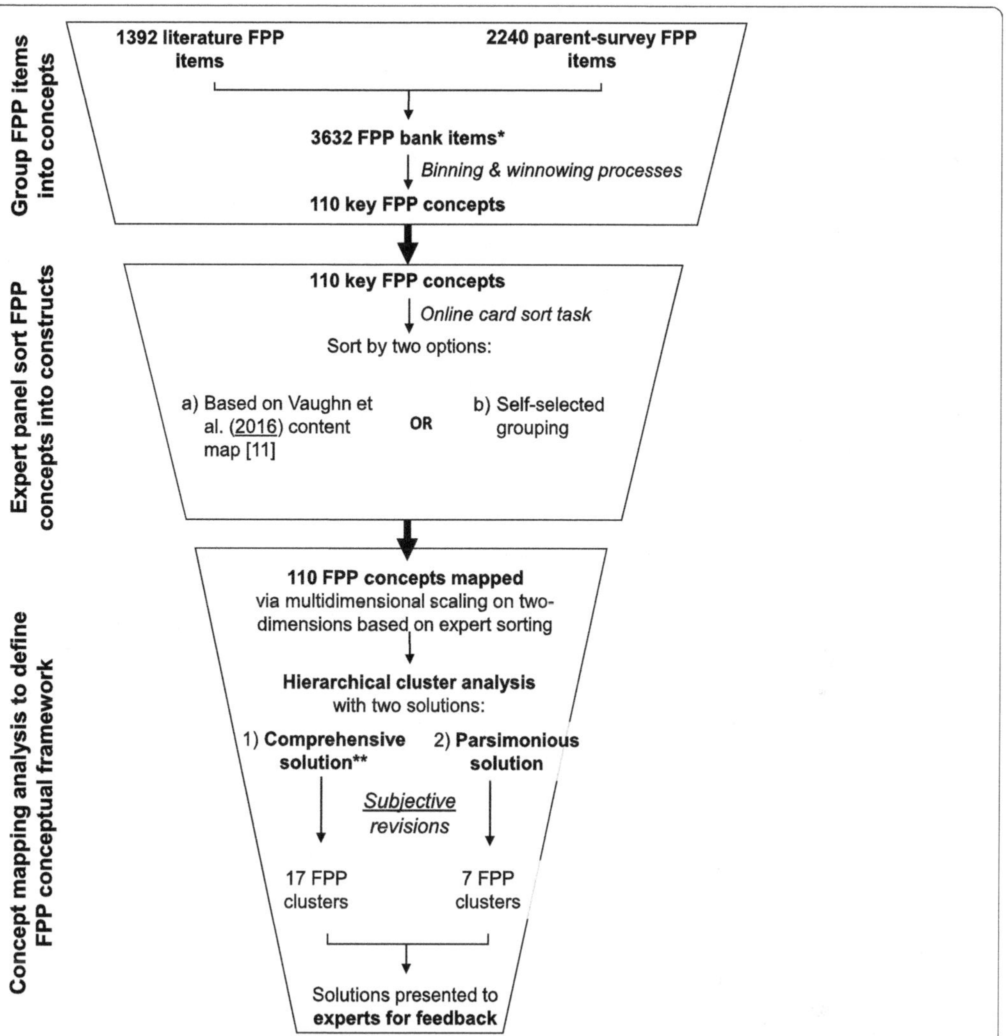

Fig. 1 Overview of the Methods to Develop the Food Parenting Practice (FPP) Concept Map. *Based on systematic item bank and first round of binning/winnowing published by O'Connor et al. [4]. **Based on content map published by Vaughn et al. [11]

the review compared to the ultimate target age range of the item bank (5–12 year old children) was selected in order to capture a wide range of items. A total of 79 measures were identified consisting of 1392 items measuring food parenting practices [4]. To ensure data saturation of food parenting practices for the item bank, 135 parents who reflected the socio-economic and ethnic diversity specific to Canada and the US, were surveyed by an online polling firm (YouGovPolimetrix, USA) about food parenting practices they have used or think other parents use [4]. They contributed 2240 valid (1985 unique, after removal of duplicates) food parenting practices, many that overlapped with published items [4]. To reduce the 3632 food parenting practice items identified from the published literature and parent reports and make the sorting task manageable for the experts, the binning and winnowing process, developed by the NIH PROMIS initiative was used [9, 10]. "Binning," or grouping similar food parenting practice items, consisted of assigning the items from the literature review and responses from the parent survey to one of 19 primary codes and a subsequent secondary code [4]. "Winnowing" or removing redundant items consisted of reviewing each bin and consolidating redundant items. The binning and winnowing process was conducted by two research members independently with all discrepancies triangulated by two other members of the research team until a consensus was reached among all four. Two rounds of binning and winnowing of the initial 1392 items found in the literature and the 2240 parent responses took place (see previously published work for first round) [4] and the final round resulted in 110 key parenting practice concepts. A food *parenting practice concept* could represent a number of food parenting practice *items*. For example, one food parenting practice concept was "I reward my child with something tasty (e.g., dessert) as a way to get him/her to eat [food]" where food could represent "healthy food", "all his dinner", or "fruits and vegetables". This concept represented a total of 43 items from the published literature or statements from parent report. The food parenting practice concepts were then grouped into food parenting practice *constructs* via Expert Panel sorting.

The participating experts were invited to sort the 110 key food parenting practice concepts into meaningful groups or constructs using the web-based Concept Mapping software (Concept Systems Inc., Ithaca, NY). To take advantage of existing substantial conceptual interpretation of food parenting practices, each expert was provided a copy of the previously published Vaughn et al. 2016 content map [11] prior to sorting and instructed to a) utilize the framework to guide their sorting and/or b) to propose a different grouping of food parenting practice concepts. The published content framework grouped food parenting practices into 19 constructs stemming from three larger domains: control, structure and autonomy promotion based on the authors' critical appraisal of the literature [11].

In addition to sorting the concepts into meaningful groups, the experts were asked to name the groups they created. They were also instructed to not group unique practices together (i.e., create a miscellaneous group of leftover practices), but instead create groups of single food parenting practice concepts if only one practice fit within the group. The sorting conducted by the experts was reviewed to ensure that each expert sorted all 110 statements and that no miscellaneous group was formed. One expert did create a miscellaneous group of 10 food parenting practice concepts. Follow up with this expert, resulted in all those concepts being sorted into existing or new categories.

Analysis

Analysis of the sorting was conducted using non-parametric multidimensional scaling (MDS) [14]. A two-dimensional solution was used to assign each food parenting practice concept an x/y coordinate on a point map. Food parenting practice concepts that appeared spatially closer to one another on the point map were grouped by the experts closer together and therefore may represent a similar construct. Acceptable stress values for MDS analysis typically range from 0.205 to 0.365 when used to develop a conceptual framework [15], as opposed to when used in controlled psychometric evaluations, which typically necessitate lower stress values (note that the MDS stress value for our solution was 0.267 and within acceptable range) [16].

A hierarchical cluster analysis was then conducted to identify clusters of food parenting practice concepts from the MDS derived point map. Specifically, the hierarchical cluster analysis was carried out on the x/y coordinates which were obtained from the MDS analysis. The concept mapping software utilizes the Ward's algorithm for the cluster analysis because it: 1) retains the location of the x/y coordinates in the final solution; 2) creates non overlapping constructs; and 3) merges clusters based on the distance of all individual statements instead of using the centroid of a cluster [14].

We adapted the procedure outlined by Trochim [14] to identify the appropriate number of clusters to retain in our solution. Trochim's approach to identify the number of clusters retained in the solution is iterative but essentially starts by: 1) reviewing an initial cluster solution that is derived statistically with more clusters that would be anticipated; 2) adding more clusters one at a time until it makes no theoretical sense to combine clusters; 3) qualitatively reviewing the statistical solution to refine and fine-tune the shape of the clusters; and 4) having experts review the solution and provide further input into the analyses. As we aimed to identify two potential solutions, we refined this process for the following two solutions: 1) a parsimonious solution and 2) a solution that approximated the Vaughn et al., 2016 content map [11] (referred herein as the comprehensive solution). The parsimonious solution was identified by first evaluating the simplest cluster analysis-generated solution and determining whether adding another cluster based on the cluster analysis made conceptual sense. This process iteratively continued and stopped when it did not make sense to add further clusters. This solution was not constrained by a pre-determined conceptual framework but aimed to identify a parsimonious solution, meaning we looked for larger clusters that contained related food parenting practice concepts. The solution was then examined and subjectively modified to integrate the team's consensus solution of the two-dimensional point map. Specifically, the content of each cluster was examined, with emphasis on food parenting practice concepts at the border of each cluster to assess whether it could better fit with another cluster, prioritizing neighboring clusters when appropriate. This iterative process continued until the final solution was obtained.

We identified the comprehensive solution by using the Vaughn et al. 2016 content map [11] to initially examine a larger than expected cluster solution. We arbitrarily started by examining the 28-cluster solution and then determined whether reducing the cluster analysis derived solution into fewer clusters made conceptual sense based on the Vaughn's content map. We proceeded until merging could no longer be supported by the framework. Again, after we identified a statistical solution (potential number of clusters to retain), we subjectively reviewed the solution to determine an optimal solution that integrated the MDS results and the subjective evaluation of the two-dimensional point map using the same procedure described above. Three members of the research team (TO, LCM & AT) independently conducted these subjective analyses and their consensus solution was presented to the primary team of investigators (SH, MB, and TB) who provided initial feedback for modification and agreed on a solution to be presented to the Expert Group. We presented the two solutions to the Expert Group who were asked to select their preferred solution and provide feedback and suggestions on that solution. One last round of modifications to both solutions was conducted based on the expert's feedback until consensus was reached among the authors.

Results

Expert sorting

The 28 participating Experts sorted the food parenting practice concepts into 3–28 categories, with a mean (standard deviation) of 18.1 (6.5) and mode of 19 food parenting practice categories. Six Experts sorted the food parenting practices concepts into 19 categories, the same number as presented by the Vaughn et al. 2016 content map [11]. Of those, there was overlap in the names of 5–19 constructs (mean 14.7, stand dev 5.8) with the content map, with only two having exactly the same structure (19/19 constructs) as the proposed content map [11]. It is not known how many elected to use the published content guide to inform their sorting. However, in reviewing the names of categories proposed by the Experts, many used at least some of the same construct names while adding to and/or deleting food constructs for their final solution.

Expert preference for proposed solutions

Both the parsimonious and the comprehensive concepts map solutions were presented to the original experts who participated in the sorting task. Of the 27 eligible expert respondents (TMO was excluded because she managed the responses), 23 responded (85.2%). The comprehensive concept map informed by the published content map [11] (Fig. 2) was preferred by 52% of experts, and another 35% preferred to present both solutions. Based on these preferences, we include the comprehensive concept map informed by the published content map within this article,

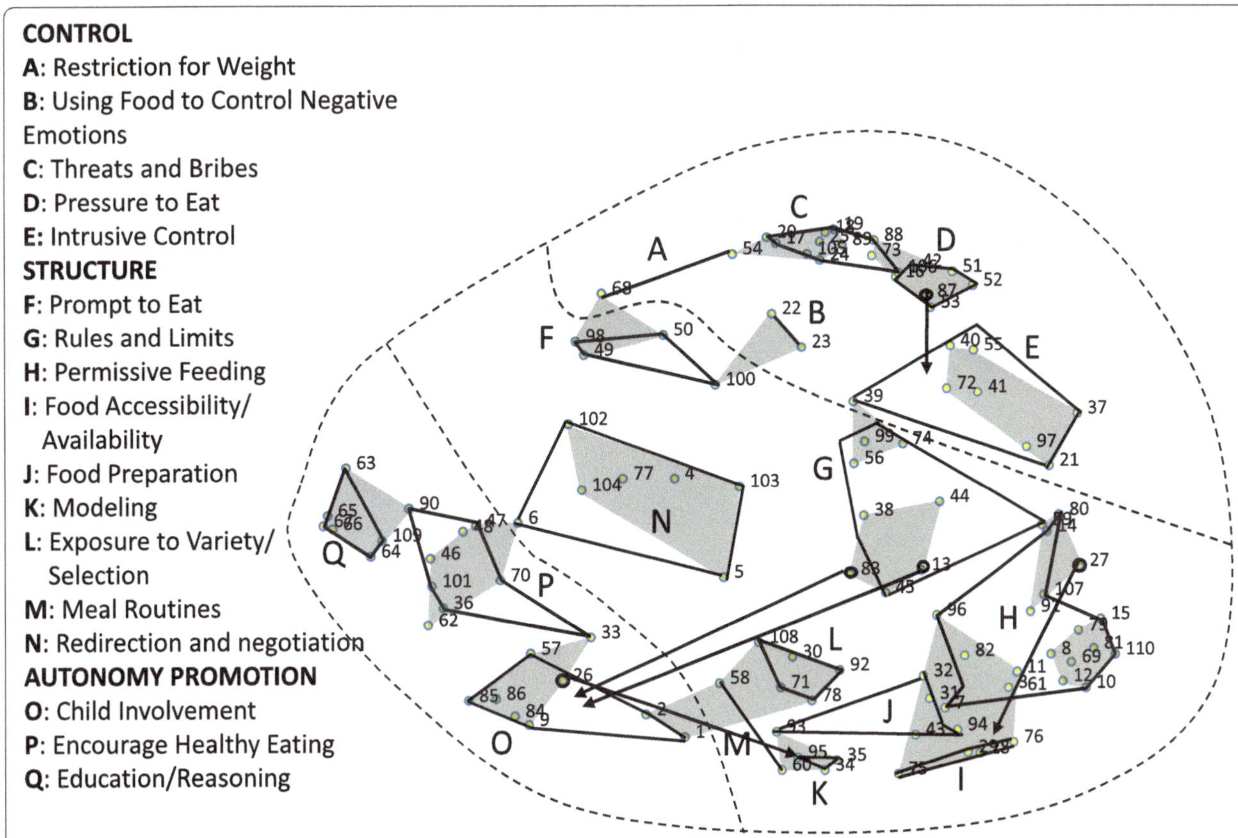

The point map was generated from hierarchical cluster analysis and non-parametric multidimensional scaling of categories generated by 28 experts in food parenting from a list of 110 parenting concepts. Gray shaded regions demonstrate the original 16 cluster solution proposed by the cluster analysis, and the black outlined areas define the proposed 17 clusters.

Fig. 2 Comprehensive solution for food parenting statements subjectively grouped into clusters, informed by the hierarchical cluster analysis and a published framework (Vaughn et al. [11]).

but have made the parsimonious solution available online in an Additional file 1.

Experts reported they preferred the comprehensive solution because it was more theoretically based and the specific differentiation of food parenting practices had promise for better informing which food parenting practices were most important in influencing child eating behaviors. The most common reason for preferring to present both solutions was that the two frameworks had the potential for serving different purposes, with the comprehensive solution being more applicable to researchers in this area and the parsimonious solution being useful for those who try to operationalize promoting these practices in obesity prevention programs or policy statements. A few experts suggested future work may be able to integrate the two models into one model, with a more parsimonious global solution and detailed "sub-factors" embedded within the parsimonious constructs.

The Comprehensive conceptual framework of food parenting practices

The comprehensive food parenting practices concept map based on the published content map [11] resulted in an 17-cluster solution from a statistically derived 16 cluster solution (see Fig. 2 with concepts, construct names, and definitions listed in Table 1) with subjective modifications. Vaughn et al., proposed grouping food parenting practices into three larger overarching domains: Control, Structure, and Autonomy Promotion [11]. Figure 2 illustrates how the comprehensive concept map potentially supports these same three overarching dimensions.

Most of the food parenting practice constructs under each dimension defined by Vaughn and colleagues' content map [11] appear to also cluster on the comprehensive concept map (Fig. 2). All four Coercive Control constructs identified on the content map were spatially close and therefore labeled to belong to Control on the comprehensive concept map: Restriction (A), Using Food to Control Negative Emotions (B), Threats & Bribes (C), and Pressure to Eat (D). One notable difference in our solution was the construct of Restriction (A) was specific for controlling weight, whereas in the content map Restriction was a more general concept. Another difference was the addition of a new construct under Control, termed Intrusive Control (E). This construct included demanding and directive concepts where the parent dictated what and how much the child should eat. These demanding and directive concepts were distinct from pressuring the child to eat more, as seen in Pressure to Eat (D), and from the guidelines and boundaries that parents set, found in the Rules and Limits construct (G) under the Structure dimension. Intrusive Control was therefore made into a new construct. It was included in the Control domain because the focus was on parents dictating to the child without child input.

The proposed content map [11] identified nine constructs under Structure, of which six were identified in the comprehensive concept map solution: Rules and Limits (G), Food Availability and Accessibility (I), Food Preparation (J), Modeling (K), Meal Routines (M), and Permissive (H) (or "unstructured practices" as termed by Vaughn et al. [11].) The Availability and Accessibility construct was separated into two constructs by Vaughn et al. [11], however, the comprehensive concept map solution collapsed it into one construct. In the comprehensive concept map, there was a lack of a distinct Monitoring category in the Structure dimension as defined by the published content map, which may be due to the multiple published items on monitoring being condensed down into one monitoring concept (# 38) for this sorting task. In the solution presented here it falls into the Rules and Limit construct, but future studies will need to assess whether it should be a separate construct in the Structure dimension.

Different from Vaughn's et al. content map, three new categories were identified in the comprehensive concept map under the Structure dimension: Prompt to Eat (F), Exposure to a Variety/Selection (L) and Redirection & Negotiation (N). Upon review of the solution, some experts identified similarities of the concepts clustered in Prompt to Eat to concepts clustered under Pressure to Eat. However, the two clusters were spatially separate from each other on the map. Therefore, Prompt to Eat was identified as a distinct construct from Pressure to Eat and reflected more gentle reminders for a child to eat, as opposed to pushing the child to eat beyond satiety as seen in Pressure to eat. This difference suggests that the Experts may distinguish varying degrees of how parents remind or push their child to eat and some Experts felt that Prompt to Eat was a form of Structure instead of Control. Exposure to a Variety/Selection was not identified by the published content map but concepts that clustered into this construct spatially fell into the Structure dimension on the comprehensive concept map. On face validity, these concepts may be an extension of availability, but the concepts were spatially separate from the Availability and Accessibility construct on the map and therefore made into a new construct. Redirection & Negotiation was also not a construct in the content map proposed by Vaughn et al., but does have some overlap with the content map's Limited/Guided Choices (which was not present in the solution presented in Fig. 2). Future work will need to explore the overlap and differences between these two constructs.

The Autonomy Promotion dimension had the most differences between the comprehensive concept map and the previously proposed content map [11]. Similar

Table 1 110 food parenting concepts grouped into 17 clusters based on qualitative cluster assignment informed by published Food Parenting Framework [11] of expert's sorting (corresponds with Fig. 2)

Concept Number	Food Parenting Practice Concept	Hierarchal Analysis Point MapCluster Assignment[a]	Qualitative Content Map Cluster Assignment	Definition
Control				
54	I restrict my child's food intake to control his/her weight.	3	A: Restriction for Weight	Due to concern for child's weight, parent restricts access to or discourages consumption of certain foods, large portions, multiple servings, or frequent snacks.
68	I tell my child to avoid certain food or drinks as they can make him/her fat.	1		
22	I use food to soothe my child.	2	B: Using Food to Control Negative Emotions	"Parent uses food to manage or calm the child when he/she is upset, fussy, angry, hurt, or bored." [11]
23	I give my child food to keep him/her occupied.	2		
17	I reward my child with something tasty (e.g. dessert) as a way to get him/her to eat [food/healthy food/all his/her dinner].	3	C: Threats and Bribes	Parent threatens to take or takes something away for misbehavior or promises/offers something to the child to coerce them into desired behavior. Threats and bribes related to food include those used to manage child's general behavior by using food as reward or threat; or using threats or bribes to influence the child's eating behaviors. (modified from Vaughn et al.) [11]
18	I tell my child that I will take away privileges (e.g., screen time) if s/he does not eat (./healthy food type).	3		
19	I punish my child (e.g., send away from table, spank) if s/he does not want to finish his/her plate, taste a food, or eat fruit or vegetables.	3		
20	I promise my child [unhealthy food] as a reward for good behavior.	3		
24	I scold or show disapproval when my child eats too much.	3		
25	I show disapproval by arguing with or yelling at my child for not eating [healthy food].	3		
73	I use scare tactics to discourage my child from eating unhealthy foods.	4		
88	I use threats to get my child to eat.	4		
89	I make my child feel guilty when s/he doesn't eat vegetables or finish his/her meal.	3		
105	I withhold dessert as a consequence for bad behavior.	3		
106	I discipline my child if s/he consumes an unhealthy food/drinks without my permission.	4		
16	I make sure my child eats [all their dinner/all their fruits/vegetables] before s/he can have dessert.	4	D: Pressure to Eat	Parent is forceful or demanding in order to push the child to eat food, when child is either not interested in eating, not hungry, or does not want to eat or taste the food that is served during a meal or snack. The parent does not take into consideration the child's current hunger or satiety, nor the child's food preferences. (modified from Vaughn et al.) [11]

Table 1 110 food parenting concepts grouped into 17 clusters based on qualitative cluster assignment informed by published Food Parenting Framework [11] of expert's sorting (corresponds with Fig. 2) *(Continued)*

42	I beg my child to eat (./at least something from his/her plate).	4		
51	I make my child eat all the food on his/her plate.	4		
52	I get my child to eat more vegetables, even if s/he says "I'm not hungry."	4		
53	I insist/force my child to "try one bite" or taste a [food/healthy food].	4		
21	I trick my child into eating [healthy food] by mixing it with other food or disguising it.	5	E: Intrusive Control	Parent dictates how and what the child should eat. Parent tells their child what to do and expects their child to comply without question. (NEW)
37	I tell my child to eat [healthy food] or not eat [unhealthy food/drinks] but do not follow this myself.	5		
39	I decide what my child should eat (./at meals/snacks).	6		
40	I don't allow my child to eat more than I think s/he should.	5		
41	I make my child eat [healthy food] every day.	5		
55	If my child eats more than usual at one meal, I try to restrict his/her eating at the next meal.	5		
72	I make my child eat his/her fruit and vegetables first at mealtimes or snacks.	5		
87	I criticize my child about the food s/he eats.	4		
97	I decide when my child eats his/her meals and snacks.	5		
Structure				
49	I have to strongly encourage my child to eat foods that are good for him/her.	1	F: Prompt to Eat	Parent suggests to the child or prompts the child to eat food without being forceful and without consequence. There is no focus on eating beyond satiety. There is an emphasis on promoting to eat nutritious food. (NEW)
50	I encourage my child to eat all the food on his/her plate.	1		
98	I try to convince my child to eat fruit or vegetables instead of cake or candy.	1		
100	I tell my child to eat fruit and vegetables.	2		
38	I monitor or keep track of the [healthy/unhealthy food/drinks] my child eats/drinks.	7	G: Rules and Limits	Parent has and makes known expectations, guidelines, or boundaries for how much or what kind of foods the child eats, maintains the timing or routine of meals, or promotes a certain order in which foods are eaten. The parent can monitor whether the child sticks to the rules. (modified from Vaughn et al.) [11]

Table 1 110 food parenting concepts grouped into 17 clusters based on qualitative cluster assignment informed by published Food Parenting Framework [11] of expert's sorting (corresponds with Fig. 2) *(Continued)*

44	I do not allow my child to eat or drink an hour before meals or after a certain hour of the day.	7		
45	I ask others not to give my child unhealthy food (candy, sweets, salty snacks).	7		
56	I limit or do not allow my child to eat/drink certain [unhealthy food/drinks].	6		
59	I insist my child eat meals/snacks at the table.	8		
74	If I allow my child an unhealthy meal/snack the next meal snack must be healthy.	6		
99	If my child eats junk food, s/he must also include something healthy.	6		
11	I allow my child to have whatever sweets and snacks s/he chooses at social occasions or to celebrate an achievement.	10	H: Permissive Feeding	"Parent allows child complete control of their eating, including timing and frequency of meals and snacks, and amount and type of foods eaten." [11] Parent does not impose limits and will provide different foods for the child from what the rest of the family eats based on the child's preferences and whims. Parent facilitates less nutritious food selection by keeping those in the home or taking the child place those foods are served.
14	I serve dessert to my child if s/he is no longer hungry for her/his main dish but is willing to eat dessert.	8		
61	I take my child to eat at fast food places.	10		
79	I serve/offer unhealthy foods [at meals/snacks/for dessert].	9		
91	I offer my child seconds.	8		
96	I eat/drink unhealthy foods/drinks with my child.	10		
3	I give my child money to buy food (snacks, treats, or meals).	10		
7	I allow my child to eat whenever s/he is hungry or shows signs of hunger.	10		
8	I allow my child to buy [unhealthy food type] if s/he wants it as a snack or meal.	9		
10	I serve what my child demands at meals.	9		
12	I make or allow my child to make something else if s/he does not like what is served.	9		
15	I give into my child's food demands (./after saying no)	9		

Table 1 110 food parenting concepts grouped into 17 clusters based on qualitative cluster assignment informed by published Food Parenting Framework [11] of expert's sorting (corresponds with Fig. 2) *(Continued)*

69	I allow my child to eat unhealthy when we are away from home (e.g., doing errands, driving to practices).	9		
80	I allow my child to have seconds if s/he finishes foods from his/her plate at dinner.	8		
81	I let my child eat unhealthy food whenever s/he wants.	9		
82	I let my child substitute a food s/he does not like for one s/he likes.	10		
107	I allow my child to skip meals.	8		
110	I allow my child to eat unhealthy when we are on vacation.	9		
27	I hide or intentionally keep less [healthful food/drinks] out of my child's reach.	27	I: Food Accessibility/ Availability	The amount and types of foods that a parent brings into the home; or how readily accessible the parent makes healthy and unhealthy foods in the home. Accessibility includes making foods ready and easy to eat, such as washing, cutting up and making food easy to see and reach for the child. (Modified from Vaughn et al.) [11]
28	I keep or have ready to eat fruits and vegetables in the fridge for my child to eat (e.g., pre-cut, clean).	10		
29	I avoid having [unhealthy food/drinks] available at home.	10		
75	I make sure that I have healthy foods in the house (./that my child likes).	10		
76	I have unhealthy foods in the house (./that my child likes).	10		
31	I include [healthy food] in my child's lunch/snacks/meals (./that s/he likes).	10	J: Food Preparation	The planning, preparation and cooking methods that a parent employs when providing or serving meals and snacks, which may impact the healthfulness of the foods served. (Modified from Vaughn et al.) [11]
32	I balance all food groups in my child's meals.	10		
43	I plan and prepare my child's meals/school lunches (./from scratch).	10		
93	I prepare food in a low-fat or healthy way for my family.	11		
94	I use pre-packaged, convenience food for meals.	10		
26	I show enthusiasm about eating healthy foods.	14	K: Modeling	Eating specific behaviors the parent engages in themselves in front of child that may entice their child to emulate his/her eating behaviors, food choices, or amounts of food. It can either be in regards to nutritious foods or less nutritious foods. It is distinct from creating opportunities to role model eating behaviors such as having a family meal together.

Table 1 110 food parenting concepts grouped into 17 clusters based on qualitative cluster assignment informed by published Food Parenting Framework [11] of expert's sorting (corresponds with Fig. 2) *(Continued)*

34	I eat/drink [healthy food/drinks] in front of my child (./even if they are not my favorite).	11		
35	I avoid eating/drinking [unhealthy food/drinks] in front of my child.	11		
95	I take a second helping of food at dinner in front of my child.	11		
30	I serve [healthy food] multiple times and in different ways to encourage my child to develop a taste for it.	12	L: Exposure to Variety/Selection	Parent exposes the child to nutritious and/or different food on a regular basis, includes variety of ways to prepare or eat nutritious food, and may allow choice for the child. (NEW)
71	I expose my child to a variety of fruits and vegetables (./since s/he was little).	12		
78	I serve/offer [healthy food type] (./each day, for snacks, for a side-dish, for breakfast/ for dinner/for dessert)	12		
92	To ensure my child eats a particular food (e.g., vegetables), I serve it with food my child likes.	12		
108	I suggest places to eat out that have healthy selections for my child.	12		
58	I try to minimize distractions during mealtimes (e.g., watching TV, answering phone calls, texting, playing with toys).	12	M: Meal Routines	"Parent implements consistency and predictability around meals and snacks with regard to their location, timing, presence of family members, conversational tone, and presence/ absence of distractions." [11]
60	I make sure my family eats together as often as possible.	11		
4	I give my child small portions to get him/her to eat a particular food or new foods.	13	N: Redirection and Negotiation	"Parent engages with child to come to an agreement about what or how much the child will eat. Negotiation allows for resolution of different opinions between parent and child by finding an acceptable compromise." [11] Parent uses tactics to take the child's mind off of certain foods or drinks, provides them with alternatives, or shares food to decrease portion size. The tactics are not forceful and there are no consequences if not successful.
5	I offer/provide my child healthy options when s/he asks for unhealthy food or treats.	13		
6	I negotiate with my child about how much unhealthy or healthy food s/he eats or drinks.	15		
77	I encourage my child to eat [vegetables] by playing games with my child at meals times or by challenging him/her to eat it.	13		
102	I encourage my child to drink water when s/he feels hungry.	13		

Table 1 110 food parenting concepts grouped into 17 clusters based on qualitative cluster assignment informed by published Food Parenting Framework [11] of expert's sorting (corresponds with Fig. 2) *(Continued)*

103	To discourage my child from eating a particular food, I give him/her something else to do.	13		
104	I encourage my child to control his/her intake of unhealthy food/drinks by sharing it.	13		
Autonomy Support				
1	I take into account the [healthy food/drinks] my child likes when shopping for food or preparing meals.	12	O: Child involvement	Parent acknowledges the child is an independent individual and takes into consideration the preferences and wants of the child by actively involving the child during meal planning, grocery shopping, meal preparation, or mealtime, with the goal to motivate more nutritious intake (modified from Vaughn et al.) [11]
2	I allow my child to serve him/herself and decide how much food s/he eats.	12		
9	I let my child have a lot of say in what is eaten or prepared for meals.	14		
13	I let my child season the vegetables, such as adding ketchup or cheese sauce, to make them taste better.	7		
57	I talk to my child during meals.	14		
62	I ask my child to suggest how s/he can eat more healthy food.	15		
83	If my child does not want to taste a food, I do not try to make him/her eat it.	7		
84	I let my child prepare his/her lunch/snacks.	14		
85	I involve my child in meal and snack preparation.	14		
86	I let my child choose fruits and vegetables while grocery shopping.	14		
33	I encourage my child to eat [healthy food] by making the food interesting (e.g., cutting into shapes, preparing it in a variety of ways, or seasoning it).	14	P: Encourage Health Eating	Non-directive methods to suggest that the child try or eat a healthy food, but is not forceful and does not have consequences associated with child not following through. These non-directive methods include gentle verbal cues or reminders, non-verbal methods by making food more appealing or interesting for child. It also includes promoting self-regulation of intake by children to not eat beyond satiety. (Modified from Vaughn et al.) [11]
36	I tell my child how much I like a food to encourage him/her to eat it.	15		
46	I encourage my child to eat/drink/ try [healthy food] (./but do not force him/her to do so)	15		
47	I encourage my child to eat/drink [healthy food/drinks] instead of or before [unhealthy food/drinks].	15		

Table 1 110 food parenting concepts grouped into 17 clusters based on qualitative cluster assignment informed by published Food Parenting Framework [11] of expert's sorting (corresponds with Fig. 2) *(Continued)*

48	I tell my child that his/her friends/ sibling(s)/favorite characters like the [healthy food] as a way to encourage him/her to eat it.	15		
70	I remind/encourage my child to stop eating or to not take more food when s/he feels full.	15		
90	I praise my child for eating healthy food or fruit and vegetables.	16		
101	I help my child set a goal to eat more fruit and vegetables.	15		
63	I persuade my child to eat healthy food by explaining why it's important (e.g., you will feel better, good for you, you'll grow big and strong, do better at school).	16	Q: Education/Reasoning	Explanations given by parent to child to educate the child about foods' nutritional qualities, such as the benefits of eating healthy foods or the consequences of eating unhealthy ones. Parent uses logic or explanations to persuade the child to change his or her eating behavior (modified form Vaughn et al.) [11]
64	I teach my child that certain food/drinks should only be consumed in moderation.	16		
65	I tell my child that certain food or drinks are not good for his/her health or teeth.	16		
66	I use mealtimes to teach my child about healthy eating.	16		
67	I teach my child about healthy eating by reading food labels and playing educational games.	16		
109	I give my child ideas on how to eat healthier (e.g., eating more fruits and vegetables).	16		

[a]This refers to the cluster the item was assigned based on the original 16-cluster solution identified by the cluster analysis. This is visually depicted in Fig. 2 as the gray shadow clusters and illustrates how many subjective changes were made to generate the proposed 17 cluster solution

to the proposed framework, Child Involvement (O) was a distinct construct under Autonomy Promotion. However, the two proposed constructs of Praise and Encouragement were combined into a single Encourage Healthy Eating (P) construct, while the two proposed Nutrition Education and Reasoning constructs were combined into a single Education/Reasoning (Q) construct. Lastly, the proposed construct Negotiation, which Vaughn et al. suggested belonged in Autonomy Promotion [11] was instead collapsed with Redirection in the Structure dimension (Fig. 2).

Five concepts (13, 26, 27, 83, and 87- Fig. 2) were grouped with clusters spatially removed from their closest cluster on the point map, because the research team deemed they fit better conceptually. Food parenting practice concepts 13 (I let my child season the vegetables, such as adding ketchup or cheese sauce, to make them taste better) and 83 (If my child does not want to taste a food, I do not try to make him/her eat it), were spatially closest to Rules and Limits and Permissive Feeding, respectively. However, the team proposed both concepts fit better into Child Involvement, which includes concepts that allow the parent to consider their child as an individual when motivating them to eat more nutritious foods. Concepts 26 (I show enthusiasm about eating healthy foods.) was spatially within Child involvement (P), but was moved into Modeling (M), to capture the concept of enthusiastic modeling [17], as per recommendation of Experts. Concept 27 (I hide or intentionally keep less [healthful food/drinks] out of my child's reach) has sometimes been classified as a form of covert control, but several experts felt it better fit into J: Availability/Accessibility. Concept 87 (I criticize my child about the food s/he eats.), was initially grouped with Pressure to Eat concepts, but it did not promote eating more food like the other concepts in Pressure to Eat. It was therefore moved to the adjacent new construct Intrusive Control which focused on directive and intrusive parental control of their child.

The parsimonious conceptual framework of food parenting practices

The parsimonious solution was derived from the 4-cluster statistical solution which expanded to a 7-cluster solution after it was subjectively reviewed and endorsed as part of the consensus process. The final model can be found in Additional file 1: Figure A (online) with construct names, definitions and corresponding concepts found in Additional file 1: Table A (online). The subjective separation of clusters was performed because the increased number into 5, 6 or 7 clusters resulting from the hierarchical cluster solution did not fit based on face validity. Instead, subjective modifications to the 4-cluster solution were based on the research team's current understanding of the published literature. The first modification was due to one of the 4 clusters containing unique concepts for different forms of coercive control (e.g. punitive restriction and pressure to eat). Prior research suggests that parents use pressure to eat more with picky eaters or underweight children, and it has been associated with lower weight status among children in several cross-sectional and longitudinal studies [18–21]. On the other hand, restriction has been more commonly associated with higher child weight status in cross-sectional and longitudinal studies and may be a response to children who are heavier or are more food responsive [18–21]. These divergent outcomes associated with pressure to eat and restriction suggested these two constructs may be conceptually different and should be measured independently of each other. Therefore, all the concepts in this group that reflected pushing children to eat more (whether coercive or not) were moved to the Pressure to Eat construct (Cluster 1). All the concepts that reflected the use of punishment or coercion to restrict the amount that children could eat remained in the Restriction construct (Cluster 2).

The next modification involved a large cluster that emerged from the 4 cluster solution which contained concepts related to parental Rules and Expectations (Cluster 4), along with two concepts (concepts 22 and 23) that theoretically did not belong with the others. These two concepts on the border of the cluster were more consistent with the idea of Emotional Feeding, first identified by Wardle et al. [22], and were therefore separated into a different construct named Emotional Feeding (Cluster 3).

The statistically derived 4-cluster solution included one large cluster that combined concepts for creating structure for a child with indulgent food parenting practices. Indulgent feeding style has consistently been associated with higher child weight status in cross-sectional [23] and recently in a longitudinal study [24]. However, structure is believed to be protective from excessive weight gain among children and for ensuring adequate consumption and growth for children with low weight status. It was considered whether these constructs are at the opposite ends of one spectrum, but we believed it is possible that parents can be indulgent with or without structure. The last modification therefore involved separating these two constructs into Indulgence (Cluster 5) and Structure (Cluster 6). The final cluster identified in the statistically derived 4-cluster solution contained strategies that involved parental Active Encouragement for Nutritious Eating by their child, and remained intact (Cluster 7). Based on expert input on the solution, items that may require further evaluation for fitting within each construct are identified for future studies in Additional file 1. A comparison of the two solutions can be found in Additional file 1: Figure B (online).

Discussion

An international expert panel of researchers involved in food parenting practices research helped guide the development of a new Concept Map for Food Parenting Practices. Both of the final two Food Parenting Practices Concept Maps presented here were derived from a MDS point map of the spatial relationships of 110 food parenting concepts based on the sorting task of 28 food parenting experts from around the world. One of the concept maps (Fig. 2, Table 1) is a subjective clustering of the food parenting practice concepts point map that retains a more comprehensive structure and was informed by the developmental psychology literature cited by Vaughn et al. [11] This comprehensive concept map should allow researchers to evaluate the impact of each of the proposed food parenting practice constructs on child outcomes, how parents use these practices in combination [25, 26], and whether child characteristics moderate the impact of each construct. This detailed solution will also allow researchers to select specific constructs when testing hypothesis or developing or evaluating interventions. The other concept map (Additional file 1: Figure A and Table A) was informed by the hierarchical cluster analysis solution and took a parsimonious approach as we aimed at identifying fewer clusters or constructs. This latter approach may help scientists enhance their measurement of food parenting practice by reducing the burden of measurement, while assessing more global and potentially predictive constructs. After they were given the opportunity to review both solutions, over half of the experts preferred the comprehensive solution. They felt this model allows for a better distinction of which constructs are most predictive of child behavior and health outcomes and have a greater impact to move this area of research forward.

Both the comprehensive and parsimonious solutions required subjective modifications to the statistically derived cluster solutions from the MDS point map. The difficulty in interpreting any of the hierarchical cluster analysis solutions without modifications, suggest that there was not great consensus among these experts for how to conceptualize a framework for food parenting practice, despite being provided with a published content map that several of the investigators and experts in this study helped develop. Of note, the cluster analysis of the MDS solution of only those experts that participated in the development of the published content map [11] and this sorting task was also explored, with no clearer solution apparent. One expert suggested that the comprehensive solution may be sub-factors within the more global parsimonious solution. Unfortunately, the current solutions do not fully support this as illustrated in Additional file 1, where there is not always clear overlap between the constructs defined in the two solutions. It is possible that future studies can help further refine both solutions such that the relationships between the two can be better delineated.

In this study, an international group of experts helped develop a concept map for food parenting practices using a systematic approach to identify the food parenting practice concepts, by allowing them to sort the concepts into categories and interpret their sorting using statistical analysis. This is distinct from the approach taken to develop Vaughn et al.'s content map [11], for which an overlapping group of experts were asked to collaboratively propose a framework for food parenting practices based on their own research and review of the literature. This published content map currently lacks validation. While the intent of this study was not to validate the published content map, the team felt it was important to allow the experts access to it. Since the food parenting content map was not published at the time the experts were asked to complete the sorting task, it was provided to allow them to use all possible resources. They were instructed to use the framework only if it worked with their own conceptual approach to the sorting task. It is not known how many elected to do so.

The work presented here was based on an item bank developed from published instruments of food parenting practice instruments systematically identified in 2013 [4]. Since that time, additional studies have been published that adapted or tested the psychometrics of food parenting practice scales already included in the item bank, to new populations [27–31]. In addition, several important new instruments of food parenting practices have been published that could not be included in the item bank to inform the Experts' tasks. These include the Parental Feeding Practices (PFQ) scale for Mexican American families [32], the Vegetable Parenting Practice scale [33], Feeding Practices and Structure Questionnaire (FPSQ-28) [34], and the Structure and Control in Parent Feeding (SCPF) [35]. However, several of these instruments were developed based on previously published scales and had much overlap with items already included in the item bank and would likely integrate with the concepts we identified. The extent to which these newer items fit within our existing concepts will be tested empirically in the future.

The goal of this study is ultimately to improve the measurement of food parenting practices to allow for a more standardized assessment of food parenting practice constructs and better comparisons of results across studies. The team is currently iteratively developing items to cover the constructs presented in the comprehensive food parenting practice solution using existing or modified items from published scales. Future work will include testing the resulting questionnaire in English with parents via cognitive interviews, and then assessing parents' use of the food parenting practices in a large cross-sectional study for classical test theory and advanced psychometric analysis (e.g. item response modeling). This will allow psychometric testing of the proposed comprehensive model. If the comprehensive model is a poor fit which cannot be improved with minor alterations, the parsimonious model will be tested instead. Ultimately, the goal is to create a calibrated item bank that can be used for computer assisted testing in observation and interventions studies. The psychometric analysis will help achieve this by assessing whether items are stable across participant characteristics (e.g. income and education) via differential item functioning within a Canadian sample. Future work will need to assess the stability of items across different cultural racial and ethnic groups and in different languages. The improvements in measuring food parenting practices will hopefully result in more consistent use of instruments across studies and better understanding of the impacts of food parenting practices on child outcomes, and whether child characteristics or behaviors moderate these findings.

Strengths and limitations

This study has several strengths including a systematic approach to identifying food parenting practice concepts, engaging an international sample of experts in food parenting and child feeding in a sorting task, and using both quantitative and subjective approaches to interpret the resulting point map solution of food parenting practices. Limitations of this methodology should also be acknowledged. The item bank is based on instruments published before March 2013, and therefore does not include instruments developed after this time. Experts varied by how much they relied on the previously published content map [11] to inform their own sorting, which may have influenced the final analysis. The cluster analysis derived solution of food parenting practice clusters also suggested there was variability in how the Experts operationalized each construct. Another limitation in measuring food parenting practice concepts is they are typically operationalized as unidirectional behaviors of parents aimed at their child. This may imply the assumption that we can fully understand the impact of food parenting practice on child dietary behavior by applying the Concept Map in observational and intervention studies. It should be acknowledged that food parenting practice is embedded in a more complex family context, including the back-and-forth interactions between a parent and a child, as well as sibling and marital relationships, with reciprocal influences between all family members. Thus, it is likely that food parenting practices can be best understood in the context of interactions within the family as a whole.

Conclusion

In summary, the comprehensive food parenting practice concept map derived from the experts' sorting of food parenting practice concepts provides a conceptual map and the roadmap for the selecting and developing of items for each construct. These will in turn be tested to eventually develop a calibrated item bank of food parenting practices, which will help standardize the measurement of food parenting practice in future observational and intervention studies.

Abbreviations

FPP: Food Parenting Practices; IRM: Item Response Modeling; ISBNPA: International Society of Behavioral Nutrition and Physical Activity; MDS: Multidimensional Scaling; NIH: National Institute of Health

Acknowledgements

We want to thank the full set of experts who participated in this study. Without their thoughtful input this study would not be possible. Expert panel members were given the option of contributing as an author or being acknowledged for their contribution to this work. All who requested to be an authors reviewed several versions of the solutions, approved the proposed solution, and provided important feedback on the manuscript. All the authors have reviewed and approved this manuscript. We also want to express our sincere thank you to Drs. Karen Campbell, Jennifer Fisher, Lori Francis, Erin Hennessy, Susan Johnson, Megumi Murashima, Dara Musher-Eizenman, Angela Odoms-Young, Heather Patrick, Natalie Pearson, Ana Bertha Pérez Lizaur, Thomas G. Power, Carola Ray, Georgina Russell, Heather Ullrich-Kitzman, Dianne Ward and one expert who wished to remain anonymous, for participating as experts and for making important contributions to this study.

Funding

The project described was supported by award number MOP-119359 from the Canadian Institute of Health Research (CIHR); LCM received salary support from the BC Child's Hospital Research Institute (BCCHRI); AWW received post-doctoral support from CIHR; and AT received post-doctoral support from BCCHRI and the Michael Smith Foundation for Health Research.
This work is also a publication of the US Department of Agriculture (USDA/ARS) Children's Nutrition Research Center, Department of Pediatrics, BCM funded in part by the USDA/ARS (Cooperative Agreement 58-3092-5-001). The contents of this publication do not necessarily reflect the views or policies of the USDA, nor does mention of organizations imply endorsement from the US government.

Authors' contributions

LCM, TMO, SOH, MRB and TB designed the study. LCM oversaw the data collection. TMO, LCM, AWW, and TP conducted the binning and winnowing to generate the food parenting concepts. LCM and AWT performed the statistical analyses. TMO, LCM, ATW, SOH, MRB, and TB provided subjective input in the analyses. TMO managed the expert feedback, revisions of the solutions, and drafted the manuscript. All authors critically assessed drafts of the concept solutions and the manuscript. The authors have read and approved the final manuscript.

Competing interests

The authors declare that they have no competing interests.

Author details

[1]USDA/ARS Children's Nutrition Research Center, Baylor College of Medicine, 1100 Bates St, Houston, TX, USA. [2]BC Children's Hospital Research Institute, School of Population and Public Health, University of British Columbia, Vancouver, BC, Canada. [3]Child & Family Research Institute, School of Population and Public Health, University of British Columbia, Vancouver, BC, Canada. [4]Division of Epidemiology and Community Health, School of Public Health, University of Minnesota, Minneapolis, MN, USA. [5]School of Kinesiology, University of British Columbia, Vancouver, BC, Canada. [6]Department of Family Medicine and Community Health, University of Minnesota Medical School, Minnesota, MN, USA. [7]Family Resilience Center, Department of Human Development and Family Studies, University of Illinois at Urbana-Champaign, Urbana, IL, USA. [8]Sansom Institute for Health Research (PHRC), School of Pharmacy and Medical Sciences, University of South Australia, Adelaide, Australia. [9]Department of Nutritional Sciences, College of Agriculture and Life Sciences, University of Arizona, Tucson, AZ, USA. [10]NUTRIM School of Nutrition and Translational Research in Metabolism, Maastricht University Medical Center, Maastricht, The Netherlands. [11]Department of Pediatrics, University of California, San Diego, CA, USA. [12]School of Psychology, Deakin University, Melbourne, Australia. [13]Department of Nutrition, Gillings School of Global Public health, University of North Carolina, Chapel Hill, NC, USA.

References

1. Mitchell G, Farrow C, Haycraft E, Meyer C. Parental influences on children's eating behaviour and characteristics of successful parent-focused interventions. Appetite. 2013;60:85–94.
2. Larsen J, Hermans R, Sleddens E, Engels R, Fisher J, Kremers S. How parental dietary behavior and food parenting practices affect children's dietary behavior. Interacting sources of influence? Appetite. 2015;89:246–57.
3. Berge J, Wall M, Bauer K, Neumark-Sztainer D. Parenting characteristics in the home environment and adolescent overweight: a latent class analysis. Obesity. 2010;18(4):818–25.
4. O'Connor T, Pham T, Watts A, et al. Development of an item bank for food parenting practices on published instruments and reports from Canadian and US parents. Appetite. 2016;103:386–95.
5. Baranowski T, O'Connor T, Hughes S, et al. Houston. .. We have a problem! Measurement of parenting. Child Obes 2013;9(Suppl 1):S1-S4.
6. Masse L, Watts A. Stimulating innovations in the measurement of parenting constructs. Childhood Obesity. 2013;9(S1):S5–S13. PMC3746250
7. Gevers DW, Kremers SP, de Vries NK, van Assema P. Clarifying concepts of food parenting practices. A Delphi study with an application to snacking behavior. Appetite. 2014;79:51–7.
8. Hughes S, Frankel L, Beltran A, et al. Food parenting measurement issues: working group consensus report. Childhood Obesity. 2013;9(Suppl):S95–102.
9. Revicki D, Cella D. Health status assessment for the twenty-first century: item response theory, item banking and computer adaptive testing. Qual Life Res. 1997;6(595):600.
10. DeWalt D, Rothrock N, Yount S, Stone A. Evaluation of item candidates: the PROMIS qualitative item review. Med Care. 2007;45:S12–21.
11. Vaughn A, Ward D, Fisher J, et al. Fundamental constructs in food parenting practices: a content map to guide future research. Nutr Rev. 2016;74(2):98–117.
12. de Lauzon-Guillain B, Oliveira A, Charles M, et al. A review of methods to assess parental feeding practices and preschool children's eating behaviors: the need for further development of tools. J Acad Nutr Diet. 2012;112(10):1578–602.

13. Vaughn A, Tabak R, Bryant M, Ward D. Measuring parent food practices: a systematic review of existing measures and examination of instruments. Int J Behav Nutr Phys Act. 2013;10(61):PMC3681578.
14. Kane M, Trochim W. Concept mapping for planning and evaluation. Thousand Oaks: Sage Publications; 2007.
15. Trochim W. The reliability of concept mapping. [serial online] 1993. https://www.socialresearchmethods.net/research/Reliable/reliable.htm.
16. Kruskal J, Wish M. Multidimensional scaling. Beverly Hills: Sage Publications; 1978.
17. Hendy HM, Raudenbush B. Effectiveness of teacher modeling to encourage food acceptance in preschool children. Appetite. 2000; 2000;34(1):61-76.
18. Ventura AK, Birch LL. Does parenting affect children's eating and weight status? Int J Behav Nutr Physical Activity. 2008;5:15.
19. Faith MS, Scanlon KS, Birch LL, Francis LA, Sherry B. Parent-child feeding strategies and their relationships to child eating and weight status. [review] [61 refs]. Obes Res. 2004;12(11):1711–22.
20. Hurley K, Cross M, Hughes S. A systematic review of responsive feeding and child obesity in high-income countries. J Nutr. 2011;141(3):495–501.
21. Shloim N, Edelson L, Martin N, Hetherington M. Parenting styles, feeding styles, feeding practices, and weight status in 4-12 year-old children: a systematic review of the literature. Front Psychol. 2015;6:1849.
22. Wardle J, Sanderson S, Guthrie CA, Rapoport L, Plomin R. Parental feeding style and the inter-generational transmission of obesity risk. Obes Res. 2002; 10(6):453–62.
23. El-Behadli A, Sharp C, Hughes S, Obasi E, Nicklas T. Maternal depression, stress and feeding styles: towards a framework for theory and research in child obesity. Br J Nutr. 2015;113(Suppl1):S55–71.
24. Hughes S, Power T, O'Connor T, Fisher J, Chen T. Maternal feeding styles and food parenting practices as predictors of longitudinal changes in weight status in hispanic preschoolers from low-income families. J Obes. 2016;7201082:9. Article ID 7201082.
25. Gevers DW, Kremers SP, D Vries NK, Assema PV. Patterns of food parenting practices and Children's intake of energy-dense snack foods. Nutrients. 2015;7(6):4093–106.
26. O'Connor T, Hughes S, Watson K, et al. Parenting practices are associated with fruit and vegetable consumption in preschool children. Public Health Nutr. 2010;13(1):91–101.
27. Afonso L, Lopes C, Servo M, et al. Bidirectional association between parental child-feeding practices and body mass index at 4 and 7 y of age. Am J Clin Nutr. 2016;103(3):861–7.
28. Al-Qerem W, Ling J, AlBawab A. Validation of the comprehensive feeding practice questionnaire among school aged children in Jordan: a factor analysis study. Int J Behav Nutr Phys Act. 2017;14(1):23.
29. Schmidt R, Richter R, Brauhardt A, Hiemisch A, Kiess W, Hilbert A. Parental feeding practices in families with children aged 2-13 years: psychometric properties and child age-specific norms of the German version of the child feeding questionnaire (CFQ). Appetite. 2017;109:154–64.
30. Warkentin S, Mais L, Latorre MR, Carnell S, Taddei J. Validation of the comprehensive feeding practices questionnaire in parents of preschool children in Brazil. BMC Public Health. 2016;16:603.
31. Canals-Sans J, Blanco-Gomez A, Lugue V, et al. Validation of the child feeding questionnaire in Spanish parents of school children. J Nutr Educ Behav. 2016;48(6):383–91.
32. Tschann J, Gregorich S, Penilla C, et al. Parental feeding practices in Mexican American families: initial test of and expanded measure. Int J Behav Nutr Phys Act. 2013;10:6. PMC3552721
33. Baranowski T, Chen TA, O'Connor T, et al. Dimensions of vegetable parenting practices among preschoolers. Appetite. 2013;69:89–93.
34. Jansen E, Mallan K, Daniels L. Extending the validity of the feeding practices and structure questionnaire. Int J Behav Nutr Phys Act. 2015;12:90.
35. Savage J, Rollins B, Kugler K, Birch L, Marini M. Development of a theory-based questionnaire to asses structure and control in parent feeding (SCPF). Int J Behav Nutr Phys Act. 2017;14(1):9.

14

Bidirectional associations between activity-related parenting practices, and child physical activity, sedentary screen-based behavior and body mass index: a longitudinal analysis

Ester F. C. Sleddens[1], Jessica S. Gubbels[1*], Stef P. J. Kremers[1], Eline van der Plas[1] and Carel Thijs[2]

Abstract

Background: It has been generally assumed that activity-related parenting practices influence children's activity behavior and weight status. However, vice versa parents may also change their parenting behaviors in response to their perceptions of their child's activity behavior and weight status. This study examined the bidirectional relationships between activity-related parenting practices, and physical activity, sedentary screen-based behavior, and body mass index (BMI) between children's age of 5 and 7 years.

Methods: Three scales of the Activity-related Parenting Questionnaire (i.e. 'restriction of sedentary behavior', 'stimulation of physical activity', and 'monitoring of physical activity') were completed by 1694 parents of the Dutch KOALA Birth Cohort Study at the child's age of around 5 and again around age 7. Physical activity, sedentary screen-based behavior and BMI were measured at both ages as well. Linear regression models were used to estimate the bidirectional associations between each parenting practice and the child's physical activity levels, sedentary screen-based behavior and BMI z-scores.

Results: Several parenting practices at age 5 predicted child physical activity, sedentary screen-based behavior, and BMI z-scores at age 7. Restriction of sedentary behavior positively predicted child BMI and sedentary screen-based behavior, whereas this practice negatively predicted child physical activity. In addition, stimulation of physical activity at age 5 was significantly associated with higher levels of child physical activity at age 7. The following child factors at age 5 predicted parenting practices at age 7: Child physical activity positively predicted parental stimulation of physical activity and monitoring activities. Sedentary screen-based behavior was associated with lower parental stimulation to be active.

Conclusions: Findings generally revealed that parents and children mutually influence each other's behavior. A reinforcing feedback loop was present between parental stimulation of physical activity and child physical activity. Bidirectional parent-child interaction should be considered in future research in order to properly inform parenting-related intervention programs aimed at preventing or treating childhood overweight or obesity. System dynamic methods to explore the existence of reinforcing or balancing loops are needed in this regard.

Keywords: Activity-related parenting practices, Bidirectional associations, Body mass index, Children, Physical activity, Sedentary screen-based behavior

* Correspondence: jessica.gubbels@maastrichtuniversity.nl
[1]Department of Health Promotion, NUTRIM School of Nutrition and Translational Research in Metabolism, Maastricht University, Maastricht University Medical Center, P.O. Box 616, 6200 MD Maastricht, the Netherlands
Full list of author information is available at the end of the article

Background

Parenting practices are content-specific acts of parenting [1], such as rules about activity behaviors. The literature on parenting and childhood obesity is dominated by studies about specific food-related parenting practices [2], whereas physical activity-related parenting practices are less studied but gaining interest during the last few years. Xu, Wen & Rissel [3] conducted a review about associations of parental influences with children's physical activity and screen time, and found that parental encouragement and support increase children's physical activity. In addition, reducing parents' own screen time can lead to decreased child screen time. Earlier, two reviews were conducted on the then available activity-related parenting practices measures and associations with either physical activity or screen time [4, 5]. They found mixed evidence regarding the association between activity-related parenting practices and child physical activity and screen time [4, 5]. Despite limitations in existing studies, findings from a previous systematic review concluded based on their systematic review that supporting physical activity behaviors (including modeling) were positively related to children's physical activity levels [5]. However, previous research hypotheses have been largely unidirectional, assuming that parenting practices induce child behaviors. In addition, most of these studies were cross-sectional in nature and therefore causality could not be assessed [5].

'The chicken or the egg' causality issue has hardly been addressed in the study of parent-child interactions in the development of childhood obesity. A few researchers tried to disentangle this issue in the parental feeding domain (e.g., [6–9]) (although solely with child BMI as a predictor and outcome and not dietary behavior), but studies that address microsystem dynamics with regard to activity-related parenting are lacking to date. The studies of parent-child interaction in the feeding domain found that food parenting practices were often influenced by the child's weight status, in addition to the food parenting practice influencing the child's weight gain [7–9]. Despite these findings, the energy balance-related parenting literature is dominated by studies characterizing parents as the agents acting upon the child, without considering children's influence on parents [10, 11].

The aim of this study was to examine bidirectional associations between activity-related parenting practices (i.e., restriction of sedentary behavior, stimulation of physical activity, and monitoring of child physical activity), child physical activity and sedentary screen-based behavior, and parental perception of child weight status at age 5 and age 7. Based on previous food-parenting studies, we hypothesized parenting practices to be a response to child activity behavior and Body Mass Index (BMI), in addition to being a cause. The longitudinal design made it possible to examine the bidirectional nature of the parent-child dynamics: whether activity-related parenting practices predicted change in child activity behavior and BMI; or whether child activity behavior and BMI predicted change in activity-related parenting practices.

Methods

Data collection and participants

Data were collected within the KOALA Birth Cohort Study in the Netherlands (described elsewhere) [12]. Briefly, from 2000 onwards, healthy pregnant women from the general population who participated in an existing cohort study on pregnancy-related pelvic girdle pain were recruited (N = 2343; referred to as the 'conventional' recruitment group). In addition, healthy pregnant women with an 'alternative' lifestyle with regard to dietary habits (e.g., preferring organic foods), vaccination programs and/or antibiotics use (N = 491; referred to as the 'alternative' recruitment group) were recruited through several 'alternative' circles like anthroposophical physician offices and midwives, and organic food shops. All participants (N = 2834) were enrolled between 14 and 18 weeks of gestation and completed questionnaires during pregnancy and at regular intervals after birth. Informed consent was signed by all parents, and ethical approval was obtained from the Maastricht University/University Hospital Maastricht medical ethics committee.

For the current study we used data from the measurements around the child's age of 5 and again around age 7. In total, 2061 participants (72.7% of the initial cohort) completed the questionnaire around age 5 and 1810 participants (63.9% of the initial cohort) completed the questionnaire around the child's age of 7. Of those, 1694 completed the child's parent-reported physical activity behavior questions and/or the activity-related parenting practices at both measurements. Children that were included in the final analyses had a somewhat higher BMI z-score at age 7 compared to children not included (−0.32 vs. -0.53, p-value = 0.03). There was no other selective drop-out (all p-values >0.05) with regard to recruitment group or other child or parental background characteristics. Child mean (SD) age during the first measurement around age 5 was 5.00 (0.53) years (range 3 to 6 years), and during the second measurement around age 7 was 7.17 (0.65) years (range 5 to 8 years).

Measures

At both measurements similar questions were asked regarding activity-related parenting practices, child physical activity behavior and child weight and height.

Activity-related parenting practices

We used the Activity-related Parenting Questionnaire [13], which was based on the Child Feeding Questionnaire

[14] and adapted to assess physical activity and sedentary screen-based behavior parenting practices. Three scales from this questionnaire were used for the current study: 'restriction of sedentary behavior' (assessing the extent to which parents restrict their child's access to sedentary activities; 7 items), 'stimulation to be physically active (assessing the extent to which parents encourage their child to be physically active; 3 items)' and 'monitoring activity (assessing the extent to which parents oversee their child's physical activity; 2 items)'. In the current study we decided to delete the item 'As a reward for good behavior, I put on a nice video/DVD/computer game for my child' originally belonging to the scale labeled 'restriction of sedentary behavior'. This item was dropped prior to the analyses based on potential mismatch with this scale. For all three scales, a five-point Likert scale has been used ranging from 1 (*Completely disagree*) to 5 (*Completely agree*) for 'restriction of sedentary behavior' and 'stimulation to be active', and ranging from 1 (*Never*) to 5 (*Always*) for 'monitoring activity'. The items used to assess these activity-related parenting practices and the corresponding Cronbach's alphas at both measurements are listed in Table 1. Intercorrelations between the different parenting practices were low to moderate, ranging from 0.19 to 0.33.

Child activity behavior and body mass index

Children's activity behavior was assessed using questions based on a standard questionnaire for measuring activity behavior, used in Dutch Youth Health Care [15]. Parents were asked on how many days in a normal week during the last 4 weeks their child went to school by bicycle or on foot, had played sports at a sports club, and had played outside (outside school hours). A second question assessed the average duration of each of these activities, with five predefined answering categories ranging from half an hour or less, to 3 h or more. Based on the assumption that there is a linear association between physical activity and parenting practices [5], we recoded the answer scale to calculate the average time of these activities. Half an hour or less was recoded into 15 min, half an hour to 1 h into 45 min, 1 to 2 h into 90 min, 2 to 3 h into 150 min and finally, 3 h or more into 181 min. For the item 'child went to school by bicycle or on foot' answering categories were similar as above for age 7, but different for the measurement at age 5. The answering categories at age 5 for this item were: shorter than 10 min (recoded into 5 min), 10–20 min (recoded into 15 min), 20–30 min (recoded into 25 min), half an hour-1 h (recoded into 45), and more than 1 h (recoded into 61 min). The duration and number of days were multiplied to calculate the number of minutes spent on a particular activity per week. The number of minutes spent on the various activities were then added up to calculate the total number of minutes of physical activity per week, which was divided by 7 to get the average time (in minutes) the children were physically active per day. Sedentary screen-based behavior was assessed in a similar manner, asking parents about their child's television watching (including videos and DVDs) and computer playing (including game consoles). A similar approach was followed as for physical activity to calculate the number of screen hours per day.

During both measurements, parents were asked to report their child's weight and height (measured without shoes and clothes, specified to one decimal), in order to calculate the child's BMI (weight (kg)/(height (m)^2). BMI was then recoded into BMI z-scores compared to the 1997 national reference population (i.e., the Fourth Dutch National Growth Study) [16]. BMI z-score > 85th percentile was considered to indicate overweight and a BMI z-score > 95th percentile was considered to indicate obesity [17]. Anthropometric scores were systematically checked for plausibility using the following procedure. All outliers (z-scores >3, i.e. more than 3 standard deviations from the mean) for height, weight and BMI were

Table 1 Descriptive and scale information of the activity-related parenting practice scales (*N* = 1694)

Activity-related parenting practices	Cronbach's alpha; Mean (SD)	
	Age 5 years	Age 7 years
Restriction of sedentary behavior	0.71; 3.00 (0.76)	0.72; 3.12 (0.75)
- I have to be sure that my child does not…		
* …watch too much television.		
* …play too many computer games.		
- If I did not guide or regulate my child's activity behavior, (s)he would..		
* watch too much television or play too many computer games.		
* not get enough physical activity.		
* be sedentary a lot (or play without being physically active).		
- I intentionally keep my child away from the television or computer.		
Stimulation to be active	0.58; 4.26 (0.65)	0.56; 4.45 (0.53)
- If my child says "I don't feel like walking or bicycling to there", I try to get him/her to do this anyway.		
- I have to be careful that my child gets enough exercise.		
- I make sure that my child travels actively on foot or by bicycle (with or without me) as often as possible.		
Monitoring activity	0.64; 3.94 (0.79)	0.57; 4.00 (0.67)
How much do you keep track of…		
- ..the amount of television your child watches and how many computer games (s)he plays?		
- ..the amount of physical activity your child has?		

The Corrected-Item Total Correlations for each of the items were above 0.30; The item 'as a reward for good behavior, I put on a nice video/DVD/computer game for my child' originally belonging to the scale labeled 'restriction of sedentary behavior' was already dropped prior to the analyses based on theory; response scale ranging from 1 (*Completely disagree*) to 5 (*Completely agree*) for 'restriction of sedentary behavior' and 'stimulation to be active', response scale ranging from 1 (*Never*) to 5 (*Always*) for 'monitoring activity identified. In addition, longitudinal anthropometric data were checked for inconsistencies and impossible and highly unlikely changes (e.g. a child shrinking in height). The outliers and inconsistencies were then checked with the original paper questionnaires. If the outlier could not be corrected based on this check, it was recoded into a missing value.

Background variables

As child covariates we included birth weight (in grams) and gender. With regard to parental covariates we included employment (i.e., the number of working hours per week) of the questionnaire completer and partner, their country of birth, and the highest parental educational level attained in the household at the child's age of 5. Educational level was recoded into three levels (low, medium and high), in line with international classification systems [18]. Country of birth was recoded into 'Netherlands' versus 'other'. We additionally included the recruitment group ('conventional' versus 'alternative') as a covariate in all analyses.

Data analyses

Statistical analyses were performed using the statistical software package IBM Statistics 21. Descriptive statistics were used for the background characteristics of the sample. Both internal reliability coefficients (Cronbach's α) and Corrected Item–Total Correlations (CITC) were calculated for the scales of the Activity-related Parenting Questionnaire at both ages. A cut-off point of 0.50 for Cronbach's α was used [19]. CITC values above 0.30 were regarded as 'good' [20].

To assess the bidirectional associations between activity-related parenting practices and the child's physical activity, sedentary screen-based behavior and BMI, two sets of linear regression models were conducted. Each set of models examines one of the two assumed directions of the association. The first set of models (A) examined the association between each of the activity-related parenting practices at age 5 and child's physical activity, sedentary screen-based behavior and BMI z-scores at age 7. The second set (B) examined the associations between the child's physical activity, sedentary screen-based behavior, and BMI at age 5 and each of the parenting practice scales at age 7. For both directions, three models are presented: Model 1: an unadjusted model; Model 2: a model adjusted for covariates (recruitment group; child birth weight and gender; parental employment, country of birth and educational level); and Model 3: a model adjusted for covariates and additionally for either baseline physical activity, sedentary screen-based behavior, or BMI z-score (in the models examining parenting practices as a predictor of child behavior and BMI (A)), or for baseline parenting practices (in the models examining child behavior as a predictor for later parenting practices (B)). Controlling for these baseline scores at age 5 in this third model allows for examination of the effect of changes within the dependent variable between ages 5 and 7 years, independent of the child's baseline scores on the dependent variable.

Results

Sample characteristics

The percentage boys and girls taking part in the study were about equally distributed (Table 2). Most families were included in the category with the highest education level achieved (67.8%). The majority of the questionnaires were completed by mothers (97.6%). The majority of participants were of Dutch origin (more than 96% for both female and male caregivers). The children's mean (*SD*) physical activity in minutes per week was 610.81 (394.25) at age 5 and increased to 904.48 (375.42) at age 7. For sedentary screen-based behavior this was 363.16 (292.19) minutes per week at age 5 and increased to 553.08 (351.69) at age 7. Mean (*SD*) BMI z-score at age 5 was −0.26 (0.99), compared to −0.32 (0.91) at age 7. To specify, 8.9% of the children were identified as being overweight/obese at age 5, whereas this decreased to 6.4% at age 7.

Associations between activity-related parenting practices at age 5 and child BMI/physical activity/sedentary screen-based behavior at age 7

For a visual inspection of the significant associations found between activity-related parenting practices at age 5 and child BMI, physical activity and sedentary screen-based behavior development up to age 7 we refer to Fig. 1a. The parenting practice 'restriction of sedentary behavior' showed positive associations with BMI z-score and sedentary screen-based behavior at age 7 (Table 3), even after correction for potential confounders and for the child's behavior at age 5 (i.e., for BMI z-score at age 5 when BMI at age 7 was predicted and for child sedentary screen-based behavior at age 5 when sedentary screen-based behavior at age 7 was predicted). In the final model (model 3), the association with sedentary screen-based behavior was marginally significant ($p = 0.055$). Restriction of sedentary behavior was negatively associated with the child's physical activity level at age 7. Stimulation to be active was only related to the child's physical activity. Higher scores on stimulation to be active were significantly associated with an increase of mean scores of the child's physical activity 2 years later. In addition, parental monitoring of their child's activity was not associated with children's BMI, physical activity levels or sedentary screen-based behavior.

Associations between child BMI/physical activity/sedentary screen-based behavior at age 5 and activity-related parenting practices at age 7

For a visual inspection of the significant associations found between physical activity-related variables at age 5

Table 2 Sample Characteristics (N = 1694)

Description				Age 5 years			Age 7 years		
		n	%	*n*	%	Mean (SD)	*n*	%	Mean (SD)
Child gender	Boy	868	51.2						
	Girl	826	48.8						
Questionnaire completer	Mother			1652	97.5		1619	95.6	
	Father			38	2.2		40	2.4	
	Unknown/other/NA			4	0.3		35	2.1	
Partner questionnaire completer	Mother			33	1.9		39	2.3	
	Father			1492	88.1		1436	84.8	
	Unknown/other/NA			169	9.9		219	12.9	
Working hours questionnaire completer						21.25 (9.25)			
Working hours partner questionnaire completer						36.71 (12.84)			
Education level (highest in household)	Low			72	4.3				
	Medium			472	27.9				
	High			1145	67.8				
Birth country female caregiver	Netherlands			1634	96.9				
	Other			52	3.1				
Birth country male caregiver	Netherlands			1622	96.3				
	Other			62	3.7				
Recruitment channel	Conventional	1372	81.0						
	Alternative	322	19.0						
Total physical activity (minutes per week)				1676		610.81 (394.25)	1623		904.48 (375.42)
Active transport to school (minutes per week)				1679		45.10 (53.11)	1659		108.99 (106.12)
Sports (minutes per week)				1694		42.94 (50.82)	1655		127.62 (110.23)
Playing outside (minutes per week)				1677		522.42 (385.30)	1661		669.08 (319.46)
Total sedentary screen-based behavior (minutes per week)				1679		363.16 (292.19)	1659		553.08 (351.69)
Television watching (minutes per week)				1679		315.71 (258.45)	1671		417.06 (263.44)
Computer playing (minutes per week)				1681		47.39 (91.23)	1665		137.26 (163.50)
Body Mass Index z-scores				1585		−0.26 (0.99)	1446		−0.32 (0.91)
Weight categories	Underweight			132	8.3		102	7.1	
	Normal-weight			1312	82.8		1251	86.5	
	Overweight			97	6.1		67	4.6	
	Obesity			44	2.8		26	1.8	

Missings educational level 5, missings BMI (5 years) 109, missings BMI (7 years) 248, missings physical activity (5 years) 18, missing physical activity (7 years) 71, missing sedentary screen-based behavior (5 years) 15, missings sedentary screen-based behavior (7 years) 35, missings birth country female caregiver 8, missings birth country male caregiver 10

and activity-related parenting practices development up to age 7 we refer to Fig. 1b. For child BMI z-score (Table 4), significant associations were only found with the parenting practice 'restriction of sedentary behavior': this association was positive in the unadjusted model (model 1) and the model adjusted for covariates (model 2). The child's physical activity was significantly related to all three activity-related parenting practices: positive for 'stimulation to be active' and 'monitoring activity', and negative for 'restriction of sedentary behavior'. The association between physical activity and restriction of sedentary behavior at age 7 attenuated after adjustment for restriction of sedentary behavior at age 5, indicating that physical activity did not influence change of this parenting practice between age 5 and 7. The child's sedentary screen-based behavior only had a significant association with stimulation to be active. Parents of children that were sedentary at age 5 were less likely to stimulate their child to be physically active at age

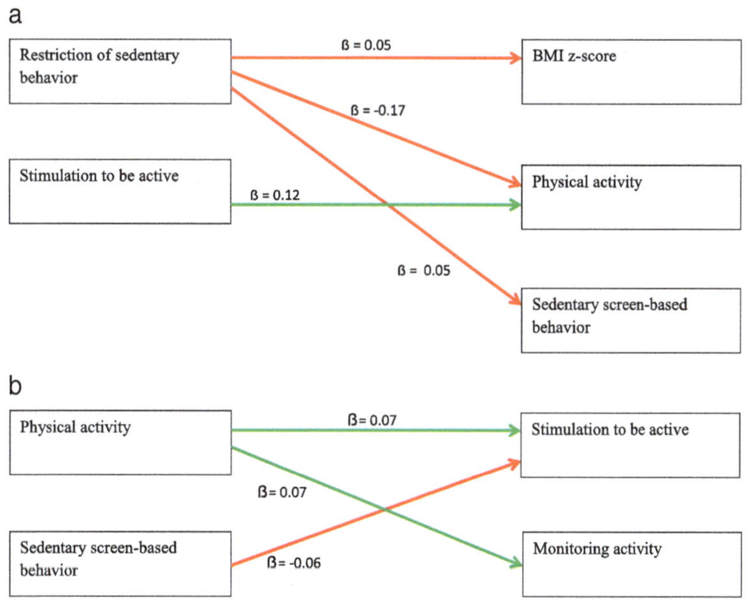

Fig. 1 **a** A visual representation of the significant associations between activity-related parenting practices at age 5 and child's BMI, physical activity and sedentary screen-based behavior development up to age 7. *Legend:* The direction of the standardized regression coefficient is presented in the figure, only for the third model (adjusted for covariates 'recruitment group (conventional vs alternative), child gender and birth weight, parental educational level, employment and country of birth' and in addition for BMI z-score at age 5 in parenting practice-BMI associations, and for either physical activity sedentary screen-based behavior in the parenting practice-physical activity/sedentary screen-based behavior associations; red line: unintended effects, green line: intended effects. **b** A visual representation of the significant associations between physical activity-related variables at age 5 and activity-related parenting practices development up to age 7. *Legend:* The direction of the standardized regression coefficient is presented in the figure, only for the third model (adjusted for covariates 'recruitment group (conventional vs alternative), child gender and birth weight, parental educational level, employment and country of birth' and in addition for restriction of sedentary screen-based behavior at age 5 in the activity-related variables & BMI-restriction of sedentary screen-based behavior association, and for either stimulation to be active or monitoring activity in the activity-related variables & BMI- stimulation to be active or monitoring activity parenting practice associations; Green line: reinforcing effect, red line: reactance effect

7. This association remained significant after correcting for potential confounders and considering the parenting practice 'stimulation to be active' at age 5.

Discussion

This study examined the bidirectional associations between activity-related parenting practices (i.e., restriction of sedentary behavior, stimulation to be active, and monitoring activity) and the child's BMI, physical activity levels, and sedentary screen-based behavior. To date, the focus in the literature has very much been on activity-related parenting practices as a risk factor for low levels of physical activity and high levels of sedentariness among children or high body weight. Our study reveals that children influence parenting as much as the other way around behavior.

In this study we found that child sedentary screen-based behavior negatively influenced stimulation of physical activity. In cross-sectional studies such a finding could easily be misinterpreted as parental stimulation to be active having a detrimental impact on children's sedentary screen-based behavior, for example when they push children too much. However, our results suggest the reverse is true. It thus seems that parents of children with high levels of sedentary screen-based behavior do not stimulate their children (anymore) to be physically active. Parents might reach a point where unsuccessful efforts te decrease their child's sedentary time in the past, have led to decreased self-efficacy to address the child's behavior, which in turn influences their parenting practices [21]. Alternatively, parents might not consider sedentarity as a problem, or perceive it as an unchangeable trait of the child.

Parents are additionally responding to child physical activity levels; parents were more likely to monitor their child's activity when the child was already physically active. These parents are probably enthusiastic about their child's willingness to be physically active and therefore supporting and motivating their child, which could be characterized by increased monitoring of their child's activity behavior.

In addition, we found that stimulation of physical activity led to higher levels of physical activity, but also that physical activity was positively related to stimulation of physical activity. This process can be characterized as a reinforcing or positive feedback loop. A feedback loop

Table 3 Association between activity-related parenting practices at age 5 and child's BMI, physical activity and sedentary screen-based behavior development up to age 7

Activity-related parenting practices	Model	Standardized regression coefficients (β) BMI z-score	Physical activity	Sedentary screen-based behavior
Restriction of sedentary behavior	1	0.13***	−0.25***	0.07*
	2	0.13***	−0.23***	0.08**
	3	0.05*	−0.17***	0.05[a]
Stimulation to be active	1	−0.02	0.16***	0.00
	2	−0.02	0.15***	−0.03
	3	−0.02	0.12***	0.01
Monitoring activity	1	−0.04	−0.01	−0.05
	2	−0.04	−0.02	−0.03
	3	0.00	−0.03	0.00

* $p < 0.05$, ** $p < 0.01$, *** $p < 0.001$; a the p-value was marginally significant: $p = 0.055$; model 1: unadjusted; model 2: adjusted for recruitment group (conventional vs alternative), child gender and birth weight, parental educational level, employment and country of birth; model 3: adjusted for covariates from model 2 and in addition for BMI z-score at age 5 in parenting practice-BMI associations, and for either physical activity or sedentary screen-based behavior at age 5 in the parenting practice-physical activity/sedentary behavior associations; Explained variances (R2): for BMI: Model 1 = 0.01, Model 2 = 0.06, Model 3 = 0.39; for Physicalactivity: Model 1 = 0.08, Model 2 = 0.13, Model 3 = 0.21; for Sedentary screen-based behavior: Model 1 = 0.01, Model 2 = 0.13, Model 3 = 0.38

Table 4 Association between physical activity-related variables at age 5 and activity-related parenting practices development up to age 7

Physical activity related variables	Model	Standardized regression coefficients (β) Restriction of sedentary behavior	Stimulation to be active	Monitoring activity
BMI z-score	1	0.08**	0.04	0.02
	2	0.08**	0.04	0.02
	3	0.03	0.03	0.02
Physical activity	1	−0.11***	0.11***	0.07*
	2	−0.12***	0.11***	0.07*
	3	−0.03	0.07**	0.07*
Sedentary screen-based behavior	1	0.00	−0.07**	−0.05
	2	0.02	−0.09**	−0.04
	3	0.00	−0.06*	−0.03

* $p < 0.05$, ** $p < 0.01$, *** $p < 0.001$; model 1: unadjusted; model 2: adjusted for recruitment group (conventional vs alternative), child gender and birth weight, parental educational level, employment and country of birth; model 3: adjusted for covariates from model 2 and in addition for restriction of sedentary behavior at age 5 in the activity-related variables & BMI-restriction of sedentary behavior association, and for either stimulation to be active or monitoring activity in the activity-related variables & BMI-stimulation to be active or monitoring activity parenting practice associations. Explained variances (R^2): for Restriction of sedentary behavior: Model 1 = 0.02, Model 2 = 0.06, Model 3 = 0.31; for Stimulation to be active: Model 1 = 0.02, Model 2 = 0.04, Model 3 = 0.20; for Monitoring activity: Model 1 = 0.01, Model 2 = 0.01, Model 3 = 0.16

is a path along which information can be traced from one point in a system, and back to the point of origin. Feedback loops are an essential feature of system dynamics modeling [22]. In the current study, we found strong indications for the existence of such positive feedback loops. This is notable, since traditional health behavior theories often assume homeostasis or negative feedback loops: low levels of child PA would lead to parental stimulation, which would lead to more PA. The existence of positive feedback loops like those uncovered in the current study, may particularly explain non-linearity of environment – behavior relationships in the area of childhood obesity [23]. It may accurately describe the process where parents and children unintentionally become caught into a negative spiral from which it is hard to escape (i.e. more sedentary behavior leading to less stimulation to be active, in turn leading to even more sedentary behavior, and so on). However, the findings with regard to stimulation of physical activity and actual physical need to be interpreted with caution, as both concepts have a slightly different focus as regards the type of physical activity (i.e. focus on active travel versus on physical activity in general, respectively).

Restriction of sedentary behavior was found to have a detrimental impact on child activity-related and BMI outcomes; it was associated with an increase of child BMI and a decrease in child physical activity behavior. In accordance with the literature about restriction in the feeding domain, where food restriction could lead to an increase of children's desire and intake of forbidden foods [24], it could be that children who are restricted in the amount of screen time increase their preferences for these behaviors and act upon that by being less physically active. However, we did not find that parents adapted their restrictive parenting practices to deviations in child outcomes (i.e. BMI z-score, physical activity, and sedentary screen-based behavior). It thus seems that parents do not (further) restrict their child's sedentary behavior when their child is overweight or less active.

Study strengths and limitations

This study is unique in its study design. Data were prospectively collected in a large cohort, and activity-related parenting practices and child physical activity-related variables were measured similarly on two time points. Although the questionnaires that were used were previously validated [13, 15], they have been used in only a few studies. We recommend replication studies using other parenting questionnaires, investigating the bidirectionality of the association between child outcomes and other parenting practices (such as parental modeling of activities). Also as regards behavior other questionnaires, including measures of other behaviours, might be worthwhile, as our study was limited to screen-based sedentary activities. Other sedentary behaviors such as reading are an understudied topic. Parental efforts decrease sedentary time might merely cause shifts from one type of sedentary behavior to another. Our study is further limited as it relies on self-reports. This systematic bias may produce spurious results. For instance, parents are likely to underestimate their children's weight and overestimate height, especially if their child was overweight or obese, whereas parents of underweight children tended to overestimate weight [25]. This could be a reason why our study reported lower percentages of overweight/ obesity (8.9% at age 5 and 6.4% at age 7) compared to the Dutch reference population of children aged 5–7 (2009: ranging from 12.8% and 18.8% for overweight and from 2.0% to 3.4% for obesity) [26]. It is likely that the present study yielded underestimates of associations between the activity-related parenting practice scales and child physical activity-related and BMI variables and vice versa, because of the parental reported nature of this study. This dilution of effects could also be due to imprecision of measurements and possible misspecification of models through assumptions of linearity. Future efforts should address more measurement points. While mutual influence between parent and child is a repeated, continuous process of interactions and adaptations, this process may likely be non-linear. Future studies could also establish whether the time lag of activity-related parenting practices that influence child physical activity-related variables is similar or different from the time lag for child physical activity-related variables to influence activity-related parenting practices.

Conclusions

This study addresses the importance of conducting longitudinal research to get insight into the bidirectional nature of parent-child relations with regard to activity-related behavior. Parents and children are continuously adapting to each other and future efforts should make further progress in this area by addressing system dynamics in the home setting. The mutual influence between parents and children in influencing their activity-related behaviors could lead parents to unintentionally and unconsciously become caught into a negative spiral from which it is hard to escape (i.e., reinforcing causal loop chains). It is important to give those parents support as regards raising awareness for such processes and parenting practices that they could apply to get their child to become more physically active.

Abbreviations

BMI: Body Mass Index; CITC: Corrected Item–Total Correlations; PA: Physical activity

Acknowledgements

Not applicable.

Funding

This work was supported by the Netherlands Heart Foundation (E.F.C.S., grant number 2014 T037); and the Netherlands Organization for Scientific Research (NWO), Division for the Social Sciences (MaGW), the Netherlands (J.S.G., grant number 016.145.091). Financial support for the follow-up of the KOALA Birth Cohort Study at age 5 was provided by the Dutch Ministry of Economic Affairs, the Dutch Ministry of Health, Welfare and Sports, FrieslandCampina and the Dutch Sugar Bureau, all in the Netherlands.

Authors' contributions

ES and JG conceptualized the study. ES, JG and CT were involved in data collection, ES conducted the statistical analyses, interpreted the data, and drafted the manuscript. All authors reviewed draft versions of the manuscript and provided feedback. JG revised the manuscript after peer review. All authors read and approved the final manuscript.

Competing interests

The authors declare that they have no competing interests.

Author details

[1]Department of Health Promotion, NUTRIM School of Nutrition and Translational Research in Metabolism, Maastricht University, Maastricht University Medical Center, P.O. Box 616, 6200 MD Maastricht, the Netherlands. [2]Department of Epidemiology, Maastricht University, CAPHRI Care and Public Health Research Institute, P.O. Box 616, 6200 MD Maastricht, the Netherlands.

References

1. Darling N, Steinberg L. Parenting style as a context: an integrative model. Psychol Bull. 1993;113:487–98.
2. Vaughn AE, Tabak RG, Bryant MJ, Ward DS. Measuring parent food practices: a systematic review of existing measures and examination. Int J Behav Nutr Phys Act. 2013;10:61.
3. Xu H, Wen LM, Rissel C. Associations of parental influences with physical activity and screen time among young children: a systematic review. J Obes. 2015;2015: 546925.
4. Jago R, Edwards MJ, Urbanski CR, Sebire SJ. General and specific approaches to media parenting: a systematic review of current measures, associations with screen-viewing, and measurement implications. Child Obes. 2013;9:S51–72.
5. Sleddens EFC, Kremers SPJ, Hughes SO, Cross MB, Thijs C, De Vries NK, et al. Physical activity parenting: a systematic review of questionnaires and their associations with child activity levels. Obes Rev. 2012;13:1015–33.
6. Afonso L, Lopes C, Severo M, Santos S, Real H, Durão C, et al. Bidirectional associations between parental child-feeding practices and body mass index at 4 and 7 y of age. Am J Clin Nutr. 2016;103:861–7.
7. Jansen PW, Tharner A, van der Ende J, Wake M, Raat H, Hofman A, et al. Feeding practices and child weight: is the association bidirectional in preschool children? Am J Clin Nutr. 2014;100:1329–36.
8. Rhee KE, Coleman SM, Appugliese DP, Kaciroti NA, Corwyn RF, Davidson NS, et al. Maternal feeding practices become more controlling after and not before excessive rates of weight gain. Obesity (Silver Spring). 2009;17:1724–9.
9. Webber L, Cooke L, Hill C, Wardle J. Child adiposity and maternal feeding practices: a longitudinal analysis. Am J Clin Nutr. 2010;92:1423–8.
10. Berge JM. A review of familial correlates of child and adolescent obesity: what has the 21st century taught us so far? J Adolesc Med Health. 2009;21:457–83.
11. Patrick H, Hennessy E, McSpadden K, Oh A. Parenting styles and practices in children's obesogenic behaviors: scientific gaps and future research directions. Child Obes. 2013;9:S73–86.
12. Kummeling I, Thijs C, Penders J, Snijders BE, Stelma F, Reimerink J, et al. Etiology of atopy in infancy: the KOALA birth cohort study. Pediatr Allergy Immunol. 2005; 16:679–84.
13. Gubbels JS, Kremers SPJ, Stafleu A, De Vries SI, Goldbohm RA, Dagnelie PC. Association between parenting practices and children's dietary intake, activity behavior and development of body mass index: the KOALA birth cohort study. Int J Behav Nutr Phys Act. 2011;8:18.
14. Birch LL, Fisher JO, Grimm-Thomas K, Markey CN. Confirmatory factor analysis of the child feeding questionnaire: a measure of parental attitudes, beliefs and

practices about child feeding and obesity proneness. Appetite. 2001;36:201–10.
15. Monitor Jeugdgezondheid: Standaard Vraagstelling Bewegen (Standard Questionnaire Physical Activity). GGD Nederland, Rijksinstituut voor Volksgezondheid en Milieu (RIVM) and Actiz organisatie van zorgondernemers; 2009.
16. Fredriks AM, van Buuren S, Wit JM, Verloove-Vanhorick SP. Body index measurements in 1996–1997 compared with 1980. Arch Dis Child. 2000;82:107–12.
17. Barlow SE. Expert committee recommendations regarding the prevention, assessment, and treatment of child and adolescent overweight and obesity: summary report. Pediatrics. 2007;120(S4):S164–S92. Aappublications. org/content/120/Supplement_4
18. Eurostat. Task force on Core social variables. Final report. Luxembourg: European Communitees; 2007.
19. Portney LG, Watkins MP. Foundations of clinical research: applications to practice. 2nd ed. Upper Saddle River, NJ: Prentice Hall;2000.
20. Bernstein IH, Nunnally J. Psychometric theory. New York: McGraw-Hill; 1994.
21. Gerards SMPL, Hummel K, Dagnelie PC, De Vries NK, Kremers SPJ. Parental self-efficacy in childhood overweight: validation of the lifestyle behavior checklist in the Netherlands. Int J Behav Nutr Phys Act. 2013;10:7.
22. Sterman JD. Business dynamics: systems thinking and modeling for a complex world. New York: Irwin/McGraw-Hill; 2000.
23. Hamid TKA. Thinking in circles about obesity: applying systems thinking to weight management. New York: Springer; 2009.
24. Jansen E, Mulkens S, Jansen A. Do not eat the red food!: prohibition of snacks leads to their relatively higher consumption in children. Appetite. 2007;49:572–7. doi:10.1016/j.appet.2007.03.229.
25. Scholtens S, Brunekreef B, Visscher TLS, Smit HA, Kerkhof M, De Jongste JC, Gerritsen J, Wijga AH. Reported versus measured body weight and height of 4-year-old children and the prevalence of overweight. Eur J Pub Health. 2007;17:369–74.
26. Schönbeck Y, Talma H, van Dommelen P, Bakker B, Buitendijk SE, Hirasing RA, van Buuren S. Increase in prevalence of overweight in Dutch children and adolescents: a comparison of nationwide growth studies in 1980, 1997 and 2009. Plos One. 2011;6:e27608. doi:10.1371/journal.pone.0027608.

15

Pathways through which higher neighborhood crime is longitudinally associated with greater body mass index

Andrea S. Richardson[1*], Wendy M. Troxel[1], Madhumita Ghosh-Dastidar[1], Gerald P. Hunter[1], Robin Beckman[1], Natalie Colabianchi[2], Rebecca L. Collins[1] and Tamara Dubowitz[1]

Abstract

Background: Although crime and perceived safety are associated with obesity and body mass index (BMI), the pathways are less clear. Two likely pathways by which crime and perceived safety may impact obesity are through distress and physical activity.

Methods: We examined data from 2013 to 2014 for 644 predominantly African-American adults (mean age 57 years; 77% female) living in low-income Pittsburgh, PA neighborhoods, including self-reported perceptions of safety and emotional distress, interviewer-measured height/weight, and physical activity measured via accelerometry. We used secondary data on neighborhood crime from 2011 to 2013. We built a structural equation model to examine the longitudinal direct and indirect pathways from crime to BMI through perceived safety, distress and physical activity.

Results: Long-term exposure to crime was positively associated with lack of perceived safety ($\beta = 0.11$, $p = 0.005$) and lack of perceived safety was positively associated with BMI ($\beta = 0.08$, $p = 0.03$). The beneficial association between physical activity and BMI ($\beta = -0.15$, $p < 0.001$) was attenuated by a negative association between crime and physical activity ($\beta = -0.09$, $p = 0.01$). Although crime was associated with distress we found no evidence of a path from crime to BMI via distress.

Conclusions: Our findings suggest decrements in perceived safety and physical activity are important processes that might explain why neighborhood crime is associated with greater BMI.

Keywords: Obesity, Crime, Physical activity, Neighborhood, Perceived safety, Structural equation modeling

Background

African Americans are disproportionately affected by obesity [1] and more likely to live in neighborhoods with higher crime rates than whites [2, 3]. Neighborhood crime and perceived lack of safety have been associated with psychological distress [4, 5], poor health [6–9], limited physical activity [10–14], and obesity [15, 16]. Literature on objective crime measures and their association with obesity, BMI and physical activity supports associations between neighborhood safety and activity [12, 17, 18]. However, the role of crime, varying degrees of perceived safety and the intersection of these factors in influencing resident distress, physical activity, and BMI are not well understood (see reviews [19–21]), especially in low-income, African American populations [22, 23].

Neighborhoods provide environments that may promote or limit health-related behaviors [24]. Increasing evidence has shown objectively measured crime and perceived lack of safety to increase stress, limit physical activity because of safety concerns, and therefore influence obesity [12, 25]. Several plausible pathways exist through which neighborhood crime could influence obesity. Chronic activation of the physiologic stress system resulting from crime exposure could lead to obesity, given how cortisol production increases BMI [26–29]. Another path from crime to obesity could operate through perceived lack of safety to physical activity. Understanding residents' perceptions of neighborhood

* Correspondence: arichard@rand.org
[1]RAND Corporation, Health Division, 4570 Fifth Avenue, Pittsburgh, PA 15213, USA
Full list of author information is available at the end of the article

safety and their role in resident health could help identify ways to support resilience in disadvantaged neighborhoods [30]. Much of the existing evidence is based on self-reported physical activity and anthropometry, which are subject to reporting bias [31, 32]. Furthermore, much of the cross-sectional research focuses on direct associations between crime/perceived safety and obesity/BMI without considering two mediating pathways through distress and physical activity.

Among the few studies examining pathways, Roman et al., used structural (SEM) equation modeling with data from two deprived Chicago neighborhoods (n = 328, mean age 47 years) to examine the direct and indirect pathways from perceptions of neighborhood violence and disorder to obesity through fear of walking [5]. Perceived violence was positively associated with fear of walking but not with physical activity or obesity. However, this cross-sectional study relied on self-reported anthropometry and physical activity. A cross-sectional study of 864 adults from a low-income and ethnically mixed neighborhood in Salt Lake City, UT used objectively measured anthropometry and physical activity [11]. They found that low perceived safety was associated with high BMI and that lower moderate-to-vigorous physical activity partially explained the relationship between safety and BMI. Yet the authors were unable to examine how crime may relate to perceived safety.

It remains unclear how peoples' perceptions of crime impact their sense of safety, in part, because no consensus exists on whether the location and timing of crime incidents influences resident perceptions. Understanding the types, location and timing of crimes and their relationship with perceptions of safety is necessary in order to robustly model an indirect pathway whereby crime influences BMI through perceived safety using the objective measure that is most strongly associated with perceived safety.

Prior studies have examined crime across a wide range of geographic areas (e.g., census block group [33], census tract [15], half-mile [15], and 1-mile [13]) surrounding residents' homes in association with physical activity, diet and BMI. But it is unknown how proximity from crimes, or the timing at which crimes occurred, may be associated with physical activity and health. In one study, agreement was poor between objective measures of crime and perceived fear across 1-, half-, and eighth-mile buffers but agreement appeared to increase with decreasing buffer size [18]. This study was limited by small sample size (n = 303) and crimes were aggregated to an annual rate, ignoring more detailed timing of the occurrences (e.g., a month versus a year ago). In addition, much of the research on the role of crime in neighborhoods has not considered influences on health from crimes occurring with varying degrees of proximity [34].

In sum, limitations of research on neighborhood crime, perceptions, behaviors, obesity, and distress include the lack of studies that use objectively measured data (crime, physical activity, and BMI), to examine longitudinal pathways to resident health, and to examine patterns of association with crime across different levels of crime aggregation (over space and time). To address these gaps, this longitudinal study examined how proximity and timing of crime related to perceptions of safety in two predominantly African American low-income Pittsburgh neighborhoods. We then derived a long-term measure of neighborhood crime based on these associations. In a SEM, we tested direct and indirect pathways from long-term exposure to neighborhood crime (prior 2 years) to BMI a year later through perceived safety and the two likely additional mediating pathways, distress and physical activity.

Methods

Study population and participants

Pittsburgh Research on Neighborhoods, Exercise and Health (also known as 'PHRESH Plus') was designed to document and evaluate neighborhood investments in greenspace and housing on physical activity and active transport in lower-income African American neighborhoods in Pittsburgh. The sample includes randomly selected households from two communities who are part of a cohort followed over time. The Hill District neighborhood has and continues to undergo neighborhood economic investments, including renovation of greenspace for recreational activities. Homewood, the comparison neighborhood, although experiencing some investment and change, did not experience the same degree of investment. This study uses the PHRESH Plus baseline data (collected Spring 2013), prior to major greenspace and housing renovations, and follow-up data on the same cohort members from a sister PHRESH study (collected in Spring 2014). Data collection included neighborhood-level built and social characteristics, and detailed individual-level data. All study protocols were approved by the institution's Institutional Review Board.

Outcome variable: Body mass index (BMI) (2014)

Interviewers measured height (without shoes) to the nearest eighth inch using a carpenter's square and an 8-ft folding wooden ruler marked in inches. Weight was measured to the nearest tenth of a pound using the SECA Robusta 813 digital scale. BMI was calculated as weight in kg divided by height in m^2.

Exposure variable: Neighborhood-level crime (2011–2013)

Incident-level crime data was provided by the City of Pittsburgh police department which contained comprehensive lists of all reported crimes in Pittsburgh for 2 years preceding the household survey administration (i.e., 2011–2013). We calculated street network distances from each household to crime locations for all types (e.g., robbery, assault, etc.) using ArcGIS 10.2. We geocoded 95% of the incidents using address information. To assess how different crime measures are associated with perceived safety we first calculated them across varying distances from the residents' homes, summing the number of crimes that occurred within 1/10-, 1/4-, 1/2-, and 3/4-mile radial distances from each household address. To assess how timing of the criminal activity is associated with perceived safety we summed the number of crimes that occurred within 1 month, 3 months, 6 months, 1 year and 2 years prior to the date the respondent was interviewed in 2013. We created 20 crime measures total (e.g., crimes that occurred within last month and ½ mile of the residents' residence) for each combination of timing and proximity. Because the crime measures are aggregated to buffers surrounding the respondents' residence they are respondent-based exposures (i.e., a crime can be counted multiple times in the sample for different individuals depending on their residential location). Thus, we used counts of crime rather than neighborhood population-based rates.

To assess long-term exposure to neighborhood crime we used the measure that was most sensitive to perceived safety and averaged it over the 2 years preceding the interview date.

Intermediate variables (2013)

Perceived safety

Study interviewers administered questionnaires and residents answered the question "Your neighborhood is safe from crime" using a five-point disagree-agree scale. We reverse coded responses so that higher values reflected lack of perceived safety because of neighborhood crime.

Psychological distress

The Kessler 6 (K6) psychological distress scale is a self-report instrument to assess psychological distress [35]. We chose the K6 because it is a well-validated measure of psychological distress that can detect the presence of mild to severe psychological problems with high levels of sensitivity and specificity in a wide variety of populations [36]. As such, it has indeed been linked with cortisol in prior research [37]. Data collectors asked residents the frequency with which they experienced distress symptoms (e.g., "feel hopeless"; "feel restless or fidgety") in the last 30 days. Responses were on a five-point scale. Scores were summed into a single score where high values reflect distress. K6 scores can be interpreted as no or low distress = 0–4 points, moderate distress = 5–12 points, or severe distress = 13–24 points [38].

Objectively measured physical activity

Participants were given a tri-axial accelerometer (i.e., ActiGraph GT3X+) and asked to wear the device on their non-dominant wrist for 7 consecutive (24 h) days. Data were sampled at 30 hz and summarized into 60 s epochs. Non-wear was determined based on the Choi algorithm using vector magnitude values [39]. Sleep intervals were identified from daily bed and wake times reported by the participant. When these times were not available or irregular (e.g., > 12 h or < 3 h sleep interval; suspected inaccurate date recorded by the participant), further visual inspection of the raw accelerometer signal was used to supplement the recorded data. All sleep interval data was removed from analyses. Further, because participants did not report their bed times on the first day the monitor was worn, the first full 24 h of recording was removed to ensure that no sleep time was included in vector magnitude calculations. Vector magnitude is the square root of the sum of the three squared axes [e.g., $(x^2 + y^2 + z^2)^{1/2}$]. Data were processed in ActiLife v6.13.1. The daily average of vector magnitude counts per minute was averaged across all days with at least 10 h of wear time. A participant was included in the analysis if he/she had at least 3 days of valid wear and their vector magnitude counts were analyzed continuously. While no vector magnitude cut points for the ActiGraph wrist exist yet for sedentary activity, a 2000 counts per minute cut point was identified in 94 older women to be very low activity [40].

Individual-level covariates (2013)

Below, we describe the variables we used as covariates in models. Residents provided information on date of birth, gender, education (categorized into at least some college/bachelor's degree versus less than college), and marital/cohabitation status (married or living with a partner versus living alone). We also included annual income per capita (we imputed missing values $n = 45$). We did not control for race/ethnicity because the majority of the sample (92%) self-identified as Black or African American. To capture physical activity limitation we used their responses to the question "Does your health limit you when walking one block?" which we dichotomized to "a little or a lot" versus "not at all." To account for unmeasured differences across neighborhoods that could confound associations between crime and obesity, we controlled for neighborhood, using a binary indicator of Hill District versus Homewood. Social networks may mitigate negative effects of crime on health and well-being [7] by providing positive support and social cohesion [41] and might also influence whether crimes occur in one's neighborhood. Therefore, we also controlled for social network size which was measured using a previously validated scale [42]. Participants reported the number of people they knew (e.g., family, close friends, neighbors, etc.). The number of people in each category was summed to compute each participant's social network size.

Analytic sample

We excluded residents if they did not live in Hill District or Homewood at the time of the 2013 interview (n = 27) (i.e., if they had moved out of the neighborhood from initial enrollment into the study), were missing accelerometry data (n = 98), had less than 3 valid (≥ 10 h) accelerometer days (n = 15), were lost to follow up in 2014 when the BMI outcome was collected (n = 248), were missing crime data (n = 8), or were missing response to the question about perceived safety (n = 198). The final analytic sample included 644 adults who wore the accelerometer for an average of 5.7 ± 0.6 days. We calculated T-tests (continuous variables) and Chi-Square tests (categorical variables) to compare the included versus excluded (n = 397) residents. We compared all covariate, intermediate and, outcome variables between excluded individuals and individuals included, and only age and social network size differed. Those individuals excluded were younger (mean age 53 years vs 57 years among the included, p = < 0.001) and had fewer social network members (mean 28 vs 48 among the included, p = < 0.001).

Statistical analyses

We performed descriptive analyses and tested multivariable models using Stata 14.0 (StataCorp, College Station, TX). We calculated means and standard deviations (continuous variables) and percentages (categorical variables) of individual-level – and neighborhood-level crime. To identify the timing and proximity of crime most sensitive (based on relative magnitude of association) to perceived safety, we used logit models to predict perceived safety as a function of 20 different crime measures. We estimated separate models for counts of crime by time and proximity. We controlled for age, gender, education, married or living with a partner, physical limitation, neighborhood, social network size, and household income in these crime-safety tests. To illustrate the magnitude of the associations we plotted a three-dimensional bar graph of the logit estimates (y-axis) by crime timing (x-axis) and distance (z-axis).

To examine longitudinal indirect pathways from crime to later BMI through perceived safety, psychological distress and physical activity, we used Mplus version 7.11 [43] to build a SEM. We used the measure of crime that emerged as the best predictor of perceived safety in the above analyses and averaged it over the 2 years preceding the respondents' interview to derive a measure that is sensitive to perceived safety and also captures long-term exposure to crime. We allowed for a direct pathway from crime to BMI. Given that there may be bidirectional associations between distress and physical activity [44, 45], we also tested whether distress and physical activity covaried (double-headed curved arrow in Fig. 1). Figure 1 presents our conceptual model. We controlled for the above-mentioned covariates to address confounding of associations between: (1) crime and BMI (exposure to outcome); (2) perceived safety, physical activity, and BMI (mediators to outcome); (3) crime, perceived safety, distress, and physical activity (exposure to mediators) that were not likely to be affected by crime [46]. A statistically non-significant Chi-Square test statistic [47], Root Mean Square Error of Approximation (RMSEA) < 0.06 [48], and Comparative Fit Index (CFI) values approaching 1.0 [49] imply the model fits the data well.

Results

In 2013, the analytic sample was on average 57 years of age, low-income (mean per capita income $13,400), burdened with low mobility, and overweight in 2014 (mean body mass index (kg/m^2) was 31 kg/m^2 (Table 1).

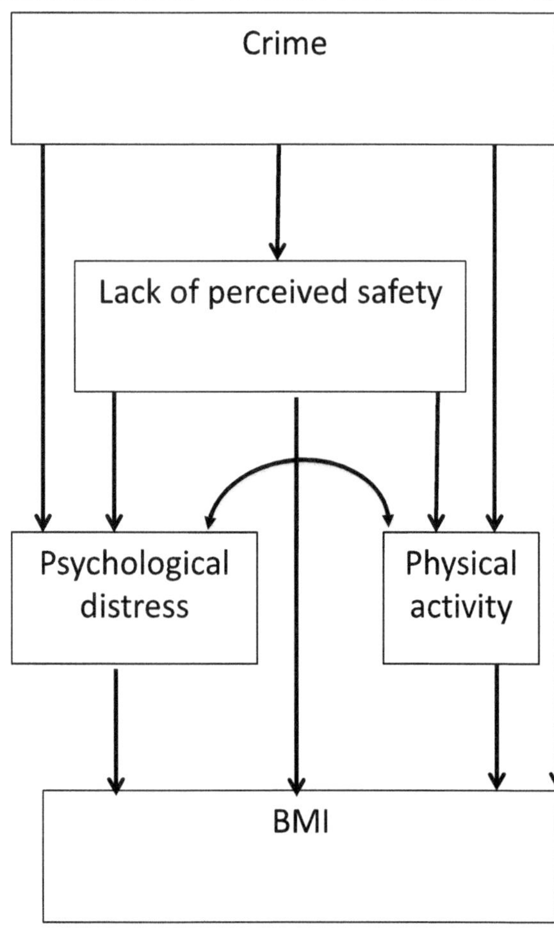

Fig. 1 Conceptual model of direct and indirect paths from crime to BMI

Table 1 Study population characteristics in 2013 and body mass index in 2014, $n = 644$

	Mean (SD) or percentage
Body mass index (kg/m^2)	31.1 (7.6)
Physical activity (vector magnitude[a] [counts/min])	2139.6 (777.0)
Kessler psychological distress score (K6)[b]	4.3 (4.6)
Lack of perceived safety in neighborhood	3.8 (1.0)
Age (years)	57.0 (15.4)
Male sex	23.0%
Mean per capita annual income (in $1000)	13.5 (13.2)
Social network size	47.5 (50.4)
Education (at least some college/bachelor's degree)	45.0%
Married or living with partner	18.9%
Any physical limitation walking 1 block	28.7%
Neighborhood	
Hill District	69.4%
Homewood	30.6%

[a]Based on 3–7 days of accelerometry data using a 1-min epoch
[b]Responses were on a five-point scale. Scores were summed into a single score (0–24) where high values reflect psychological distress

Table 2 Number of reported crimes (of any kind) by distance from resident's home and time frame[a] (2011–2013), $N = 644$

	Mean (SD)
Within last month	
Within 1/10 mile	1.9 (0.1)
Within 1/4 mile	8.8 (0.2)
Within 1/2 mile	31.0 (0.7)
Within 3/4 mile	64.2 (1.2)
Within last 3 months	
Within 1/10 mile	5.6 (0.2)
Within 1/4 mile	25.2 (0.6)
Within 1/2 mile	88.6 (2.0)
Within 3/4 mile	183.3 (3.1)
Within last 6 months	
Within 1/10 mile	10.8 (0.4)
Within 1/4 mile	47.8 (1.2)
Within 1/2 mile	167.2 (3.6)
Within 3/4 mile	346.9 (5.7)
Within last year	
Within 1/10 mile	21.4 (0.7)
Within 1/4 mile	93.6 (2.2)
Within 1/2 mile	333.5 (7.1)
Within 3/4 mile	695.5 (14.3)
Within 2 years	
Within 1/10 mile	44.4 (1.4)
Within 1/4 mile	191.9 (4.5)
Within 1/2 mile	685.2 (14.3)
Within 3/4 mile	1424.1 (21.9)

[a]Counts of crimes obtained from Pittsburgh Police Department and aggregated by timing preceding interview and radial distance from resident household

About one fifth of the cohort was married or living with a partner (19%), and an average vector magnitude of 2140 cpm suggests very low activity [40, 50]. The cohort reports relatively low distress with a mean of 4.3. The average number of crime exposures ranged from about 2 to 1424 depending on distance from residence and time frame (Table 2).

We associated 1) residents' perceived neighborhood safety with 2) counts of crimes in varying time frames preceding the 2013 interview and 3) distance from the residence. Figure 2 shows plots of the magnitude of the logit beta estimates (y-axis) across the time frame of the crimes (x-axis) and the distance from residents' residence (z-axis). Most estimates were statistically significant ($p < 0.05$, data not shown). Magnitude of the association between crime and perceived safety increased as distance between crime and participants' residence decreased and as timing was closer to the interview. Perceived safety was most strongly associated with crimes that occurred within 1/10-mile from the resident's home, and those that that happened within the month preceding the interview. Although the correlation between perceived safety and crimes within 1/10-mile and 1 month was not significant (Pearson's correlation coefficient = 0.06, $p = 0.11$), which is likely due to the small number of crimes that occurred within 1/10 mile and the 1 month timeframe.

To address temporality, we created an average of crime over a longer period of time. First, we derived a monthly count of crime for each respondent for each month over 2 years (2011–2013) preceding the date of the resident's interview (2013). Next, we averaged the monthly counts across the 2 years by summing the counts and dividing by 24 (mean = 1.84 crimes per month SD = 1.5). This captures the importance of crime timing to concurrent perceptions of safety, while providing an indicator of such over a longer period of time in order to better predict slow-changing BMI.

In our initial model, the covariance path between distress and physical activity was not statistically significant ($p = 0.35$) and model fit was not ideal (RMSEA = 0.00, CFI = 1.00, Chi-Square = 0.00 (0 df) $p = < 0.001$). The SEM model deleting this path fit the data well (RMSEA = 0.00, CFI = 1.00, Chi-Square = 0.02 (1 df) $p = 0.88$. Figure 3 presents this result. For clarity, we present only associations that were statistically significant ($p < 0.05$). Long-term exposure to crime was indirectly associated with BMI through perceived safety. We saw a positive association between the average monthly number

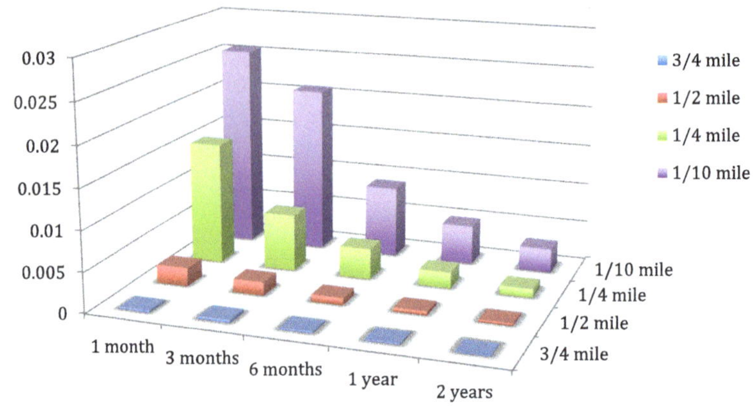

Fig. 2 Logit coefficients from 20 models estimating lack of perceived safety as a function of crime measures that vary by time frame and distance from residents' home

of nearby crimes and lack of perceived safety (β = 0.11, p = 0.005) and lack of perceived safety was positively associated with BMI a year later (β = 0.08, p = 0.03). Physical activity also appeared to serve as an indirect pathway between crime and later BMI. Crime was associated with reduced physical activity (β = −0.09, p = 0.009), and physical activity was negatively associated with BMI (β = −0.15, p < 0.001). Crime was also associated with distress, but because distress was not predictive of BMI, distress does not serve as a pathway between crime and this outcome, nor does it explain associations between perceived safety and BMI. Finally, we find no direct association between crime and BMI, suggesting that the indirect paths through perceived safety and physical activity, account entirely for the association between these two variables.

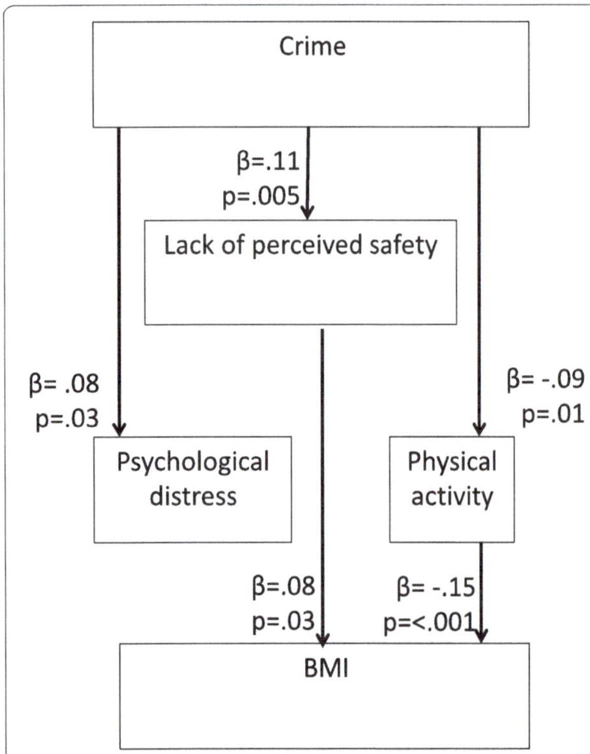

Fig. 3 Longitudinal SEM model testing direct and indirect paths from crime to BMI, N = 644

Discussion

We found that objectively measured long-term exposure to crime is associated with higher BMI at a later point in time through two separate paths, lack of perceived safety and decreased physical activity. Unexpectedly, distress did not explain associations between objectively measured crime, lack of perceived safety and BMI, suggesting other processes could be at play along this particular path. Future work may be warranted exploring other potential pathways. For example, lack of perceived safety may impact neighborhood cohesion or disorder and subsequently have downstream impacts on BMI via social fragmentation and isolation [51–53] that promote poor dietary behaviors. Our covariate measure of social network size may not have adequately captured such a process.

Lack of perceived safety appeared to mediate the pathway between objective crime and BMI. Thus, it is possible that perception of crime is more acutely relevant to BMI than objectively reported crime events in one's neighborhood. This is consistent with other studies showing that perceptions of neighborhood conditions are more strongly associated with health outcomes than objective measures [54–56].

Perceived safety was not associated with physical activity, contradicting prior findings indicating that residents who felt safe in their neighborhood were more likely to walk [12, 57, 58] and be physically active [11]. However, some studies have found no association between safety perceptions and physical activity [10]. One of the first studies to examine how changes in crime and perceptions associated with walking over time found little evidence that perceived safety or police-reported crime associated with walking [13]. Fear is another reaction to crime and is a distinct construct from perceived safety, although the two constructs are correlated and both empirically linked with health [59]. Given the apparent links between neighborhood crime, fear and health [8, 60], fear may be more salient to physical activity than perceived safety. A longitudinal study in Perth, Australia, (n = 531) among adults (mean age 40 years) reported that perceived safety was associated with increased time walking [12]. Yet, in an earlier publication this same group reported that fear of crime was also associated with walking time and the effect size was stronger for fear than for perceived safety (22 min/wk. vs 20 min/wk). Future research should test whether fear is more salient to ones' decision to engage in physical activity than perceived safety. While future research should examine pathways through which both perceived safety and fear may mediate associations between crime, and BMI, it is beyond the scope of this paper. Our survey asked the residents how safe their neighborhood was from crime so we opted to use this specific measure of perceived safety.

Our study population is urban, low-income, predominantly African American and sedentary so findings may not be generalizable. Given uncertainty in cut points, we analyzed vector magnitude as a continuous variable where vector magnitude is a volume measure of activity that may (or not) happen in the neighborhood. The average vector magnitude in our study was 2124.7 which is not much more than the 2000 cut point identified in 94 older women as sedentary [40]. Nonetheless, it is an important group of interest to both the study of crime and the study of overweight.

Another issue underlying inconsistencies may be the approaches used to quantify feeling safe in prior studies, such as using composite scores that include questions about walking at night and aesthetics [61, 62], unattended dogs, and safety jogging [63], or worry about being attacked [64]. These measures may tap into slightly different aspects of perceived safety or they may confound perceived safety with other variables. That is, composite measures of perceived safety may conflate other safety-related issues with safety specific to crime. For this reason, we opted to use a single-item measure that directly asked how safe their neighborhood was from crime.

Our finding that lack of perceived safety was associated with higher BMI is consistent with other studies [65–67]. Of the few that examine both physical activity and BMI [11, 66, 68, 69], perceived social nuisances (e.g., incivilities) among 14,836 English adults were positively associated with obesity but it was not mediated by physical activity [69]. While the strengths of Poortinga's study include measured anthropometry and examination of mediation by physical activity they lacked objective measures of crime and physical activity. Another study among 9252 American adults living in urban areas found a positive association between county-level crime and BMI but not between county-level crime and walking [70]. Yet, this study was limited by variation within counties and by modeling physical activity and BMI separately, which does not address potential mediating pathways. Our pathway findings do support the theory that African American adults living in deprived neighborhoods are obese because crime deters physical activity [19] since we found associations between crime, perceived safety, and physical activity.

Some research suggests that people living in deprived areas with high crime rates experience stress that translates into dysregulation of the hypothalamic-pituitary-adrenal that can cause higher BMI [27, 71]. Our findings suggest that high levels of crime increase distress. In another large longitudinal study of older Australian adults that used objective measures of crime an increase in risk of experiencing distress was associated with an increase in neighborhood crime [72]. However, this study did not include perceptions of safety and our findings suggest that distress does not play a role in pathways from crime to BMI.

We also found that the association between number of crimes and lack of perceived safety got progressively stronger as the reference period was defined closer in time to interview and distance from residents' homes was smaller. We provide evidence that when and where crimes occur is important to consider in studies that link objective measures of crime with resident perceptions of safety. Thus, researchers might not need a long reference period or wide area of assessment in studies of crime and perceived safety. However, in the case when the study outcome is slow to change, such as with BMI, it is also important to consider a method of aggregating such a measure to tap a longer history of immediate (proximal in time and space) exposure.

No consensus exists about the geographic area that best represents a neighborhood [73] and to our knowledge only one study examined how counts of crime aggregated within different distances from residents homes associated with perceived safety [18]. Among 303 adults living in Winston-Salem, NC the number of police service calls within 1-, 1/2-, and 1/8-mile and normalized by population size had low agreement with perceived safety (weighted kappas [95% CI]: 1-mile, .12 [.04–.20]; half-mile, .18 [.10–.26]; eighth-mile, .22 [.14–.30]). However, agreement appears to have been highest when using the crime rate within the closest distance. To our knowledge, no study has explored how the timing of when crimes occur influences perceptions of safety and key health outcomes.

Our study is longitudinal, capturing changes in environment, perceptions, behaviors or health. However, this study has limitations. We could not control for how long participants lived at their current address, which could contribute to a mismeasurement of their crime exposure. However, we did collect information regarding years lived in neighborhood of residence. The participants in our study are a stable population. Only 6% reported living in their neighborhood for less than a year, while 80% of the residents reported living in their neighborhood for over 5 years, and 50% of the residents reported living in their neighborhood for 20 years or more. Participants excluded from this analysis were younger which may have biased our results. Residential location choice is complex and driven by more than health-related preferences. Yet, individual behaviors and health may be tied to unobserved characteristics (e.g., health consciousness [74]) that underlie an individual's residential location. Thus, residential selection could bias our results. We lacked dietary data at this assessment, so we were unable to test alternate pathways through energy balance. Lastly, our participants were mostly sedentary, so the lack of variation may have limited our ability to detect associations with physical activity.

Despite these limitations we present longitudinal data from a low-income and predominantly African American cohort living in underserved urban neighborhoods that includes historic crime data combined with individual-level perceptions, behaviors, and objectively measured anthropometry and physical activity. Accelerometry is superior to self-report where over-reporting can bias estimates [75]. Similarly, measured heights and weights are less vulnerable to reporting bias than self-report [32]. Further, our study population is often at increased risk of residing in disadvantaged neighborhoods [2, 3], limited physical activity [75, 76] and suffering higher rates of inactivity-related cardiometabolic conditions [77–79]. To our knowledge, this is the first analysis linking objective measures of crime and perceived safety, to psychological distress, accelerometry-derived activity, and measured anthropometry in an older, disadvantaged, and predominantly African American population.

Conclusion

This work adds evidence that among African Americans living in urban low-income neighborhoods, lack of perceived safety in one's neighborhood because of high crime rates is associated with higher BMI, independent of physical activity and distress. Importantly, crime is also associated with higher BMI through less physical activity, but this process is a separate one. Neighborhood investments that reduce crime and improve resident perception of safety remain critical for the wellbeing of communities. Public health professionals and policy makers may consider crime and perception of safety as salient neighborhood factors that could exacerbate obesity in the United States.

Abbreviations

BMI: Body mass index; CFI: Comparative fit index; RMSEA: Root mean square error of approximation; SEM: Structured equation modeling

Acknowledgments

The authors express sincere appreciation and gratitude to La'Vette Wagner, field coordinator of the Pittsburgh Hill/Homewood Research on Eating, Shopping, and Health study and the data collection staff. The authors thank the Hill House Association, Operation Better Block, and Homewood Children's Village. Without their participation, the study could not have happened.

Funding

Funding was provided by the National Cancer Institute (Grant No. R01CA164137 "Impact of Greenspace Improvement on Physical Activity in a Low Income Community" and National Heart Lung Blood Institute (Grant No. R01 HL122460 "Neighborhood Change: Impact on Sleep and Obesity-Related Health Disparities").

Authors' contributions

ASR conceptualized, performed statistical analyses, and drafted the manuscript. TD and WT acquired the data. RB and GPH created variables and data sets. NC, MGD, RLC, WT and TD made substantial contributions to conception and design of the study. All authors involved in drafting the manuscript, revising critically for important content, agreed to be accountable for all aspects of the work in ensuring that questions related to the accuracy or integrity of any part of the work are appropriately investigated and resolved, and approved the final manuscript.

Competing interests

The authors declare that they have no competing interests.

Author details

[1]RAND Corporation, Health Division, 4570 Fifth Avenue, Pittsburgh, PA 15213, USA. [2]University of Michigan, School of Kinesiology, Ann Arbor, MI 48109-2013, USA.

References

1. World Health Organization: WHO global Infobase. 2011.
2. White K, Borrell LN. Racial/ethnic residential segregation: framing the context of health risk and health disparities. Health Place. 2011;17(2):438–48.
3. Williams DR, Collins C. Racial residential segregation: a fundamental cause of racial disparities in health. Public Health Rep. 2001;116(5):404–16.

4. Roberts B, Stickley A, Petticrew M, McKee M. The influence of concern about crime on levels of psychological distress in the former soviet union. J Epidemiol Community Health. 2012;66(5):433–9.
5. Roman CG, Knight CR, Chalfin A, Popkin SJ. The relation of the perceived environment to fear, physical activity, and health in public housing developments: evidence from Chicago. J Public Health Policy. 2009;30(Suppl 1):S286–308.
6. Kitchen P, Williams A. Quality of life and perceptions of crime in Saskatoon, Canada. Soc Indic Res. 2010;95(1):33–61.
7. Lorenc T, Clayton S, Neary D, Whitehead M, Petticrew M, Thomson H, Cummins S, Sowden A, Renton A. Crime, fear of crime, environment, and mental health and wellbeing: mapping review of theories and causal pathways. Health Place. 2012;18(4):757–65.
8. Ross CE, Mirowsky J. Neighborhood disadvantage, disorder, and health. J Health Soc Behav. 2001;42(3):258–76.
9. White M, Kasl SV, Zahner GEP, Will JC. Perceived crime in the neighborhood and mental-health of women and children. Environ Behav. 1987;19(5):588–613.
10. Bracy NL, Millstein RA, Carlson JA, Conway TL, Sallis JF, Saelens BE, Kerr J, Cain KL, Frank LD, King AC. Is the relationship between the built environment and physical activity moderated by perceptions of crime and safety? Int J Behav Nutr Phys. 2014;11 https://doi.org/10.1186/1479-5868-1111-1124.
11. Brown BB, Werner CM, Smith KR, Tribby CP, Miller HJ. Physical activity mediates the relationship between perceived crime safety and obesity. Prev Med. 2014;66:140–4.
12. Foster S, Hooper P, Knuiman M, Christian H, Bull F, Giles-Corti B. Safe RESIDential environments? A longitudinal analysis of the influence of crime-related safety on walking. Int J Behav Nutr Phys Act. 2016;13:22.
13. Kerr Z, Evenson KR, Moore K, Block R, Diez Roux AV. Changes in walking associated with perceived neighborhood safety and police-recorded crime: the multi-ethnic study of atherosclerosis. Prev Med. 2015;73:88–93.
14. Van Dyck D, Cerin E, De Bourdeaudhuij I, Salvo D, Christiansen LB, Macfarlane D, Owen N, Mitas J, Troelsen J, Aguinaga-Ontoso I, et al. Moderating effects of age, gender and education on the associations of perceived neighborhood environment attributes with accelerometer-based physical activity: the IPEN adult study. Health Place. 2015;36:65–73.
15. Mujahid MS, Diez Roux AV, Shen M, Gowda D, Sanchez B, Shea S, Jacobs DR Jr, Jackson SA. Relation between neighborhood environments and obesity in the multi-ethnic study of atherosclerosis. Am J Epidemiol. 2008;167(11): 1349–57.
16. Pham do Q, Ommerborn MJ, Hickson DA, Taylor HA, Clark CR. Neighborhood safety and adipose tissue distribution in African Americans: the Jackson heart study. PLoS One. 2014;9(8):e105251.
17. McDonald NC. The effect of objectively measured crime on walking in minority adults. Am J Health Promot. 2008;22(6):433–6.
18. McGinn AP, Evenson KR, Herring AH, Huston SL, Rodriguez DA. The association of perceived and objectively measured crime with physical activity: a cross-sectional analysis. J Phys Act Health. 2008;5(1):117–31.
19. Foster S, Giles-Corti B. The built environment, neighborhood crime and constrained physical activity: an exploration of inconsistent findings. Prev Med. 2008;47(3):241–51.
20. Van Cauwenberg J, De Bourdeaudhuij I, De Meester F, Van Dyck D, Salmon J, Clarys P, Deforche B. Relationship between the physical environment and physical activity in older adults: a systematic review. Health Place. 2011; 17(2):458–69.
21. Ding D, Gebel K. Built environment, physical activity, and obesity: what have we learned from reviewing the literature? Health Place. 2012;18(1):100–5.
22. Feng J, Glass TA, Curriero FC, Stewart WF, Schwartz BS. The built environment and obesity: a systematic review of the epidemiologic evidence. Health Place. 2010;16(2):175–90.
23. Kumanyika SK, Gary TL, Lancaster KJ, Samuel-Hodge CD, Banks-Wallace J, Beech BM, Hughes-Halbert C, Karanja N, Odoms-Young AM, Prewitt TE, et al. Achieving healthy weight in African-American communities: research perspectives and priorities. Obes Res. 2005;13(12):2037–47.
24. Sallis JF, Bauman A, Pratt M. Environmental and policy interventions to promote physical activity. Am J Prev Med. 1998;15(4):379–97.
25. Rachele JN, Ghani F, Loh VH, Brown WJ, Turrell G. Associations between physical activity and the neighbourhood social environment: baseline results from the HABITAT multilevel study. Prev Med. 2016;
26. Barrington WE, Stafford M, Hamer M, Beresford SA, Koepsell T, Steptoe A. Neighborhood socioeconomic deprivation, perceived neighborhood factors, and cortisol responses to induced stress among healthy adults. Health Place. 2014;27:120–6.
27. Champaneri S, Xu X, Carnethon MR, Bertoni AG, Seeman T, DeSantis AS, Diez Roux A, Shrager S, Golden SH. Diurnal salivary cortisol is associated with body mass index and waist circumference: the multiethnic study of atherosclerosis. Obesity. 2013;21(1):E56–63.
28. Karb RA, Elliott MR, Dowd JB, Morenoff JD. Neighborhood-level stressors, social support, and diurnal patterns of cortisol: the Chicago community adult health study. Soc Sci Med. 2012;75(6):1038–47.
29. Do DP, Diez Roux AV, Hajat A, Auchincloss AH, Merkin SS, Ranjit N, Shea S, Seeman T. Circadian rhythm of cortisol and neighborhood characteristics in a population-based sample: the multi-ethnic study of atherosclerosis. Health Place. 2011;17(2):625–32.
30. Ball K, Abbott G, Cleland V, Timperio A, Thornton L, Mishra G, Jeffery RW, Brug J, King A, Crawford D. Resilience to obesity among socioeconomically disadvantaged women: the READI study. Int J Obes. 2012;36(6):855–65.
31. Helmerhorst HJ, Brage S, Warren J, Besson H, Ekelund U. A systematic review of reliability and objective criterion-related validity of physical activity questionnaires. Int J Behav Nutr Phys Act. 2012;9:103.
32. Villanueva EV. The validity of self-reported weight in US adults: a population based cross-sectional study. BMC Public Health. 2001;1:11.
33. Roman CG, Chalfin A. Fear of walking outdoors. A multilevel ecologic analysis of crime and disorder. Am J Prev Med. 2008;34(4):306–12.
34. Morenoff JD. Neighborhood mechanisms and the spatial dynamics of birth weight. Am J Sociol. 2003;108(5):976–1017.
35. van Hees VT, Gorzelniak L, Dean Leon EC, Eder M, Pias M, Taherian S, Ekelund U, Renstrom F, Franks PW, Horsch A, et al. Separating movement and gravity components in an acceleration signal and implications for the assessment of human daily physical activity. PLoS One. 2013;8(4):e61691.
36. Arnaud B, Malet L, Teissedre F, Izaute M, Moustafa F, Geneste J, Schmidt J, Llorca PM, Brousse G. Validity study of Kessler's psychological distress scales conducted among patients admitted to French emergency Department for Alcohol Consumption-Related Disorders. Alcohol Clin Exp Res. 2010;34(7): 1235–45.
37. Berger M, Leicht A, Slatcher A, Kraeuter AK, Ketheesan S, Larkins S, Sarnyai Z: Cortisol awakening response and acute stress reactivity in first nations people. Sci Rep-Uk. 2017. 7 Digital ObjectIdentifier. doi:10.1038/srep41760.
38. Kessler RC, Barker PR, Colpe LJ, Epstein JF, Gfroerer JC, Hiripi E, Howes MJ, Normand SL, Manderscheid RW, Walters EE, et al. Screening for serious mental illness in the general population. Arch Gen Psychiatry. 2003;60(2):184–9.
39. Choi L, Ward SC, Schnelle JF, Buchowski MS. Assessment of wear/nonwear time classification algorithms for triaxial accelerometer. Med Sci Sports Exerc. 2012;44(10):2009–16.
40. Kamada M, Shiroma EJ, Harris TB, Lee IM. Comparison of physical activity assessed using hip- and wrist-worn accelerometers. Gait Posture. 2016;44:23–8.
41. Ross CE, Jang SJ. Neighborhood disorder, fear, and mistrust: the buffering role of social ties with neighbors. Am J Community Psychol. 2000;28(4):401–20.
42. Vardavas E, Marcum SC. Modeling influenza vaccination behavior via inductive REasoning games. In: d'Onofrio A, editor. Modeling the interplay between human behavior and spread of infectious disease. Manfredi P: Springer; 2012.
43. Muthén LK, Muthén BO. Mplus User's Guide. Los Angeles, CA: Muthén & Muthén; 1998-2010.
44. Stults-Kolehmainen MA, Sinha R. The effects of stress on physical activity and exercise. Sports Med. 2014;44(1):81–121.
45. Perales F, Pozo-Cruz JD, Pozo-Cruz BD. Impact of physical activity on psychological distress: a prospective analysis of an Australian national sample. Am J Public Health. 2014;104(12):e91–7.
46. Valeri L, Vanderweele TJ. Mediation analysis allowing for exposure-mediator interactions and causal interpretation: theoretical assumptions and implementation with SAS and SPSS macros. Psychol Methods. 2013;18(2):137–50.
47. Bollen KA. Front Matter, in Structural Equations with Latent Variables. Hoboken: Wiley; doi:10.1002/9781118619179.fmatter.
48. Hu L, Bentler PM. Cutoff criteria for fit indexes in covariance structure analysis: conventional criteria versus new laternatives. Struct Equ Model. 1999;6(1):1–55.
49. Tucker LR, Lewis C. Reliability coefficient for maximum likelihood factor-analysis. Psychometrika. 1973;38(1):1–10.
50. Koster A, Shiroma EJ, Caserotti P, Matthews CE, Chen KY, Glynn NW, Harris TB. Comparison of sedentary estimates between activPAL and hip- and wrist-worn ActiGraph. Med Sci Sports Exerc. 2016;
51. Ross CE. Fear of victimization and health. J Quant Crim. 1993;9:159–75.

52. Kawachi I, Kennedy BP, Wilkinson RG. Crime: social disorganization and relative deprivation. Soc Sci Med. 1999;48(6):719–31.
53. Sampson RJ, Raudenbush SW, Earls F. Neighborhoods and violent crime: a multilevel study of collective efficacy. Science. 1997;277(5328):918–24.
54. Weden MM, Carpiano RM, Robert SA. Subjective and objective neighborhood characteristics and adult health. Soc Sci Med. 2008;66(6): 1256–70.
55. Mackenbach JD, Lakerveld J, Van Lenthe FJ, Teixeira PJ, Compernolle S, De Bourdeaudhuij I, Charreire H, Oppert JM, Bardos H, Glonti K, et al. Interactions of individual perceived barriers and neighbourhood destinations with obesity-related behaviours in Europe. Obes Rev. 2016; 17(Suppl 1):68–80.
56. Troxel WM, Shih RA, Ewing B, Tucker JS, Nugroho A, D'Amico EJ. Examination of neighborhood disadvantage and sleep in a multi-ethnic cohort of adolescents. Health Place. 2017;45:39–45.
57. Foster C, Hillsdon M, Thorogood M. Environmental perceptions and walking in English adults. J Epidemiol Community Health. 2004;58(11):924–8.
58. Jack E, McCormack GR. The associations between objectively-determined and self-reported urban form characteristics and neighborhood-based walking in adults. Int J Behav Nutr Phys Act. 2014;11:71.
59. Hinkle JC. Emotional fear of crime vs. perceived safety and risk: implications for measuring "fear" and testing the broken windows thesis. Am J Crim Justice. 2015;40(1):147–68.
60. Stafford M, Chandola T, Marmot M. Association between fear of crime and mental health and physical functioning. Am J Public Health. 2007;97(11): 2076–81.
61. Chandola T. The fear of crime and area differences in health. Health Place. 2001;7(2):105–16.
62. Craig CL, Brownson RC, Cragg SE, Dunn AL. Exploring the effect of the environment on physical activity - a study examining walking to work. Am J Prev Med. 2002;23(2):36–43.
63. Wilson DK, Kirtland KA, Ainsworth BE, Addy CL: Socioeconomic status and perceptions of access and safety for physical activity. Ann Behav Med 2004, 28(1):20-28.
64. Jackson J. A psychological perspective on vulnerability in the fear of crime. Psychol Crime Law. 2009;15(4):365–90.
65. Tamayo A, Karter AJ, Mujahid MS, Warton EM, Moffet HH, Adler N, Schillinger D, Hendrickson O'Connell B, Laraia B. Associations of perceived neighborhood safety and crime with cardiometabolic risk factors among a population with type 2 diabetes. Health Place. 2016;39:116–21.
66. Christian H, Giles-Corti B, Knuiman M, Timperio A, Foster S. The influence of the built environment, social environment and health behaviors on body mass index. Results from RESIDE. Prev Med. 2011;53(1–2):57–60.
67. Lange D, Wahrendorf M, Siegrist J, Plachta-Danielzik S, Landsberg B, Muller MJ. Associations between neighbourhood characteristics, body mass index and health-related behaviours of adolescents in the Kiel obesity prevention study: a multilevel analysis. Eur J Clin Nutr. 2011;65(6):711–9.
68. Lovasi GS, Bader MD, Quinn J, Neckerman K, Weiss C, Rundle A. Body mass index, safety hazards, and neighborhood attractiveness. Am J Prev Med. 2012;43(4):378–84.
69. Poortinga W. Perceptions of the environment, physical activity, and obesity. Soc Sci Med. 2006;63(11):2835–46.
70. Doyle S, Kelly-Schwartz A, Schlossberg M, Stockard J. Active community environments and health: the relationship of Walkable and safe communities to individual health. J Am Plan Assoc. 2006;72(1):19–31.
71. Daniel M, Moore DS, Decker S, Belton L, DeVellis B, Doolen A, Campbell MK. Associations among education, cortisol rhythm, and BMI in blue-collar women. Obesity. 2006;14(2):327–35.
72. Astell-Burt T, Feng X, Kolt GS, Jalaludin B. Does rising crime lead to increasing distress? Longitudinal analysis of a natural experiment with dynamic objective neighbourhood measures. Soc Sci Med. 2015;138:68–73.
73. Diez Roux AV, Mair C. Neighborhoods and health. Ann N Y Acad Sci. 2010; 1186:125–45.
74. Cervero R. Transit-oriented development's ridership bonus: a product of self-selection and public policies. Environ Plan A. 2007;39(9):2068–85.
75. Tucker JM, Welk GJ, Beyler NK. Physical activity in U.S.: adults compliance with the physical activity guidelines for Americans. Am J Prev Med. 2011; 40(4):454–61.
76. Parks SE, Housemann RA, Brownson RC. Differential correlates of physical activity in urban and rural adults of various socioeconomic backgrounds in the United States. J Epidemiol Community Health. 2003;57(1):29–35.
77. Beckles GL, Zhu J, Moonesinghe R. Centers for disease C, prevention: diabetes - United States, 2004 and 2008. MMWR Suppl. 2011;60(1):90–3.
78. May AL, Freedman D, Sherry B, Blanck HM. Obesity - United States, 1999-2010. Mmwr-Morbid Mortal W. 2013;62(3):120–8.
79. Keenan NL, Rosendorf KA. Centers for disease C, prevention: prevalence of hypertension and controlled hypertension - United States, 2005-2008. MMWR Suppl. 2011;60(1):94–7.

16

Effect of a mobile app intervention on vegetable consumption in overweight adults: a randomized controlled trial

Sarah Mummah[1,2*], Thomas N. Robinson[1,3], Maya Mathur[1], Sarah Farzinkhou[1], Stephen Sutton[2†] and Christopher D. Gardner[1†]

Abstract

Background: Mobile applications (apps) have been heralded as transformative tools to deliver behavioral health interventions at scale, but few have been tested in rigorous randomized controlled trials. We tested the effect of a mobile app to increase vegetable consumption among overweight adults attempting weight loss maintenance.

Methods: Overweight adults (n=135) aged 18–50 years with BMI=28–40 kg/m^2 near Stanford, CA were recruited from an ongoing 12-month weight loss trial (parent trial) and randomly assigned to either the stand-alone, theory-based Vegethon mobile app (enabling goal setting, self-monitoring, and feedback and using "process motivators" including fun, surprise, choice, control, social comparison, and competition) or a wait-listed control condition. The primary outcome was daily vegetables servings, measured by an adapted Harvard food frequency questionnaire (FFQ) 8 weeks post-randomization. Daily vegetable servings from 24-hour dietary recalls, administered by trained, certified, and blinded interviewers 5 weeks post-randomization, was included as a secondary outcome. All analyses were conducted according to principles of intention-to-treat.

Results: Daily vegetable consumption was significantly greater in the intervention versus control condition for both measures (adjusted mean difference: 2.0 servings; 95% CI: 0.1, 3.8, p=0.04 for FFQ; and 1.0 servings; 95% CI: 0.2, 1.9; p=0.02 for 24-hour recalls). Baseline vegetable consumption was a significant moderator of intervention effects (p=0.002) in which effects increased as baseline consumption increased.

Conclusions: These results demonstrate the efficacy of a mobile app to increase vegetable consumption among overweight adults. Theory-based mobile interventions may present a low-cost, scalable, and effective approach to improving dietary behaviors and preventing associated chronic diseases.

Trial registration: ClinicalTrials.gov NCT01826591. Registered 27 March 2013.

Keywords: mHealth, Smartphone, Mobile, Digital, Diet, Nutrition, Vegetables, Behavior change, User-centered design, Design thinking

* Correspondence: sm885@cam.ac.uk
[†]Equal contributors
[1]Department of Medicine, Stanford University School of Medicine, Stanford, CA, USA
[2]Department of Public Health and Primary Care, University of Cambridge, Cambridge, UK
Full list of author information is available at the end of the article

Background

Greater consumption of vegetables and fruits is associated with reduced risks of cardiovascular disease, stroke, cancer, and all-cause mortality [1, 2]. It has been suggested that these protective effects are greater for vegetables than for fruits [1] and follow a dose-response relationship [1–3] with benefits seen in up to 7+ servings daily [1]. However, despite current United States Department of Agriculture (USDA) recommendations to consume 5–6 servings of vegetables per day [4], United States (U.S.) adults consume an average of just 1.7 (SE = 0.03) servings of vegetables (excluding fried potatoes) each day [5]. Behavioral interventions to increase vegetable and fruit consumption have led to modest increases in daily intake [6], but typical face-to-face approaches often cannot be realistically implemented at the population level [6], particularly given the high cost of most current strategies [7] (e.g., time demands, the need for trained staff, etc.) [8].

Mobile applications (apps) present a promising means for delivering scalable behavioral interventions due to their increasing ubiquity, ability to reach individuals at nearly any time or place, and potential to deliver timely feedback, personalization, and interactivity to maximize intervention effectiveness [9]. The availability of health-promoting mobile apps has dramatically increased in recent years [10]. However, most mobile health apps have yet to undergo evaluation in randomized trials or incorporate theory-based strategies known to drive changes in health behaviors [11–13]. Among published mobile app trials, most are feasibility and pilot studies with small sample sizes [14]. Only one published study [15] sought to assess the efficacy of a stand-alone mobile app for increasing vegetable consumption, in which real-time goal setting, self-monitoring, and feedback were tested among low-income racial/ethnic-minority girls; this pilot study showed non-significant small to moderate effects and called for larger-scale testing of similar programs. Thus, the existing evidence has yet to establish whether a mobile app can increase vegetable consumption. More broadly, investigators have called for both theory-informed development and rigorous evaluation of mobile-based interventions [16, 17] using larger sample sizes [14].

A recent pilot study [18] we conducted demonstrated preliminary evidence of the efficacy of Vegethon, a stand-alone, theory-based mobile app, in increasing vegetable consumption among overweight adults [19]. While many public health interventions focus on anticipated long-term health benefits (e.g., reduced risk of cardiovascular disease) to motivate behavior change, Vegethon focuses on making the process of behavior change itself (e.g., increasing vegetable consumption) intrinsically rewarding, through the use of *process motivators* [20] such as fun, surprise, choice, control, and competition [19]. This approach has been introduced as a more effective strategy for designing public health interventions to motivate behavior change [20, 21]. The present study aimed to rigorously assess the efficacy of the Vegethon mobile app among a larger sample of overweight adults attempting weight loss maintenance.

Methods

Study design

A randomized controlled study design was used, with a 1:1 allocation ratio of intervention to wait-listed control (8-week delay). The study was conducted at a single research site in Stanford, California.

Study sample

Participants were overweight adults, recruited in two cohorts from an ongoing 12-month weight-loss trial based at Stanford University (parent trial), in which individuals were 18–50 years of age, had baseline body mass index (BMI) of 28–40 kg/m^2, were non-diabetic and non-hypertensive, had no cancer or heart, renal, or liver disease, and lived in the geographic area surrounding Stanford. We chose to design and test Vegethon among participants in a weight loss trial because they had already demonstrated motivation to alter their eating behaviors and because the parent trial provided a resource-efficient way of testing an innovative mobile intervention in the setting of a weight loss program. The added eligibility criterion for cohort 1 was ownership of an iPhone and for cohort 2 was ownership of an iPhone or Android phone (as the app became available on Android during the course of the study). This study was implemented during months 5–7 (i.e., the weight loss maintenance phase) of the 12-month parent trial. Parent trial participants were randomized to either a low-fat or a low-carbohydrate diet for 12 months and attended 22 evening classes led by a health educator, in which they were taught how to adhere to their assigned diets. Both parent trial treatment groups were encouraged to eat whole, unprocessed foods and to increase their vegetable intakes in their daily diets. Parent trial participants who chose to concurrently participate in the present study were newly randomized to receive the mobile app or to be placed on a wait-listed control condition. As a result, any potential effects of the parent trial interventions on vegetable consumption were randomly distributed across both intervention and control conditions in the present Vegethon study.

Randomization and blinding

Randomization was performed by a researcher who had no contact with participants and used a random, computer-generated allocation sequence to assign participants prospectively to each condition. The allocation sequence was designed to ensure balance across mobile intervention assignment groups as well as cohorts, diet group, and health educator within the parent trial. Because the randomized parent trial was underway at the time of the present study, cohort, diet group, and health educator were treated as existing strata, within which participants were assigned to a mobile intervention through a balanced, randomized procedure, using blocks of size 4. This assignment procedure was preferable to simple randomization because it ensured balance in mobile intervention, cohort, diet group, and health educator at any given sample size of this trial. The allocation sequence was stored electronically and concealed from participants, staff, and researchers who had contact with participants. Enrollment and communication with participants was performed by a research assistant who did not play a role in randomization or data analysis. Study staff and researchers who performed data collection (i.e., dietary recall assessors) and analysis were blinded to condition assignment. While participants could not be blinded, they were not told their condition assignment (i.e., "intervention" or "control") and were instead informed they would be assigned to use the app at parent trial month 5 or 7.

Procedures

During a pre-randomization orientation session, participants were instructed that the mobile app was intended to support them in increasing their vegetable consumption, and that it was ideally to be used for at least 1–2 min per day. Participants completing a baseline questionnaire were randomized. Those allocated to the intervention condition completed a short online tutorial that described the mobile app and its use. To prevent contamination among conditions, the app was not freely accessible via the App Store or Google Play and was made available to intervention participants through the distribution of single-use registration codes.

The user-centered, theory-based development and final version of Vegethon were shaped by extensive formative research and the Vegethon pilot study [18] and have been described in detail elsewhere [19]. Vegethon was a stand-alone mobile app that enabled goal-setting and self-monitoring of vegetable consumption. Participants set goals for daily quantity (i.e., servings) and variety (i.e., types) of their vegetable consumption and used the central app feature, *Select Veggies*, to tap on any of 30 different vegetable icons (e.g., spinach, beets) to swiftly record the types and servings of vegetables they consumed each day. Non-starchy vegetables with low energy density and high nutrient density were targeted to facilitate weight loss and weight maintenance while maximizing diet quality and nutrient adequacy in the context of the parent trial. Seven ongoing challenges were included that ranged from easy to difficult to perform (e.g., *Breakfast Champ: Eat any vegetable before 11 am*). A leaderboard engaged users in competition against "other Vegethoners" who were "most similar" to them. Just-in-time prompts to log vegetables before going to sleep were delivered most evenings at 9 p.m. through push notifications.

Overall, the app focused on making the *process* of behavior change rewarding [20] (e.g., the fun of receiving a surprise vegetable challenge; the pride in surpassing a peer's vegetable score). This process motivation strategy stands in contrast to strategies focusing on the eventual outcomes of behavior change (e.g., avoidance of a heart attack) that are often too far in the future to motivate and sustain day-to-day behavior changes [20]. As Robinson has described [20], this process motivation approach is grounded in Bandura's Social Cognitive Theory [22], which specifies that behaviors are driven by the reciprocal interactions between personal, behavioral, and environmental influences. Vegethon was therefore designed to influence users' thoughts and beliefs about eating vegetables, provide opportunities for feedback on their behaviors, and create a social environmental that promoted increasing vegetable intake. Vegethon aimed to maximize the four key processes identified by Social Cognitive Theory: attentional, retention (memory), production, and motivational. For example, attention was maximized through prompts, reminders, and a colorful, playful, interactive user interface; retention was promoted through reminders, repetition, memorable graphics and content; production (promoting the transition of thoughts into action) was supported through instructions and tips and by prompting cognitive and behavioral rehearsal with feedback; and motivation for change was maximized through internal and social comparisons, goals, and feedback.

Measures

The pre-specified primary outcome measure was average daily servings of vegetable consumption, assessed at baseline and 8 weeks post-randomization using an adapted version of the validated semi-quantitative Harvard Food Frequency Questionnaire (FFQ) [23]. The FFQ was selected as the primary outcome due to its: a) specificity to the intervention (i.e., probing each of the vegetables targeted by the intervention vs. holistic probing of all food intake); b) minimal participant burden leading to a reduced amount of missing data; c) high test-retest reliability in the target population; [18] d) evidence of sensitivity to change in the Vegethon pilot study; [18] and e) demonstrated comparable validity to 24-h recalls in measuring vegetable consumption [24]. Commonly used portion sizes for each vegetable (e.g., ½ cup of string beans) were specified, and participants were asked to indicate how often, on average, during the past week, they had consumed each type and amount of food. Eight response categories were possible, ranging from 0 to ≥6 times per day [25]. All 28 questions on vegetable consumption were included from the Harvard FFQ, supplemented by 12 further questions on the consumption of additional vegetables targeted by the intervention. Daily vegetable intake was calculated for each participant following an established method [26] in which the daily frequency of consumption for each vegetable item was multiplied by the number of servings represented by the specified portion size and subsequently combined to yield total daily vegetable servings. Vegetable subgroups were defined *a priori* based on established criteria [27] and included green leafy vegetables, cruciferous vegetables, dark yellow vegetables, tomatoes, other vegetables, and beans. All subgroups excluding beans were combined to yield overall vegetable consumption (primary outcome), and assessed individually as secondary outcomes. Beans, not targeted by the intervention, was included as a comparison measure to detect possible global vegetable reporting bias.

Secondary measures of vegetable consumption were also derived from 24-h dietary recalls at baseline and 5 weeks post-randomization, administered by trained, certified, and blinded interviewers using Nutrition Data System for Research (University of Minnesota Nutrition Coordinating Center) [28, 29]. Three unannounced 24-h recalls were attempted on nonconsecutive days (2 weekdays, 1 weekend) over 2 weeks at each of two time points, for a total of 6 recalls per participant. Average daily servings of four subgroups (dark green vegetables, deep yellow vegetables, tomato, and other vegetables) were combined to yield overall vegetable consumption. Beans was a comparison measure.

App usage was measured using inbuilt software. App usability and satisfaction were assessed using a 21-item questionnaire, administered 8 weeks post randomization to the intervention condition only, and adapted from similar surveys used by King et al. to assess user acceptability of mobile health (mHealth) interventions [30]. Participants were asked to rate their level of agreement or disagreement with each statement on a 5-point Likert-type scale.

Statistical analysis

A priori sample size estimation determined that a sample size of n = 128, or 64 per group, would provide at least 80% power to detect a medium effect size of Cohen's d = 0.5 (one-half standard deviation) [31]. Each analysis used a two-sided alpha = 0.05 threshold for statistical significance. To assess the effect of app assignment on participants' all-vegetable consumption as measured by FFQ (primary outcome), we fit a linear mixed-effects model to which each subject contributed two observations (at baseline and 8 weeks post-randomization) over the study period. The model contained main effects of app intervention status (an indicator of whether an individual was assigned to the app at the time of observation), time (baseline or 8 weeks post-randomization), sex, parent trial diet group assignment (low-carbohydrate or low-fat), parent trial health educator (4 categories), and parent trial cohort group (2 categories). The main effect of app was the primary effect of interest. To account for correlated observations within subjects, the model also included random intercepts by subject, as well as random slopes over time by subject. We assumed normally distributed error terms. An analysis following intention-to-treat principles was used with multiple imputation for missing data. Five imputed datasets were created using the chained equations method and pooled estimates using Barnard-Rubin adjusted degrees of freedom.

We conducted several pre-specified secondary analyses. We refit the primary analysis model, using alternative secondary outcome measures: [1] all-vegetable consumption as measured by 24-h recalls; [2] each of 5 vegetable subgroups as measured by FFQ; and [3] each of 4 vegetable subgroups as measured by 24-h recalls. We also performed pre-specified analyses of four potential moderators of treatment effects, baseline vegetable consumption, sex, diet group, and health educator, by adding app by possible moderator interaction terms to the model. When a statistically significant interaction was identified, it indicated a possible effect moderator, and the main effect coefficient in the model was re-examined after centering the variables [32]. To investigate the possibility of a dose-response relationship between the amount of app usage and changes in vegetable consumption, we used the Spearman rank correlation coefficient that does not assume normal distributions. Data were collected in 2014–2015 and analyzed in 2015–2016. All primary and secondary analyses followed intention-to-treat principles. Stata (v14.1, StataCorp LP, Texas) and SPSS Statistics software (v22, IBM, New York) were used.

Results

Between Nov 3, 2014 and Jan 30, 2016, 135 participants were randomized and analyzed (intervention: 68; control: 67) (Fig. 1). Participant baseline characteristics are presented in Table 1. 100% and 96% of the control condition and 100% and 94% of the intervention condition completed the primary outcome measure (FFQ) at baseline and 8 weeks post-randomization. For the secondary outcome measure (24-h recalls), 96% and 97% of the control condition and 97% and 85% of the intervention condition completed at least one recall at baseline and 5 weeks post-randomization, respectively; and 46% and 40% of the control and intervention conditions, respectively, completed all three recalls at both baseline and 5 weeks post-randomization. Of the 68 participants randomized to the intervention, 43 (63%) downloaded the app within 2 days, 17 (25%) downloaded it after 3–6 days, 6

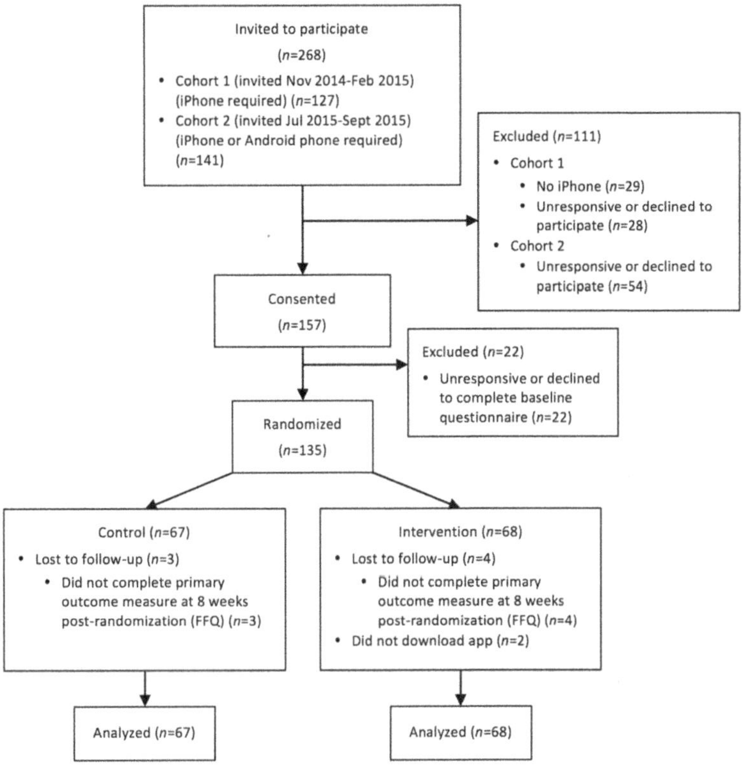

Fig. 1 CONSORT flow diagram

(9%) downloaded it after 1–5 weeks, and 2 (3%) did not download it. In addition, 51 (75%) used the app to log vegetables at least once, while 17 (25%) did not use the app to log.

Primary and secondary outcome measures of daily vegetable consumption at baseline and post-randomization and adjusted group differences are reported in Table 1. Changes in daily consumption of all vegetables are presented in Fig. 2. Daily consumption of all vegetables was significantly greater in the intervention versus control condition for both measures (adjusted mean difference: 2.0 servings; 95% CI: 0.1, 3.8, $p = 0.04$, Cohen's d = 0.18 for FFQ; and 1.0 servings; 95% CI: 0.2, 1.9; $p = 0.02$, Cohen's d = 0.20 for 24-h recalls). There was significantly greater consumption of cruciferous vegetables for FFQ (0.5 servings; 95% CI: 0.1, 0.8; $p = 0.01$) and of deep yellow vegetables for 24-h recalls (0.2 servings; 95% CI: 0.0, 0.4; $p = 0.03$). There were trends towards greater consumption of other vegetables for both measures (0.8 servings; 95% CI: -0.1, 1.7; $p = 0.06$ for FFQ; and 0.5 servings; 95% CI: -0.1, 1.1; $p = 0.08$ for 24-h recalls). Consumption of beans, a vegetable not targeted by the intervention, was not significantly different between the conditions (0.1 servings; 95% CI: -0.2, 0.3; $p = 0.64$ for FFQ; and −0.0 servings; 95% CI: -0.2, 0.1; $p = 0.60$ for 24-h recalls).

Baseline vegetable consumption was found to be a significant moderator of intervention effects ($p = 0.002$), in which the effect of the app on vegetable consumption increased as baseline vegetable consumption increased. It has been widely acknowledged in the statistical literature that ignoring a strong interaction can potentially lead to biased estimates of the main effect of treatment and to reduced power [32]. Indeed, when the model was refit including the app by baseline vegetable consumption interaction coefficient, we found substantially greater effect sizes for all vegetables (adjusted mean difference between treatment and control: 3.1 servings; 95% CI: 1.6, 4.6; $p < 0.0005$), including green vegetables (0.9 servings; 95% CI: 0.3, 1.4; $p = 0.004$) cruciferous vegetables (0.7 servings; 95% CI: 0.4, 1.0; $p < 0.0005$), dark yellow vegetables (0.3 servings; 95% CI: 0.1, 0.6; $p = 0.01$), tomatoes (0.3 servings; 95% CI: 0.1, 0.4; $p = 0.001$), and other vegetables (1.1 servings; 95% CI: 0.4, 1.9; $p = 0.002$).

Among the 51 (75%) intervention participants who used the app to log, participants logged their vegetable consumption 0.8 ± 1.1 times per day (mean ± SD). Daily frequency of vegetable logging over the course of the 8-week intervention period is presented in Fig. 3. There was a downward trend in frequency of logging behavior over time, from 0.9 ± 1.3 times per day during week one to 0.4 ± 0.8 times per day during week eight (mean ± SD). There was wide variation in logging frequency between individuals, ranging from 1.4 ± 1.2 to 0.2 ± 0.6 times per day in the upper and lower

Table 1 Baseline characteristics, primary and secondary outcome measures for vegetable consumption, and group differences

	Baseline[a]		Post-randomization[a]		Adjusted difference post-randomization[b]	
	Control	App	Control	App	Mean (95% CI)	*p* value
Female, *n* (%)	42 (62.7)	42 (61.8)				
Age, years, M (SD)	40.3 (5.8)	39.4 (6.7)				
Race/ethnicity, *n* (%)						
White	50 (74.6)	41 (60.3)				
Asian	5 (7.5)	5 (7.4)				
Black/African American	5 (7.5)	3 (4.4)				
Other	7 (10.4)	19 (27.9)				
Ethnicity, *n* (%)						
Non-Hispanic	46 (68.7)	51 (75.0)				
Hispanic	21 (31.3)	17 (25.0)				
Education, *n* (%)						
≤ Some college	13 (19.4)	16 (23.5)				
College graduate	27 (40.3)	27 (39.7)				
Post-graduate degree	27 (40.3)	25 (36.8)				
Marital Status, *n* (%)						
Married/partnered	44 (65.7)	37 (54.4)				
Single/never married	16 (23.9)	23 (33.8)				
Separated/divorced	7 (10.4)	8 (11.8)				
Phone, *n* (%)						
iPhone	60 (89.6)	61 (89.7)				
Android	7 (10.4)	7 (10.3)				
FFQ,[c] *n* (%)	67 (100)	68 (100)	64 (96)	64 (94)		
All vegetables,[d] M (SD)[g]	8.1 (8.2)	6.7 (5.2)	6.4 (4.3)	7.4 (5.4)	2.0 (0.1, 3.8)[d]	**0.04**[d]
Green leafy	2.3 (4.2)	1.6 (1.7)	1.5 (1.2)	1.5 (1.3)	0.3 (−0.5, 1.1)	0.42
Cruciferous	0.9 (1.1)	0.9 (1.5)	0.7 (0.7)	1.1 (1.0)	0.5 (0.1, 0.8)	**0.01**
Dark yellow	0.7 (1.5)	0.5 (0.6)	0.5 (0.5)	0.5 (0.6)	0.2 (−0.1, 0.5)	0.23
Tomatoes	0.8 (0.9)	0.6 (0.5)	0.6 (0.4)	0.6 (0.5)	0.1 (−0.1, 0.3)	0.23
Other	3.3 (2.8)	3.2 (2.6)	3.2 (2.5)	3.7 (3.2)	0.8 (−0.1, 1.7)	0.06
Beans (not targeted), M (SD)[g]	0.5 (1.0)	0.4 (0.8)	0.4 (0.6)	0.4 (0.5)	0.1 (−0.2, 0.3)	0.64
24-h recalls,[e] *n* (%)[f]	64 (96)	66 (97)	65 (97)	58 (85)		
All vegetables, M (SD)[g]	4.9 (3.1)	4.4 (2.9)	4.4 (2.0)	5.2 (3.9)	1.0 (0.2, 1.9)	**0.02**
Dark green	1.4 (1.6)	1.3 (1.6)	1.3 (1.1)	1.5 (1.5)	0.2 (−0.2, 0.7)	0.33
Deep yellow	0.3 (0.4)	0.4 (0.6)	0.3 (0.4)	0.5 (0.8)	0.2 (0.0, 0.4)	**0.03**
Tomato	0.9 (1.0)	0.6 (0.7)	0.7 (0.7)	0.7 (0.9)	−0.0 (−0.3, 0.2)	0.77
Other	2.4 (1.9)	2.0 (1.9)	2.1 (1.6)	2.5 (2.3)	0.5 (−0.1, 1.1)	0.08
Beans (not targeted), M (SD)[g]	0.3 (0.5)	0.3 (0.6)	0.3 (0.5)	0.2 (0.4)	−0.0 (−0.2, 0.1)	0.60

Boldface indicates statistical significance
[a]Sample sizes (*n*) for baseline and post-randomization values reported represent complete data
[b]Main effect of app from linear mixed model, using an intention-to-treat analysis with multiple imputation for missing data
[c]Measured at baseline and 8 weeks post-randomization
[d]Primary outcome defined *a priori*
[e]Measured at baseline and 5 weeks post-randomization
[f]Completed at least one recall
[g]Servings per day, unless otherwise noted

tertiles, respectively (mean ± SD). App usage was weakly correlated with changes in vegetable consumption (Spearman's rank correlation coefficient: 0.05). However, among the subgroup of intervention participants above the 50th percentile of vegetable consumption at baseline (i.e., those who benefited most from the app), there was a

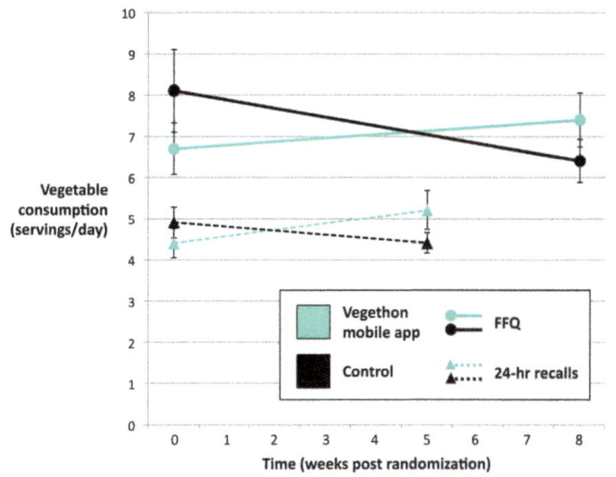

Fig. 2 Changes in daily vegetable consumption. Mean ± SE, n = 135. Measured by FFQ (baseline to 8 weeks, *solid lines*) and 24-h recalls (baseline to 5 weeks, *dashed lines*)

larger correlation between app usage and changes in vegetable consumption (Spearman's rank correlation coefficient: 0.2).

Participants who used the app at least once (n = 51) reported positive experiences with the intervention, including strongest agreement with the statements: "Vegethon has made me aware of how few vegetables I eat"; "I have found Vegethon easy to use"; and "Vegethon has helped me track my vegetable consumption" (4.1 ± 1.0, 3.8 ± 1.1, and 3.7 ± 1.1 [mean ± SD], respectively, on a 1–5 scale, with 5 = strongly agree and 1 = strongly disagree). They reported strong disagreement with the statements: "There has been too little training on how to use Vegethon"; "Overall, Vegethon was distracting"; and "Overall, using Vegethon required too much of my time" (2.1 ± 1.1, 2.3 ± 1.2, and 2.3 ± 1.1 [mean ± SD], respectively).

Discussion

The theory-based Vegethon mobile app intervention led to significantly greater daily consumption of vegetables among overweight adults attempting weight loss maintenance. Participants randomized to receive the Vegethon app reported consuming an average of two more servings per day than controls, measured with the FFQ after 8 weeks. Participants randomized to receive the Vegethon app also reported consuming an average of one more serving per day than controls when measured with 24-h dietary recalls after 5 weeks, a secondary measure of vegetable consumption. The consistency of these results using two different measures of daily vegetable consumption assessed at two time points during the study lends further credibility to the study's findings. Differences were not observed between groups in reported consumption of beans, a vegetable type not targeted by the intervention. This finding suggests the observed effects are unlikely to be explained by a differential social desirability bias leading to an over-reporting of all vegetables by participants who received the intervention. This stand-alone mobile app was evaluated in the context of an intensive weight loss trial in which consumption of high quality whole foods and vegetables was emphasized. The efficacy of the app beyond the effect of the parent weight loss intervention may suggest a potentially high degree of potency of the mobile app intervention or a synergistic effect between the two. These effects may be due to the advantages inherent to mobile-based interventions, including timely feedback, personalization, and daily interaction [9], as well as the theory-based nature of the intervention. This is the first study to demonstrate in a rigorous randomized controlled trial the efficacy of a stand-alone mobile app in increasing vegetable consumption.

Baseline vegetable consumption was a significant moderator of intervention effects, in which the effect of the mobile app on vegetable consumption was greatest among those who reported greater consumption of vegetables at baseline. This finding can inform future studies of Vegethon, and possible other interventions to increase vegetable intake, to test this observation directly by stratifying randomization on baseline vegetable consumption or by designing and testing different interventions for different groups defined by their prior vegetable consumption. Examination of the patterns of change over the course of the study suggests that, overall, the mobile app increased and maintained higher vegetable consumption in the intervention condition, compared to a reduction in vegetable consumption in the control condition (Fig. 2). This pattern may be explained because participants received the mobile app 5–7 months into a weight control program in which they had already made changes to their diets, including their vegetable intakes. It also highlights the importance of using a randomized controlled design to evaluate the efficacy of behavior change interventions, as an observational study of the mobile app may have been misleading, missing the large effect. After finding that baseline vegetable consumption moderated the impact of the intervention, an exploratory analysis including the baseline vegetable consumption by app interaction in the model showed even larger effects sizes, with significant increases in consumption of all vegetables, including green vegetables, cruciferous vegetables, dark yellow vegetables, tomatoes, and other vegetables. Future studies can be designed to account for the effect moderation of baseline vegetable intake. Given the improved health outcomes associated with greater vegetable consumption, we believe the observed effect sizes would be of clinical significance.

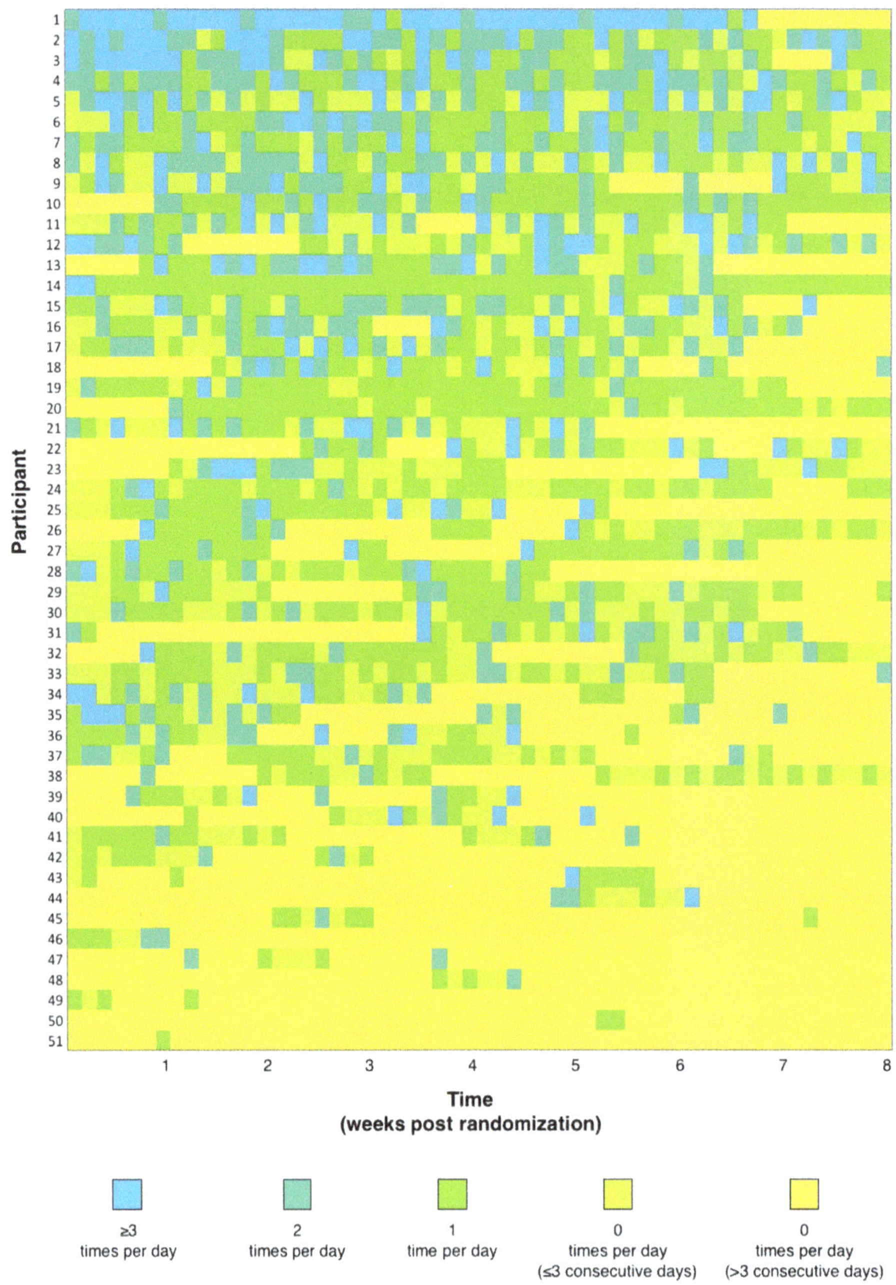

Fig. 3 Frequency of vegetable logging among intervention condition. n = 51[1]. Participants sorted in decreasing order of logging frequency.
[1]Figure excludes 17 participants who did not log

The intervention achieved reasonably high rates of engagement and was found to be easy and enjoyable to use. App usage showed a weak dose-response relationship with overall treatment effect but was more strongly associated with changes in vegetable consumption among the subgroup of participants who reported consuming more vegetables at baseline. This finding suggests that the effect of the mobile app is tied not only to frequency of use but also to individual participant characteristics.

The results of this study indicating the efficacy of the Vegethon intervention confirm those of the earlier Vegethon pilot study [18], in which increases in daily vegetable consumption among overweight adults were similarly observed. Effect sizes were substantial but smaller than those observed in the initial pilot study, as is typical when larger, more definitive trials follow small pilot studies [33]. However, they compare favorably with the only other known randomized study of a mobile app targeting vegetable consumption [15]. The theory-driven nature of the app, including goal-setting and self-monitoring behavior widely acknowledged to be critical components of behavioral mHealth interventions [11], may have led to greater behavioral changes than observed previously. These increases in vegetable consumption were observed among participants who already had a relatively high baseline vegetable consumption compared to the U.S. national average [5], due in part to their concurrent participation in a weight loss trial emphasizing healthier eating including vegetable consumption. Further studies are indicated to examine the effect of Vegethon and similar technologies among populations with lower vegetable consumption who are not concurrently enrolled in a weight loss trial. Overall, these findings align with those found in other investigations of mobile apps to change health behaviors, in which acceptability and initial efficacy has been similarly demonstrated [14].

These results warrant further research, as increases in vegetable consumption may lead to changes in overall diet composition and weight loss, even in the absence of specific guidance to decrease consumption of other foods [34]. For example, in a study among overweight adults by Norman et al., [35] a short message service (SMS) intervention that increased vegetable consumption led to weight loss. Such interventions that focus on the inherent benefits of the target behavior itself (e.g., increasing vegetable consumption) may lead to more sustained behavior changes than those focusing on longer-term goals (e.g., weight loss) [20]. Given the high and growing prevalence of overweight in the United States, and the fact that people in higher weight categories are more likely to develop chronic diseases associated with excess weight, strategies to reduce modifiable risk factors including diet among overweight adults are needed [36]. This study demonstrating the efficacy of a mobile app to increase vegetable consumption among motivated overweight adults presents one such possible strategy that warrants further investigation. Further trials of theory-driven mobile technologies to more effectively produce health behavior changes are called for.

Among the strengths of this research were the theory-based development of the app, the rigorous methods and randomized controlled study design, the use of state-of-the-art FFQ and 24-h dietary recall outcome measures, high retention rates for the primary outcome measure, and substantial sample size in comparison to most mHealth studies. This study used multiple methods of assessing vegetable consumption, which has been recommended to inform a more complete understanding of true intake [24]. Participants enrolled in the evaluation of this mobile intervention were concurrently enrolled in a weight loss trial. Generalizability of these findings to other samples that are not enrolled in a weight loss trial and/or motivated to use a mobile app to increase their vegetable consumption is unknown. Although comparable to many nutrition intervention studies, the 8-week study duration provides an assessment only of relatively short-term intervention effects. A longer trial is warranted to determine whether the observed effects increase, decrease, or are sustained over time, and whether there are effects on weight and other associated health benefits. As with all dietary assessment methods, there are inherent limitations to the adapted Harvard Food Frequency Questionnaire and 24-h recall measures including reliance on self-report. However, our finding that the differences in vegetable consumption between groups did not generalize to beans, a vegetable group not targeted by the intervention, lends support to the validity of the findings.

Conclusions

These data show that a theory-based mobile app increased vegetable consumption among overweight adults attempting weight loss maintenance. Policy makers should consider the development and implementation of theory-based mobile apps as a low-cost, scalable, and effective intervention to support dietary behavior changes among overweight adults.

Abbreviations

App: Mobile application; BMI: Body mass index; FFQ: Food Frequency Questionnaire; mHealth: mobile health; SMS: Short message service

Acknowledgements

The authors would like to thank Katherine Dotter, RDN, Dustin Yoder, Ryan Swanson, Jae Berman, RDN, Victoria Ding, MS, Haley Schmoyer, Chelsea Camara, and the team at Vendus Product Labs for their contributions to the development of Vegethon and to the design and implementation of the study. We would also like to thank the participants and staff of the Stanford *DIETFITS* parent trial.

Funding

This research was supported by a Gates Cambridge Scholarship awarded to SAM, Award Number R01DK0091831 from the National Institute of Diabetes and Digestive and Kidney Diseases (NIDDK) of the National Institutes of Health (NIH) awarded to CDG, an unrestricted gift from the Nutrition Science Initiative (NuSI) awarded to CDG, and a grant from the Stanford Child Health Research Institute awarded to TNR. This work was also supported by the Stanford Clinical and Translational Science Award (CTSA) to Spectrum (UL1 TR000093). The CTSA program is led by the National Center for Advancing Translational Sciences (NCATS) at the NIH. The funders had no role in study design, data collection and analysis, decision to publish, or preparation of the manuscript.

Authors' contributions

SAM designed the study, developed the intervention, managed data collection, conducted statistical analyses and interpretation, and wrote the manuscript. MM helped develop the intervention and statistical analysis plan. SF managed data collection. SS, TNR, and CDG contributed guidance and consultation throughout and provided feedback on the manuscript. CDG provided the study location and access to parent trial participants and data. All authors read and approved the final manuscript.

Competing interests
The authors declare that they have no competing interests.

Author details
[1]Department of Medicine, Stanford University School of Medicine, Stanford, CA, USA. [2]Department of Public Health and Primary Care, University of Cambridge, Cambridge, UK. [3]Department of Pediatrics, Stanford University School of Medicine, Stanford, CA, USA.

References

1. Oyebode O, Gordon-Dseagu V, Walker A, Mindell JS. Fruit and vegetable consumption and all-cause, cancer and CVD mortality: analysis of health survey for England data. J Epidemiol Community Health. 2014;68(9):856–62.
2. Dauchet L, Amouyel P, Dallongeville J. Fruit and vegetable consumption and risk of stroke: a meta-analysis of cohort studies. Neurology. 2005;65(8):1193–7.
3. Wang X, Ouyang Y, Liu J, et al. Fruit and vegetable consumption and mortality from all causes, cardiovascular disease, and cancer: systematic review and dose-response meta-analysis of prospective cohort studies. BMJ (Clinical research ed). 2014;349:g4490.
4. U.S. Department of Agriculture and U.S. Department of Health and Human Services. Dietary guidelines for Americans, 2010. http://health.gov/dietaryguidelines/dga2010/DietaryGuidelines2010.pdf (accessed September 19 2015).
5. Casagrande SS, Wang Y, Anderson C, Gary TL. Have Americans increased their fruit and vegetable intake? The trends between 1988 and 2002. Am J Prev Med. 2007;32(4):257–63.
6. Thomson CA, Ravia J. A systematic review of behavioral interventions to promote intake of fruit and vegetables. J Am Diet Assoc. 2011;111(10):1523–35.
7. Cobiac LJ, Vos T, Veerman JL. Cost-effectiveness of interventions to promote fruit and vegetable consumption. PLoS One. 2010;5(11):e14148.
8. Pomerleau J, Lock K, Knai C, McKee M. Interventions designed to increase adult fruit and vegetable intake can be effective: a systematic review of the literature. J Nutr. 2005;135(10):2486–95.
9. Klasnja P, Pratt W. Healthcare in the pocket: mapping the space of mobile-phone health interventions. J Biomed Inform. 2012;45(1):184–98.
10. Stephens J, Allen JK, Dennison Himmelfarb CR. "smart" coaching to promote physical activity, diet change, and cardiovascular health. The Journal of cardiovascular nursing. 2011;26(4):282–4.
11. Azar KMJ, Lesser LI, Laing BY, et al. Mobile applications for weight management: theory-based content analysis. Am J Prev Med. 2013;45(5):583–9.
12. Riley WT, Rivera DE, Atienza AA, Nilsen W, Allison SM, Mermelstein R. Health behavior models in the age of mobile interventions: are our theories up to the task? Translational behavioral medicine. 2011;1(1):53–71.
13. Pagoto S, Schneider K, Jojic M, DeBiasse M, Mann D. Evidence-based strategies in weight-loss mobile apps. Am J Prev Med. 2013;45(5):576–82.
14. Payne HE, Lister C, West JH, Bernhardt JM. Behavioral functionality of mobile apps in health interventions: a systematic review of the literature. JMIR mHealth and uHealth. 2015;3(1):e20.
15. Nollen NL, Mayo MS, Carlson SE, Rapoff MA, Goggin KJ, Ellerbeck EF. Mobile technology for obesity prevention: a randomized pilot study in racial- and ethnic-minority girls. Am J Prev Med. 2014;46(4):404–8.
16. Breton E, Fuemmeler B, Abroms L. Weight loss—there is an app for that! But does it adhere to evidence-informed practices? Translational behavioral medicine. 2011;1(4):523–9.
17. Helander E, Kaipainen K, Korhonen I, Wansink B. Factors related to sustained use of a free mobile app for dietary self-monitoring with photography and peer feedback: retrospective cohort study. J Med Internet Res. 2014;16(4):e109.
18. Mummah S, Mathur M, King AC, Gardner CD, Sutton S. Mobile technology for vegetable consumption: a randomized controlled pilot study in overweight adults. JMIR Mhealth Uhealth. (in press)
19. Mummah SA, King AC, Gardner CD, Sutton S. Iterative development of Vegethon: a theory-based mobile app intervention to increase vegetable consumption. The international journal of behavioral nutrition and physical activity. 2016;13:90.
20. Robinson TN. Stealth interventions for obesity prevention and control: motvating behavior change. In: Dubé L, Bechara A, Dagher A, et al., editors. Obesity Prevention: The Role of Brain and Society on Individual Behavior. New York: Elsevier Inc; 2010. p. 319–27.
21. Robinson TN. Save the world, prevent obesity: piggybacking on existing social and ideological movements. Obesity. 2010;18(S1):S17–22.
22. Bandura A. Social foundations of thought and action. Englewood Cliffs, NJ: Prentice-Hall; 1986.
23. Willet WC. Nutritional epidemiology. New York: Oxford University Press; 1990.
24. Resnicow K, Odom E, Wang T, et al. Validation of three food frequency questionnaires and 24-hour recalls with serum carotenoid levels in a sample of African-American adults. Am J Epidemiol. 2000;152(11):1072–80.
25. Harvard School of Public Health. Nurses Health Study II Questionnaire. 2003. http://www.channing.harvard.edu/nhs/questionnaires/pdfs/NHSII/2003.PDF (accessed September 19 2015).
26. Park SK, Tucker KL, O'Neill MS, et al. Fruit, vegetable, and fish consumption and heart rate variability: the veterans administration normative aging study. Am J Clin Nutr. 2009;89(3):778–86.
27. Liu S, Manson JE, Lee IM, et al. Fruit and vegetable intake and risk of cardiovascular disease: the Women's health study. Am J Clin Nutr. 2000;72(4):922–8.
28. Feskanich D, Sielaff BH, Chong K, Buzzard IM. Computerized collection and analysis of dietary intake information. Comput Methods Prog Biomed. 1989;30(1):47–57.
29. Johnson RK, Driscoll P, Goran MI. Comparison of multiple-pass 24-hour recall estimates of energy intake with total energy expenditure determined by the doubly labeled water method in young children. J Am Diet Assoc. 1996;96(11):1140–4.
30. King AC, Hekler EB, Grieco LA, et al. Harnessing different motivational frames via mobile phones to promote daily physical activity and reduce sedentary behavior in aging adults. PLoS One. 2013;8(4):e62613.
31. Cohen J. A power primer. Psychol Bull. 1992;112(1):155–9.
32. Kraemer HC, Wilson GT, Fairburn CG, Agras WS. Mediators and moderators of treatment effects in randomized clinical trials. Arch Gen Psychiatry. 2002;59(10):877–83.
33. Ioannidis JP. Contradicted and initially stronger effects in highly cited clinical research. JAMA. 2005;294(2):218–28.
34. Mytton OT, Nnoaham K, Eyles H, Scarborough P, Ni MC. Systematic review and meta-analysis of the effect of increased vegetable and fruit consumption on body weight and energy intake. BMC Public Health. 2014;14:886.
35. Norman GJ, Kolodziejczyk JK, Adams MA, Patrick K, Marshall SJ. Fruit and vegetable intake and eating behaviors mediate the effect of a randomized text-message based weight loss program. Prev Med. 2013;56(1):3–7.
36. Must A, Spadano J, Coakley EH, Field AE, Colditz G, Dietz WH. The disease burden associated with overweight and obesity. JAMA. 1999;282(16):1523–9.

Reducing calorie sales from supermarkets – 'silent' reformulation of retailer-brand food products

Jørgen Dejgård Jensen[1*] and Iben Sommer[2]

Abstract

Background: Food product reformulation is seen as one among several tools to promote healthier eating. Reformulating the recipe for a processed food, e.g. reducing the fat, sugar or salt content of the foods, or increasing the content of whole-grains, can help the consumers to pursue a healthier life style. In this study, we evaluate the effects on calorie sales of a 'silent' reformulation strategy, where a retail chain's private-label brands are reformulated to a lower energy density without making specific claims on the product.

Methods: Using an ecological study design, we analyse 52 weeks' sales data – enriched with data on products' energy density - from a Danish retail chain. Sales of eight product categories were studied. Within each of these categories, specific products had been reformulated during the 52 weeks data period. Using econometric methods, we decompose the changes in calorie turnover and sales value into direct and indirect effects of product reformulation.

Results: For all considered products, the direct effect of product reformulation was a reduction in the sale of calories from the respective product categories - between 0.5 and 8.2%. In several cases, the reformulation led to indirect substitution effects that were counterproductive with regard to reducing calorie turnover. However, except in two insignificant cases, these indirect substitution effects were dominated by the direct effect of the reformulation, leading to net reductions in calorie sales between −3.1 and 7.5%. For all considered product reformulations, the reformulation had either positive, zero or very moderate negative effects on the sales value of the product category to which the reformulated product belonged.

Conclusions: Based on these findings, 'silent' reformulation of retailer's private brands towards lower energy density seems to contribute to lowering the calorie intake in the population (although to a moderate extent) with moderate losses in retailer's sales revenues.

Keywords: Health promotion, Food product reformulation, Consumer demand

Background

Food product reformulation is seen as one among several tools to promote healthier eating [1–3]. By reformulating the recipe for a processed food, e.g. reducing the fat, sugar or salt content of the foods, or increasing the content of whole-grains, food manufacturers can help consumers pursue a healthier life style, even without changing their dietary behavior.

The research literature on food product reformulation aiming at health improvements has considered the size of the potentials for health promotion via product reformulation, the industry's economic incentives to reformulate, or the possible barriers for such reformulation to occur. Regarding health promotion potentials, a number of studies have considered reduction of salt content [4, 5], replacement of trans-fatty acids (TFA) [6, 7] in food products, or enhancement of whole-grain from foods [8]. Often, such studies use a static approach ignoring any behavioural adjustments to the reformulation among the consumers, and thus find that such product reformulations are promoting public health.

Studies addressing food producers' incentives to undertake product reformulation tend to fall in one of two categories [9]: supply-side incentives to reformulate driven

* Correspondence: jorgen@ifro.ku.dk
[1]University of Copenhagen, Department of Food and Resource Economics, Rolighedsvej 25, 1958 Frederiksberg C, Denmark
Full list of author information is available at the end of the article

by costs of ingredients - which in turn may be driven by e.g. agricultural policy - and demand-side incentives driven by the possibility to reap competitive advantages from consumers' demand for healthier products [10, 11]. Downs et al. [3] reviewed the literature on the effectiveness of policies to reduce the intake of TFA, such as bans or labelling. Regarding TFA in food, most of the reviewed studies found that policy interventions had led to reformulation of products to contain less TFA. The topic was also studied by Unnevehr & Jagmanaite [10] with a particular focus on stimulus to reformulate food products towards less content of TFA. Golan & Unnevehr [9] considered how food industry's incentives to undertake product reformulation may be affected by agricultural policy affecting food manufacturers' input costs. Marotta et al. [11] examined the role of product reformulation for the food industry and whether this strategy can help companies to gain a competitive advantage. They found that improved consumer information is necessary in order for such mechanisms to be effective.

As an alternative to promote reformulated products via information about their healthiness, another product reformulation strategy is to make it 'silent', i.e. not to announce the reformulation explicitly to the consumers (except on standard nutrition labels). This strategy does not have the potential competitive advantage of appealing to health-oriented consumers for the individual product. Instead, the manufacturer's or retailer's motivation to undertake such silent reformulation could be to enhance the health profile of its corporate brand, considering the reformulation as a part of its Corporate Social Responsibility (CSR) strategy. This type of reformulation strategy seems to have attracted rather little interest in the research literature, even though considerable research interest has been devoted to the potential roles of food industry self-regulation in halting the worldwide increasing trend in overweight, obesity and co-morbidities [12].

The research literature has also devoted relatively little attention to the consumers' adaptation to reformulation of food products and hence its effectiveness in reducing the consumers' intake of calories. Food reformulation towards lower fat, sugar or salt content might induce compensation effects – that the consumers perceive a need (or allowance) to compensate for the reduced contents of such substances by increasing their consumption of other products with these substances. Product reformulation might be expected to change the perceived quality of the products - and hence to affect the comparison between the reformulated product and its substitutes, for example because the reformulated product is considered to be 'unnatural' or a 'diet' product. To the extent that consumers respond to such perceived quality changes, these responses may enhance or undermine the effectiveness.

In the present analysis, consumers are assumed to make their consumption decisions regarding a product, based on their perception of the product's attributes (taste, healthiness, price,...) relative to those in potential substitute products within the same product category, but probably with slightly different characteristics. If a reformulation enhances the perception of one attribute without deteriorating other attributes, the reformulation would be expected to induce an increase in the consumption of that product. On the other hand, if the reformulation leads to a perceived improvement in some attributes but a perceived negative effect on other attributes, the sign of the demand response needs to be based on empirical analysis. It is hypothesized that such substitution effects influence the impact of the product reformulation on consumers' calorie consumption, as well as the retailer's sales value. The key research questions are, whether such substitution effects are significant and whether they are supportive of public health goals and of industry's incentive to undertake such reformulation.

We evaluate the effects of a 'silent' reformulation strategy, namely to reformulate a retail chain's private-label brands to a lower energy density without announcing the reformulation to the consumers. Such a strategy has been exercised by one of the major retail chains in Denmark. The modest changes in the food composition pursuant of the reformulation only had impact on the nutrient content, no impact on price, whilst no or insignificant changes in the sensory quality of the products. Nutrition fact labels on the products were updated as a consequence of the reformulation. If consumers have not noticed changes on the nutrition facts label nor in sensory characteristics, their product choices are hypothesized to be unaffected by the reformulation. On the other hand, if the consumers perceive a change in sensory characteristics or have noticed a changed in nutritional characteristics, their choices could be affected. The direction of such changes is however indeterminate, a priori.

We focus on the consumers' adaptation to such reformulation in eight food product categories in terms of possible changes in their composition of purchases within these categories, based on sales data from a Danish retail chain.

Methods

Study design and data

In relation to an epidemiological terminology, the study design can be characterised as an ecological design [13], where the development over time in aggregate sales of individual products is seeked explained by the development in relevant explanatory variables, such as prices and timing of product reformulation.

The dataset for the analysis consists of detailed weekly sales data from one of the larger food retail chains in Denmark for a 52-week period, from the beginning of

March 2013 till the end of February 2014. The sales data have been enriched by information about energy content in all products (kcal/100 g or kcal/100 ml).

Data concerning product reformulation for eight products were also supplied by the retail chain, including the date (week number), the character of the reformulation and its effect on the product's energy content.

Theoretical assumptions and functional form

For the empirical analysis of each product category, we have chosen the linearized Almost Ideal Demand (AID) functional specification [14]. The AID model implies that commodity i's share w_i of the product category sales value can be specified as a linear function of the logarithmic prices p and the real budget for the product category y/P (where P is the composite price index of all prices in the product category, calculated according to the Stone price index formula, $\ln P = \Sigma_i w_{it} \cdot \ln p_{it}$).

In order to investigate the potential effects of product reformulation, we have augmented the AID model with a dummy variable D, which assumes the value zero before the reformulation, and the value one after the reformulation, hence

$$w_{it} = \alpha_i + \sum_j \alpha_{ij} \cdot \ln p_{jt} + \beta_{iy} \cdot \ln(y_t/P_t) + \gamma_i \cdot D_t + \varepsilon_{it}, i = \{1, ..., n\}$$

A linear trend variable and a dummy variable representing the Christmas season (all weeks in December), were included to account for trend and seasonality effects (although the products in the study are not suspected to be subject to strong seasonal variation). Furthermore, in order to adjust for first-order autocorrelation, an autoregressive AR (1) term was included in the estimation.

Adding-up yields $\Sigma_i\alpha_i = 1$, $\Sigma_i\alpha_{ij} = 0$, $\Sigma_i\beta_{yi} = 0$, $\Sigma_i\gamma_i = 0$, given that the budget shares sum to one. At the individual consumer level, a theoretically consistent demand model should also fulfil properties of linear homogeneity and Slutsky symmetry. However, as the retailer sales data used in this study can be considered as an aggregate of several consumers, these assumptions cannot be expected to hold, and have therefore not been imposed on the econometric estimation.

Based on econometric estimation of the AID model, it is possible to separate out the effect of the reformulation dummy on the composition of product purchases at a given budget as $\Delta x_{it}|_{\Delta D} = \gamma \cdot y_t / p_{it}$. This effect reflects possible indirect within-commodity-group substitution behaviour triggered by the reformulation. The substitution effect influences both the turnover of calories and the total sales value, within the respective product categories. Other effects, such as effects of price changes, overall sales volume changes or trend development could also be separated out, but this is outside the scope of this paper and is not presented.

In addition to the indirect substitution effects of the reformulation on calorie turnover, there is also a direct effect of product reformation in terms of changed energy density of the reformulated products, Δk_i. Hence, total effect of the reformulation on calorie turnover can be determined as

$$\Delta K|_{reformulation} = \sum_i x_{it} \cdot \Delta k_i + \sum_i k_i \cdot \Delta x_{it}|_{\Delta D}$$

For sales value, the effect of the reformulation is given by:

$$\Delta R = \sum_i p_i \cdot \Delta x_{it}|_{\Delta D}$$

Products

Within the considered data period, the retail chain reformulated nine of their private label food products with the aim to lower their energy content. The nine products and their reformulations are displayed in Table 1. Two of the product reformulations were implemented simultaneously in two close substitute products (orange-flavoured yoghurt and peach melba-flavoured yoghurt), and in the subsequent analysis, this double-reformulation is analysed as one combined setting.

As appears from the table, the extent of reformulation in terms of reduction in energy density has varied across the different products. For example, for mayonnaise and fruit-flavoured yoghurt, the calorie content was reduced by 16–17%, whereas for bread products the reduction was 5–10%, and for chocolate-flavoured muesli only 2–3%.

Most of the affected product categories can be considered as 'high-frequency buys', where the possible demand effects of a reformulation would be measureable within few weeks after the reformulation has been implemented. One exception may be mayonnaise, where households' purchase frequency is likely to be lower and where it may take longer to detect an influence of the reformulation. However, as the data for mayonnaise spans more than a half year after the reformulation, we would still expect to be able to measure an effect, if any.

Results

In the following, results are presented for the eight reformulations, based on econometric estimation of the demand model outlined in the previous section. In Table 2, the reformulations' effects on calorie turnover and sales value are evaluated for the group of relatively close substitutes, which the product is presumed to belong to. Detailed econometric estimation results for each commodity category are given in Tables 3, 4, 5, 6, 7, 8, 9 and 10 in the Appendix. In general, the estimated models displayed satisfactory goodness-of-fit and only little sign of misspecification, such as heteroscedasticity, autocorrelation or non-normality in residuals.

Table 1 Overview of considered product reformulations and categories

Product	Change in energy density (%)	Date of reformulation	Category products	Reformulated product's share of category's calorie turnover	Reformulated product's share of category's sales value
	Kcal/ 100 g	Week/ year		Per cent	Per cent
Mayonnaise	720→600 (17)	36/2013	*Private-label mayonnaise,* Private-label light mayonnaise, Unbranded lemon mayonnaise, Brand 1 mayonnaise (tube), Brand 1 mayonnaise, Brand 1 lemon mayonnaise	51	38
Fruit yoghurt Orange Peach melba	93→77 (17) 90→74 (18)	14/2013	*Private-label peach melba yoghurt, Private-label orange yoghurt,* Banana/pear yoghurt, Pineapple/orange/mango yoghurt, Peach/ passion fruit yoghurt, Berry-flavoured yoghurts, Low-calorie berry-flavoured yoghurts,	15 6	11 5
Pumpkin seed rye bread	240→232 (3)	22/2013	*Private-label pumpkin seed rye bread,* Private-label sunflower seed rye bread, Brand sunflower rye bread, Brand organic sunflower rye bread	14	12
Toasting bun	280→270 (4)	36/2013	*Private-label toasting bun,* Private-label whole-grain toasting buns, Brand toasting bun	64	60
Yoghurt bread	270→250 (7)	32/2013	*Private-label yoghurt bread,* Brand1 wholemilk bread, Brand1 yoghurt bread, Brand2 wholemilk bread, Brand 3 five-grain bread	43	38
Carrot buns	310→281 (9)	22/2013	*Private-label carrot buns,* Brand1 carrot buns, Brand1 other buns, Brand 2 buns	54	46
Whole-grain rolls	260→240 (8)	22/2013	*Private-label whole-grain rolls,* Brand1 multi-grain rolls, Brand2 Sandwich rolls, Brand 2 grain rolls, Brand 3 Whole-grain rolls	35	30
Chocolate muesli	410→400 (2)	18/2013	*Private-label chocolate muesli,* Private-label regular muesli, Brand1 chocolate cereals, Brand 2 chocolate cereals, Brand 3 chocolate cereals	21	21

Note: Week numbers represent the placement of the week in the calendar year. For instance, week 36 in 2013 spanned the dates September 2–8, 2013

Table 2 Direct and indirect effects of product reformulation on calorie turnover and sales value for product groups (per cent)

	------------- Calories -------------			
	Direct reformulation	Reformulation-induced substitution	Total calorie	Sales revenue
Mayonnaise	−8.2%	0.7%	−7.5%	0.4%
Fruit yoghurt	−3.9%	0.1% N.S.	−3.8%	0.1% N.S.
Rye bread with pumpkin seeds	−0.5%	0.7% N.S.	0.2%	0.7% N.S.
Toasting buns	−2.3%	−0.7%	−3.0%	−0.5%
Yoghurt bread	−3.2%	−0.5% N.S.	−3.7%	−0.5% N.S.
Carrot buns	−4.9%	0.7% N.S.	−4.2%	0.4% N.S.
Whole-grain rolls	−2.7%	0.0%	−2.7%	−0.1%
Chocolate muesli	−0.5%	3.7% N.S.	3.1%	2.2% N.S.

N.S. Not significant

Mayonnaise

The reformulation has led to a partial decrease in calories from the reformulated mayonnaise product by 17%, as indicated in Table 1, which contributes by about 8% reduction in the total calories from the group of mayonnaise products in this retail chain. The partial substitution effect of the reformulation increased the sale of the reformulated product by 2.6% (and hence the calories from this variety) at the cost of the private-label light variety, which decreased by 0.5% due to this substitution (the latter not statistically significant, though). An interpretation of this substitution effect is that consumers tend to prefer the taste of regular mayonnaise to that of light mayonnaise, but they are also concerned about the calories in the mayonnaise. When the calorie content of the regular variety comes closer to that of the light variety, their trade-off between the two varieties becomes more in favour of the regular variety, and they become more prone to choose this variety. In total, the reformulation has led to a 7.5% reduction in calorie sales in mayonnaise.

The reformulation-induced substitution effects on sales value are identical to those on calorie turnover for the individual products. However, because effects on turnover are weighted by products' turnover shares, and effects on calories are weighted by products' calorie shares, the total percentage reformulation-induced substitution effect differs for the two outcome measures. Hence, the increase in turnover due to the reformulation per se is relatively less than the corresponding contribution to change in calorie sales - but still positive. According to these results, the retailer thus did not lose revenue due to the reformulation of the private-label mayonnaise.

Fruit yoghurt

The two reformulated yoghurts represent 11–15 and 5–6% of total fruit yoghurt sales, respectively, and neither of them could be considered as dominating in terms of sales. The direct reformulation effect constituted around 17% reduction in calorie content for both reformulated product types. Taking into account that these two products represent around 20% of total calorie sales, this direct effect amounts to 3.9% of total calorie turnover from the fruit yoghurts. The reformulation-induced substitution effects were not statistically significant, and the results in Table 2 also indicates very small contributions to the change in calorie turnover and sales value from this effect.

Rye bread with pumpkin seeds

One private-label variety of rye bread with pumpkin seeds was reformulated to contain fewer sunflower seeds and more pumpkin seeds and wholegrain rye, thus reducing the calories from 240 to 232 per 100 g. For the rye bread reformulation, the direct reformulation effect led to a 3.3% reduction in the reformulated bread, which implied a 0.5% partial reduction in the total calories from this product category. Reformulation-induced substitution effects led to a (not statistically significant) 0.7% increase in the calorie turnover - and in sales revenue. The net effect of the reformulation on calorie turnover was an insignificant 0.2 (=0.7–0.5) per cent increase, and the partial effect of the reformulation on sales value was an (insignificant) increase of 0.7%. Hence, the reduction in calorie turnover due to the reformulation could be done without reducing the sales value of this group of rye bread.

Toasting buns

One private-label 'normal' toasting bun ("krydderboller" in Danish) was reformulated to contain less fat and sugar, thus reducing the calorie content from 280 to 270 kcal per 100 g. The direct effect of the reformulation was a reduction of 3.6% calorie content in the reformulated product – which impacted the average calorie turnover in toasting buns by 2.3%. Reformulation-induced substitution effects implied a (weakly significant) shift from the reformulated private-label product to the whole-grain private-label variety, implying a net reduction in calorie turnover of 0.7%. Hence, the reformulation implied a 3% reduction in calorie turnover from toasting buns. The substitution effect also implied a reduction in sales revenue of 0.5% from these buns.

Yoghurt bread

In the category of light bread, the retailer's private label yoghurt bread was reformulated to contain more rye flour and less fat, which reduced the calorie content from 270 to 250 kcal/100 g. The direct effect of the reformulation was a 7.4% reduction in the calorie content of the reformulated product, and thus to a 3.2% reduction for the product category as a whole. Substitution effects induced by the reformulation led to (insignificant) decrease in the sale of the reformulated product and slight increases in some of the other products, leading to an overall 0.5% reduction in calorie sales, and a corresponding effect on sales value.

Buns with carrot

Private-label buns with carrot were reformulated to contain less sunflower seeds, more durum seeds, more carrot and no eggs. The direct effect of the reformulation was a reduction of the calorie content in these buns with 9.4% – and as these buns constitute about half of the considered product category, this implied a direct effect on the calorie turnover of this product category by 4.9%. Although statistically insignificant, the reformulation-induced substitution effects led to an increased sale of the reformulated buns, at the cost of another variety, and the net effect of this substitution was an increase of 0.7% in calorie turnover. Hence, the reformulation yielded a 4.2% reduction in calorie turnover, and a 0.4% increase in sales value of the buns within this product category.

Whole grain breakfast rolls

Private-label whole-grain rolls were reformulated to contain less oil, which reduced the energy density from 260 to 240 kcal/100 g. It may not be completely evident, which products are likely to be close substitutes to these rolls – and especially if this would be other types of rolls for lunch sandwiches, or other types of rolls on the breakfast table. In the case of breakfast use, the sales data contain very little substitute products within the fresh bread category, and hence the product reformulation could be expected to induce relatively little substitution in the sales, and the direct reformulation effect (i.e. a 7.7% reduction in calorie turnover from the category) would be the dominating effect.

On the other hand, if other types of sandwich rolls could substitute the reformulated rolls, we consider six products as close substitutes. The direct effect of the reformulation on the reformulated product was an 8% reduction in the calorie content. As the reformulated product represented around one third of the total sales within this category, this implies a reduction of 2.7% in the product category. Reformulation-induced substitution effects implied some shifts in the composition of this product category – however with a zero effect on total calorie turnover. Although this substitution effect was relatively small on the reformulated product, it seems to have induced a shift between some of the other product varieties. The reformulation-induced substitution effects implied a 0.1% reduction in the sales value from this product category. These somewhat peculiar substitution effects may have to do with the above considerations about which products are the actual substitutes for the reformulated whole grain rolls.

Chocolate muesli

The retailer has reformulated its private-label chocolate muesli product to contain more grains (wheat and oats) and less salt, and reduce the energy density from 410 to 400 kcal/100 g. The direct effect of the reformulation was a 2.4% reduction in calorie content of the reformulated chocolate muesli. As this product constituted around 20% of the product category, this meant a reduction in the calories from this category of 0.5%. The substitution effects of the reformulation implied an (insignificant) increase in the sales of the private-label regular muesli products, at the cost of especially one of the other brands. This substitution effect led to a 3.7% increase in calorie sales, from the product category, and hence a net increase of 3.1% in calorie turnover. The reformulation-induced substitution effect on sales value was an increase of 2.2%.

Discussion

For all products, the direct effect of product reformulation was a reduction in the sale of calories from the respective product categories. In several of the cases, the reformulation led to indirect substitution effects that to some extent were counterproductive with regard to reducing calorie turnover – but in all cases except for chocolate muesli and rye-bread, these indirect substitution effects were dominated by the direct effect of the reformulation. For all considered product reformulations, except that of toasting buns, the reformulation had either positive, zero or very moderate negative effects on the sales value of the product category to which the reformulated product belonged. Consequently, the examples suggest that silent product reformulation can be a somewhat effective and economically feasible strategy for retailers to reduce their customers' consumption of calories from their products.

It is worth noting that in most of the considered cases, the modelled reformulation did not have statistically significant effects on the composition of consumption within the respective product categories. Hence, 'silent' product reformulation does not seem to scare consumers away, nor attract new consumers. Mayonnaise is an exception from this general pattern, as the reformulation seems to have increased the demand for the reformulated private-label product, mainly at the cost of the 'light' private-label product.

Buttriss [14] pointed at some of the challenges that may have to be met in relation to food product reformulation to a lower fat or sugar content. One challenge is the constraints of food legislation for some sectors, such as minimum requirements to the fat content of e.g. a chocolate product to be marketed as such, or regulation of nutrition and health claims, which may constrain producers' publicising changes in fat content. In addition, the Danish legislation on food labelling requires that a food product to be labelled as 'light' or 'low-fat' should have an energy content of maximum 70% of the corresponding 'regular' product, which may also limit the scope and incentive for reformulation.

Another challenge is that manufacturers have an interest to retain the characteristics of the product that are attractive to consumers, making reformulation to reduce fat a costly and time-consuming exercise. Reducing sugar content also poses challenges because sugar's role in foods is often more than simply providing sweetness, and different alternative approaches may be needed to provide the products with these attributes. Some of these alternative approaches have limitations, due to e.g. regulatory constraints, potential gastrointestinal consequences associated with some alternative ingredients, consumers' resistance to foods containing many additives, or that the alternatives are often more costly than sugar.

The product reformulations considered in this study have been quite moderate, as also mentioned above. Previous studies [15–17] indeed suggest that gradual product reformations, with fairly small steps at the time and thus slowly familiarizing the consumers with changes in taste and other characteristics, can be a fruitful strategy for health-promoting product reformulations. Due to the rather moderate extent of the considered reformulations, the magnitude of the public health impact might also be limited. Nevertheless, the results of the analysis provide fairly clear indications of a reduction in calorie intake in the respective commodity groups.

Limitations of the study

In the empirical analysis, we have adopted the assumption of a "representative consumer" purchasing the range of products in the considered retail chain, and we have estimated behavioural parameters reflecting utility maximization behaviour of this representative consumer. This assumption implies that the composition of consumers – and hence the average preferences - is assumed to be stable throughout the 52-weeks data period, or develops along a linear trend.

Furthermore, we have assumed weak separability in consumption in the sense that the composition of specific products within a certain (narrow) product category (e.g. the mayonnaise category or chocolate-flavoured breakfast cereals category) is independent of the relative prices of products outside this product category [18]. This assumption has enabled us to estimate separate systems of demand equations within each product category. But the separability structure also imposes restrictions on the substitution patterns that can be detected by the analysis. In the analysis, we have considered substitution effects between the reformulated product and its close substitutes. In most cases, the range of close substitutes was relatively straightforward. However, for some of the bread products, some subjective judgement as to which products were 'close' substitutes, and which were 'less close' substitutes, was necessary. Although the delimitation of these product categories was done to the best of the authors' capabilities, this may induce some uncertainty to the results for these products.

The product reformulation was represented as a 'dummy' (or binary) variable in the econometric analysis. This approach implies the assumption that from the date of reformulation, the consumers can only buy the reformulated version of the product - and not the 'old' version. For products with a shelf life of about 1 week (such as fruit yoghurt or fresh bread), this is not an unrealistic assumption. But for chocolate muesli and mayonnaise, there may have been a longer transition period, where the individual stores have emptied their shelves with the 'old' version, before they introduced the reformulated version of the product, and this may have introduced uncertainty to the results for these two products.

The 'dummy' variable representation also assumes that the consumers either consider the reformulation in their purchase decision from day one - or do not consider it at all. Again, this may introduce some uncertainty to the results.

The econometric estimation assumes stability in the population of consumers and its composition - or as a minimum that any development in this composition can be captured by the linear trend variable included in the estimation equations. The considered retail chain has however expanded quite significantly during the 52 weeks of consideration. For this reason, this assumption could be questioned - especially if new stores have been established in areas with 'new' socio-demographic characteristics, compared to those of the 'old' stores.

The analysis is based on sales data from only this one retail chain. Thus, interpreting the results as representative for the population of consumers has to be based on an assumption that their choice of store has not been affected by the product reformulation. It might be hypothesized that changes (e.g. assortment changes, price changes, product reformulations) could induce substitution effects in the consumers' choice of store. Address of such effect across stores is however very difficult and has not been possible in this study. It might be presumed that such substitution effects would undermine the possible health promoting effects, because consumers seek 'un-reformulated' products in other stores. On the other hand, the reformulation may also attract new customers. However, as the considered reformulations are generally quite moderate, and because the chain's stores already have fairly broad assortments of relevant substitutes, such across-store substitution effects are considered to be negligible. Although this may appear a realistic assumption, it has not been verified in this study, and this may also add to the uncertainty of the results.

Conclusion

This study has evaluated the effects of 'silent' reformulating a retail chain's private-label brands to a lower energy density, based on weekly sales data for a period of 52 weeks from a Danish retail chain. The analysis distinguishes between the direct effect of the lower energy density in the reformulated product and the indirect effects due to reformulation-induced product substitution. For seven out of the eight reformulated products considered in the study, the reformulation led to a reduction in calorie sales (defined as the sum of the direct and indirect effects from the reformulation). For chocolate muesli, a counter-productive (but statistically insignificant) substitution effect outweighed the direct effect of the reformulation. In most cases, the estimated reformulation-induced substitution effects were small and statistically insignificant. Hence, the sales value was only affected to a little extent - and only negatively affected in two of the eight cases considered.

Based on these findings, 'silent' reformulation of retailer's private brands towards lower energy density, seems to be a promising strategy for the retail sector to contribute to lower calorie intake in the population, and thus supportive of public health goals and industry's incentive to undertake also modest and silent reformulations.

Appendix

Table 3 Detailed results for mayonnaise

	Brand 1, tube	Private label light	*Private label*	Unbranded lemon	Brand 1, lemon
Initial share of calories	6.2%	12.2%	50.9%	0.3%	1.9%
Initial share of sales value	13.7%	16.1%	37.6%	0.5%	1.8%
AID model estimation results					
Ln $P_{Brand\ 1,\ tube}$	0.1937	0.1072	0.5578	−0.0047	−0.0776
	(0.1669)	(0.2123)	(0.3727)	(0.0430)	(0.1428)
Ln $P_{Private\ label\ light}$	−0.1631	−0.3367	−0.5005	−0.0184	−0.1574
	(0.2208)	(0.3015)	(0.5126)	(0.0660)	(0.2053)
Ln $P_{Private\ label}$	−0.0469	−0.0145	0.3002	0.0288	−0.0221
	(0.0529)	(0.0795)	(0.1248)	(0.0175)	(0.0536)
Ln $P_{Unbranded\ lemon}$	0.0009	−0.0060	−0.0398	0.0094	0.0056
	(0.0168)	(0.0200)	(0.0361)	(0.0038)	(0.0125)
Ln $P_{Brand\ 1}$	0.0600	0.0515	0.1887	0.0026	−0.0214
	(0.0063)	(0.0064)	(0.0128)	(0.0013)	(0.0040)
Ln $P_{Brand\ 1\ lemon}$	0.0043	−0.0012	0.0187	−0.0001	0.0066
	(0.0124)	(0.0152)	(0.0274)	(0.0031)	(0.0098)
Real budget	0.0111	−0.0139	−0.0204	0.0013	0.0027
	(0.0056)	(0.0062)	(0.0117)	(0.0012)	(0.0039)
Reformulation dummy	0.0107	−0.0045	0.0260	−0.0009	−0.0094
	(0.0040)	(0.0067)	(0.0098)	(0.0016)	(0.0047)
a10	0.1123	0.0207	0.1091	0.0058	−0.0227
	(0.0412)	(0.0513)	(0.0913)	(0.0103)	(0.0343)
Trend	−0.0005	−0.0004	0.0000	0.0000	−0.0001
	(0.0003)	(0.0005)	(0.0007)	(0.0001)	(0.0003)
Christmas dummy	−0.0025	−0.0021	−0.0117	0.0007	0.0093
	(0.0049)	(0.0070)	(0.0115)	(0.0015)	(0.0047)
AR (1)	−0.0083	0.5079	0.2058	0.7861	0.6214
	(0.1816)	(0.1553)	(0.1785)	(0.1212)	(0.1336)
Intercept	−0.1459	0.6999	−0.6859	−0.0436	0.5860
	(0.2842)	(0.4293)	(0.6790)	(0.1042)	(0.2956)
Root MSE	0.0056	0.0067	0.0121	0.0014	0.0043
R^2	0.90	0.85	0.94	0.84	0.83
R^2-adj	0.86	0.80	0.92	0.78	0.78

Table 4 Detailed results, fruit yoghurt

	Private label peach melba	Private label orange	Pear/ banana	Pineapple/ orange/ mango Light	Berry-flavoured
Initial share of calories	15.4%	5.8%	44.9%	4.0%	21.4%
Initial share of sales value	11.4%	5.3%	37.1%	8.9%	20.3%
AID model estimation results					
Ln $P_{Private\ label\ peach\ melba}$	0.000006	0.000002	−0.000004	−0.000001	−0.000002
	(0.000001)	(0.000000)	(0.000001)	(0.000001)	(0.000001)
Ln $P_{Private\ label\ orange}$	0.000001	0.000002	0.000000	0.000001	−0.000004
	(0.000001)	(0.000001)	(0.000001)	(0.000001)	(0.000002)
Ln $P_{Pear/banana}$	0.000005	0.000006	0.000004	−0.000006	0.000002
	(0.000002)	(0.000001)	(0.000003)	(0.000002)	(0.000003)
Ln $P_{Pineapple/orange/mango\ Light}$	0.000001	0.000001	−0.000005	0.000015	−0.000002
	(0.000001)	(0.000001)	(0.000001)	(0.000001)	(0.000001)
Ln P_{Berry}	−0.000001	0.000001	−0.000006	−0.000001	0.000021
	(0.000002)	(0.000001)	(0.000002)	(0.000003)	(0.000003)
Ln $P_{Berry\ Light}$	−0.000002	0.000000	−0.000010	−0.000002	−0.000006
	(0.000001)	(0.000001)	(0.000001)	(0.000001)	(0.000002)
Real budget	0.000011	0.000013	−0.000010	−0.000005	0.000009
	(0.000004)	(0.000003)	(0.000005)	(0.000004)	(0.000005)
Reformulation dummy	−0.004530	0.000008	0.002339	−0.000570	0.005419
	(0.003120)	(0.002320)	(0.004070)	(0.006260)	(0.008760)
Trend	−0.000150	0.000004	−0.000130	−0.000920	0.001534
	(0.000056)	(0.000041)	(0.000073)	(0.000577)	(0.000626)
Christmas dummy	−0.001470	0.000176	−0.006100	−0.000950	0.005525
	(0.002460)	(0.001760)	(0.003190)	(0.004400)	(0.006080)
AR (1)	−0.402090	−0.186420	−0.263600	0.879930	0.862313
	(0.147000)	(0.181400)	(0.174500)	(0.093100)	(0.080600)
Intercept	0.095738	0.048126	0.362423	0.113309	0.161103
	(0.006660)	(0.004570)	(0.008380)	(0.023100)	(0.026200)
Root MSE	0.0044	0.0028	0.0053	0.0055	0.0076
R^2	0.91	0.83	0.96	0.95	0.93
R^2-adj	0.89	0.78	0.95	0.93	0.91

Table 5 Detailed results - rye bread with pumpkin seeds

	Private label pumpkin	Private label sunflower	Brand organic sunflower
Initial share of calories	13.8%	12.0%	0.0%
Initial share of sales value	11.8%	10.4%	0.0%
AID model estimation results			
$\ln P_{\text{Private label pumpkin}}$	0.0000	0.0000	0.0000
	(0.0000)	(0.0000)	(0.0000)
$\ln P_{\text{Private label sunflower}}$	0.0000	0.0000	0.0000
	(0.0000)	(0.0000)	(0.0000)
$\ln P_{\text{Brand organic sunflower}}$	0.0000	0.0000	0.0000
	(0.0000)	(0.0000)	(0.0000)
$\ln P_{\text{Brand other sunflower}}$	0.0000	0.0000	0.0000
	(0.0000)	(0.0000)	(0.0000)
Real budget	0.0000	0.0000	0.0000
	(0.0000)	(0.0000)	(0.0000)
Reformulation dummy	−0.0041	−0.0048	−0.0015
	(0.0054)	(0.0049)	(0.0034)
Trend	−0.0002	−0.0002	0.0001
	(0.0002)	(0.0002)	(0.0001)
Christmas dummy	−0.0003	0.0001	0.0006
	(0.0033)	(0.0031)	(0.0021)
AR (1)	−0.1108	−0.0573	−0.3948
	(0.2253)	(0.2215)	(0.2373)
Intercept	0.0942	0.0894	0.0251
	(0.0075)	(0.0068)	(0.0051)
Root MSE	0.0057	0.0051	0.0041
R^2	0.99	0.99	0.97
R^2-adj	0.99	0.99	0.96

Table 6 Detailed results – Toasting buns

	Private-label whole grain	*Private-label*
Initial share of calories	35.6%	0.1%
Initial share of sales value	39.9%	0.1%
AID model estimation results		
Ln $P_{\text{Private-label whole grain}}$	−0.2273	0.2328
	(0.0501)	(0.0514)
Ln P_{Brand}	0.0008	−0.0013
	(0.0043)	(0.0044)
Ln $P_{\text{Private-label}}$	0.0345	0.0110
	(0.1968)	(0.2015)
Real budget	0.1398	−0.1372
	(0.0185)	(0.0189)
Reformulation dummy	0.0245	−0.0246
	(0.0127)	(0.0130)
Trend	0.0006	−0.0006
	(0.0004)	(0.0004)
Christmas dummy	−0.0284	0.0285
	(0.0144)	(0.0147)
AR (1)	−0.1913	−0.1923
	(0.1700)	(0.1699)
Intercept	−0.6575	1.5197
	(0.5805)	(0.5942)
Root MSE	0.0256	0.0262
R^2	0.83	0.83
R^2-adj	0.80	0.79

Table 7 Detailed results - yoghurt bread

	Brand 2 Wholemilk bread	Brand 1 Wholemilk bread	*Private label yoghurt bread*	Brand 1 Yoghurt bread
Initial share of calories	0.0%	30.2%	43.2%	0.0%
Initial share of sales value	0.0%	31.8%	38.2%	0.0%
AID model estimation results				
$\ln P_{Brand\ 2\ Wholemilk\ bread}$	0.1122	−0.0442	−0.0484	0.0000
	(0.0330)	(0.0172)	(0.0182)	(0.0001)
$\ln P_{Brand\ 1\ Wholemilk\ bread}$	0.2815	−0.6210	0.2239	0.0001
	(0.0825)	(0.0430)	(0.0456)	(0.0003)
$\ln P_{Private\ label\ yoghurt\ bread}$	0.2191	0.5111	−1.1483	0.0005
	(0.3671)	(0.1913)	(0.2028)	(0.0015)
$\ln P_{Brand\ 1\ Yoghurt\ bread}$	−0.0251	0.0094	0.0058	0.0001
	(0.0181)	(0.0094)	(0.0100)	(0.0001)
$\ln P_{Brand\ 3,\ 5\text{-}grain\ bread}$	0.0612	0.1295	0.1951	0.0002
	(0.0574)	(0.0299)	(0.0317)	(0.0002)
Real budget	0.2060	−0.0789	−0.0597	−0.0002
	(0.0488)	(0.0254)	(0.0270)	(0.0002)
Reformulation dummy	−0.0013	0.0085	−0.0100	0.0000
	(0.0352)	(0.0183)	(0.0194)	(0.0001)
Trend	0.0006	−0.0005	−0.0001	0.0000
	(0.0013)	(0.0007)	(0.0007)	(0.0000)
Christmas dummy	0.0085	−0.0166	−0.0001	0.0002
	(0.0501)	(0.0261)	(0.0277)	(0.0002)
Intercept	−3.3966	1.2240	2.3714	−0.0002
	(1.2671)	(0.6603)	(0.7001)	(0.0053)
Root MSE	0.0603	0.0314	0.0333	0.0003
R^2	0.62	0.93	0.88	0.28
R^2-adj	0.53	0.92	0.85	0.11

Table 8 Detailed results - rolls with carrot

	Private label carrot rolls	Brand 1 carrot rolls	Brand 1 whole-grain rolls
Initial share of calories	53.7%	0.0%	28.2%
Initial share of sales value	45.6%	0.0%	30.0%
AID model estimation results			
$\ln P_{Private\ label\ carrot\ rolls}$	0.0000	0.0000	0.0000
	(0.0000)	(0.0000)	(0.0000)
$\ln P_{Brand\ 1\ carrot\ rolls}$	0.0007	0.0000	0.0006
	(0.0006)	(0.0000)	(0.0007)
$\ln P_{Brand\ 1\ whole\text{-}grain\ rolls}$	0.0000	0.0000	0.0000
	(0.0000)	(0.0000)	(0.0000)
$\ln P_{Brand\ 2\ linseed\ rolls}$	0.0000	0.0000	0.0000
	(0.0000)	(0.0000)	(0.0000)
Real budget	0.0000	0.0000	0.0000
	(0.0000)	(0.0000)	(0.0000)
Reformulation dummy	0.0149	0.0000	0.0151
	(0.0151)	(0.0000)	(0.0166)
Trend	−0.0012	0.0000	−0.0006
	(0.0005)	(0.0000)	(0.0005)
Christmas dummy	0.0001	0.0001	0.0001
	(0.0000)	(0.0000)	(0.0000)
Intercept	0.3657	0.0000	0.2998
	(0.0520)	(0.0001)	(0.0572)
Root MSE	0.0172	0.0000	0.0189
R^2	0.99	0.98	0.98
R^2-adj	0.98	0.96	0.96

Table 9 AID model estimation results - wholegrain rolls

	Brand 2 sandwich rolls	*Private-label wholegrain rolls*	Brand 2, grain rolls	Brand 1 multi-grain rolls
Initial share of calories	18.1%	35.1%	19.4%	27.4%
Initial share of sales value	16.1%	30.1%	20.5%	33.2%
AID model estimation results				
Ln $P_{Brand\ 2\ sandwich\ rolls}$	0.00003	−0.00001	−0.00001	−0.00001
	(0.00000)	(0.00000)	(0.00000)	(0.00000)
Ln $P_{Private\text{-}label\ wholegrain\ rolls}$	−0.00001	0.00002	−0.00001	−0.00001
	(0.00000)	(0.00000)	(0.00000)	(0.00000)
Ln $P_{Brand\ 2,\ grain\ rolls}$	−0.00001	−0.00001	0.00002	−0.00001
	(0.00000)	(0.00000)	(0.00000)	(0.00000)
Ln $P_{Brand\ 1\ multi\ grain\ rolls}$	−0.00001	−0.00002	−0.00001	0.00004
	(0.00000)	(0.00000)	(0.00000)	(0.00000)
$LnP_{Brand\ 3\ wholegrain}$	−0.00005	0.00008	0.00000	−0.00004
	(0.00006)	(0.00015)	(0.00010)	(0.00011)
Real budget	0.00000	−0.00001	0.00000	0.00001
	(0.00000)	(0.00000)	(0.00000)	(0.00000)
Reformulation dummy	−0.00615	0.00408	0.01379	−0.01164
	(0.00399)	(0.00998)	(0.00683)	(0.00756)
Trend	0.00000	0.00008	−0.00012	0.00005
	(0.00007)	(0.00018)	(0.00012)	(0.00014)
Christmas dummy	−0.00056	0.00234	0.00000	−0.00206
	(0.00534)	(0.01330)	(0.00913)	(0.01010)
AR (1)	0.22398	0.20410	0.38075	0.00000
	(0.02580)	(0.01760)	(0.01950)	(0.00000)
Intercept	0.19093	0.22398	0.20410	0.38075
	(0.01030)	(0.02580)	(0.01760)	(0.01950)
Root MSE	0.0039	0.0098	0.0067	0.0074
R^2	1.00	0.99	0.99	0.99
R^2-adj	0.99	0.99	0.99	0.99

Table 10 Detailed results - chocolate muesli

	Brand 1	Private label regular	*Private label choco*	Brand 2
Initial share of calories	5.0%	63.8%	21.3%	7.8%
Initial share of sales value	13.1%	46.7%	20.8%	14.4%
AID model estimation results				
Ln $P_{Brand\ 1}$	−0.2943	0.0960	0.0640	0.1247
	(0.0142)	(0.0313)	(0.0177)	(0.0510)
Ln $P_{Private\ label\ regular}$	0.6598	−1.2680	−0.6039	0.4600
	(0.4612)	(0.9849)	(0.5757)	(1.5450)
Ln $P_{Private\ label\ choco}$	−0.4838	0.5100	0.3138	0.1899
	(0.4055)	(0.8553)	(0.5033)	(1.3312)
Ln P_{Brand2}	0.0608	0.2019	0.1427	−0.4529
	(0.0164)	(0.0368)	(0.0205)	(0.0589)
Ln $P_{Brand\ 3}$	−0.0400	0.1023	0.1085	0.1572
	(0.0692)	(0.1513)	(0.0869)	(0.2413)
Real budget	−0.0257	−0.0966	−0.0236	0.1380
	(0.0128)	(0.0260)	(0.0149)	(0.0413)
Reformulation dummy	−0.0466	0.0570	0.0191	−0.0157
	(0.0334)	(0.0640)	(0.0383)	(0.0992)
Trend	0.0000	0.0002	0.0009	−0.0007
	(0.0008)	(0.0004)	(0.0003)	(0.0006)
Christmas dummy	0.0109	0.0096	−0.0012	0.0165
	(0.0122)	(0.0188)	(0.0126)	(0.0272)
AR (1)	0.8022	0.2210	0.4339	0.0640
	(0.1019)	(0.1694)	(0.1517)	(0.1668)
Intercept	0.7431	2.3112	0.2789	−2.4491
	(0.4261)	(0.9154)	(0.5233)	(1.4814)
Root MSE	0.0148	0.0262	0.0159	0.0413
R^2	0.94	0.85	0.81	0.89
R^2-adj	0.92	0.81	0.76	0.86

Acknowledgements

The REMA1000 retail chain is acknowledged for providing access to the data, TrygFonden is acknowledged for providing financial support for the research, and project head Gitte Laub Hansen, Danish Cancer Society is acknowledged for her constructive comments to earlier drafts of the manuscript.

Funding

The research and preparation of the paper has been funded by a research grant from TrygFonden. TrygFonden has not been involved in the analysis nor in preparation of the manuscript.

Authors' contributions

JDJ has designed and conducted the statistical analysis and drafted the manuscript. IS has collected and prepared data for the analysis and participated in planning of the study and preparation of the manuscript. Both authors read and approved the final manuscript.

Competing interests

Both authors declare to have no competing interests.

Author details

[1]University of Copenhagen, Department of Food and Resource Economics, Rolighedsvej 25, 1958 Frederiksberg C, Denmark. [2]Danish Cancer Society, Strandboulevarden 49, 4100 København Ø, Copenhagen, Denmark.

References

1. Raaij JV, Hendriksen M, Verhagen H. Potentials for improvement of population diet through reformulation of commonly eaten foods. Public Health Nutr. 2009;12(3):325–30.
2. Mancino L, Kuchler F, Leibtag E. Getting consumers to eat more whole-grains: the role of policy, information, and food manufacturers. Food Policy. 2008;33:489–96. http://www.sciencedirect.com/science/article/pii/S0306919208000535
3. Downs SM, Thow AM, Leeder SR. The effectiveness of policies for reducing dietary trans fat: a systematic review of the evidence. Bull World Health Org. 2013;91:4.
4. Webster JL, Dunford EK, Hawkes C, Neal BC. Salt reduction initiatives around the world. J Hypertens. 2011;29(6):1043–50.
5. Wyness LA, Butriss JL, Stanner SA. Reducing the population's sodium intake: the UK Food Standards Agency's salt reduction programme. Public Health Nutr. 2012;15(2):254–61.
6. Monge-Rojas R, Colón-Ramos U, Jacoby E, Mozaffarian D. Voluntary reduction of trans-fatty acids in Latin America and the Caribbean: current situation. Rev Panam Salud Publica. 2011;29(9):126. http://dx.doi.org/10.1590/S1020-49892011000200008
7. Stender S, Astrup A, Dyerberg J. What went in when trans went out? N Engl J Med. 2009;361:314–6. http://dx.doi.org/10.1056/NEJMc0903380
8. Keast DR, Rosen RA, Arndt EA, Marquart LF. Dietary modeling shows that substitution of whole-grain for refined-grain ingredients of foods commonly consumed by US children and teens can increase intake of whole grains. J Am Diet Assoc. 2011;111:1322–8.
9. Golan E, Unnevehr L. Food product composition, consumer health, and public policy: introduction and overview of special section. Food Policy. 2008;33:465–9.
10. Unnevehr L, Jagmanaite E. Getting rid of trans fats in the US diet: policies, incentives and progress. Food Policy. 2008;33:497–503.
11. Marotta G, Simeone M, Nazzaro C. Product reformulation in the food system to improve food safety. Evaluation of policy interventions, Appetite. 2014;74: 107–15.
12. Ronit K. and Jensen J.D. (2014) Obesity and industry self-regulation: a literature review, Eur J Clin Nutr , (http://www.nature.com/ejcn/journal/vaop/ncurrent/pdf/ejcn201460a.pdf).
13. Morgenstern H. (1995) Ecologic studies in epidemiology: concepts, principles and methods, annual review of public health, 16, 61-81.14.Deaton a. & Muellbauer J. An almost ideal demand system. Am Econ Rev. 1980;70(3):312–26.
14. Buttriss JL. Food reformulation: the challenges to the food industry - proceedings of the nutrition society. Cambridge Journals Online. 2012;72(1): 61–9. http://journals.cambridge.org/action/displayAbstract?fromPage=online&aid=8822959&fileId=S0029665112002868
15. Dötsch M, Busch J, Batenburg M, Lien G, Tarelius E, Mueller R, Meijer G. Strategies to reduce sodium consumption: a food industry perspective. CRC Crit Rev Food Sci Nutr. 2009;49(10):841–51.
16. Girgis S, Neal B, Prescott J, Pendergast J, Dumbrell S, Turner C, Woodward M. A one-quarter reduction in the salt content of bread can be made without detection. Eur J Clin Nutr. 2003;57:616–20.
17. Grasso S, Brunton NP, Lyng JG, Lalor F, Monahan FJ. Healthy processed meat products – regulatory, reformulation and consumer challenges, Trends in Food Science and Technology. 2014;39(1):4–17.
18. Edgerton DL. Weak separability and the estimation of elasticities in multi-stage demand systems. Am J Agri Econ. 1997;79:62–79.

PERMISSIONS

All chapters in this book were first published in IJBNPA, by BioMed Central; hereby published with permission under the Creative Commons Attribution License or equivalent. Every chapter published in this book has been scrutinized by our experts. Their significance has been extensively debated. The topics covered herein carry significant findings which will fuel the growth of the discipline. They may even be implemented as practical applications or may be referred to as a beginning point for another development.

The contributors of this book come from diverse backgrounds, making this book a truly international effort. This book will bring forth new frontiers with its revolutionizing research information and detailed analysis of the nascent developments around the world.

We would like to thank all the contributing authors for lending their expertise to make the book truly unique. They have played a crucial role in the development of this book. Without their invaluable contributions this book wouldn't have been possible. They have made vital efforts to compile up to date information on the varied aspects of this subject to make this book a valuable addition to the collection of many professionals and students.

This book was conceptualized with the vision of imparting up-to-date information and advanced data in this field. To ensure the same, a matchless editorial board was set up. Every individual on the board went through rigorous rounds of assessment to prove their worth. After which they invested a large part of their time researching and compiling the most relevant data for our readers.

The editorial board has been involved in producing this book since its inception. They have spent rigorous hours researching and exploring the diverse topics which have resulted in the successful publishing of this book. They have passed on their knowledge of decades through this book. To expedite this challenging task, the publisher supported the team at every step. A small team of assistant editors was also appointed to further simplify the editing procedure and attain best results for the readers.

Apart from the editorial board, the designing team has also invested a significant amount of their time in understanding the subject and creating the most relevant covers. They scrutinized every image to scout for the most suitable representation of the subject and create an appropriate cover for the book.

The publishing team has been an ardent support to the editorial, designing and production team. Their endless efforts to recruit the best for this project, has resulted in the accomplishment of this book. They are a veteran in the field of academics and their pool of knowledge is as vast as their experience in printing. Their expertise and guidance has proved useful at every step. Their uncompromising quality standards have made this book an exceptional effort. Their encouragement from time to time has been an inspiration for everyone.

The publisher and the editorial board hope that this book will prove to be a valuable piece of knowledge for researchers, students, practitioners and scholars across the globe.

LIST OF CONTRIBUTORS

Vanessa M. Oddo and Jessica C. Jones-Smith
Department of International Health, Center for Human Nutrition, Johns Hopkins Bloomberg School of Public Health, 615 N. Wolfe St, Baltimore, MD 21205, USA
Nutrition Sciences Program & Department of Health Services, University of Washington School of Public Health, Raitt Hall, Seattle, WA 98195, USA

Sara N. Bleich
Department of Health Policy and Management, Harvard T.H. Chan School of Public Health, 677 Huntington Avenue, Boston, MA 02115, USA

Keshia M. Pollack
Department of Health Policy and Management, Johns Hopkins Bloomberg School of Public Health, 624 N. Broadway, Baltimore, MD 21205, USA

Pamela J. Surkan
Department of International Health, Social and Behavioral Interventions Program, Johns Hopkins Bloomberg School of Public Health, 615 N. Wolfe St, Baltimore, MD 21205, USA

Noel T. Mueller
Department of Epidemiology, Johns Hopkins Bloomberg School of Public Health, 615 N. Wolfe St, Baltimore, MD 21205, USA

Mary L. Greaney
Department of Kinesiology and Health Studies, 25 West Independence Way, University of Rhode Island, Kingston, RI 02881, USA

Sandy Askew and Perry B. Foley
Duke Global Digital Health Science Center, Duke Global Health Institute, Duke University Durham, NC 27710, USA.

Sherrie F. Wallington
Georgetown Lombardi Comprehensive Cancer Center, Georgetown University, Washington, D.C. 20007, USA.

Lisa M. Quintiliani
Section of General Internal Medicine, Department of Medicine, Boston University, Boston, MA 02118, USA

Gary G. Bennett
Duke Global Digital Health Science Center, Duke Global Health Institute, Duke University Durham, NC 27710, USA.
Department of Psychology and Neuroscience, Duke University, Durham, NC 27708, USA.

Marieke De Craemer , Ilse De Bourdeaudhuij and Greet Cardon
Department of Movement and Sport Sciences, Ghent University, Watersportlaan 2, 9000 Ghent, Belgium

Maïté Verloigne
Department of Movement and Sport Sciences, Ghent University, Watersportlaan 2, 9000 Ghent, Belgium
Research Foundation Flanders, Brussels, Belgium

Odysseas Androutsos and Yannis Manios
Department of Nutrition and Dietetics, Harokopio University, School of Health Science & Education, E. Venizelou 70, 17671 Athens, Greece

Violeta Iotova
Medical University Varna, Clinic of Paediatric Endocrinology, UMHAT "St. Marina", "Hr. Smirnenski" Blvd, Varna, Bulgaria

Luis Moreno
University of Zaragoza, GENUD (Growth, Exercise, Drinking behaviour and Development), C/Corona de Aragón 42, 50009 Zaragoza, Spain

Berthold Koletzko
University of Munich Medical Centre, Dr. von Hauner Children's Hospital, Lindwurmstr.4, 80337 Munich, Germany.

Piotr Socha
Children's Memorial Institute, Al. Dzieci Polskich 20, 04–730 Warsaw, Poland

Nathalie Kliemann, Helen Croker and Fiona Johnson
Department of Behavioural Science & Health, University College London, London, England

Victoria Vickerstaff and Irwin Nazareth
Department of Primary Care & Population Health, University College London, London, England

Rebecca J. Beeken
Department of Behavioural Science & Health, University College London, London, England
Leeds Institute of Health Sciences, University of Leeds, Level 10, Worsley Building, Clarendon Way, Leeds LS2 9NL, England

Janet H.W. van den Boer, Jentina Kranendonk, Anne van de Wiel, Edith J.M. Feskens, Anouk Geelen and Monica Mars
Division of Human Nutrition, Wageningen University, P.O. Box 17, 6700 AA Wageningen, The Netherlands

S. Hawkesworth, B. Armstrong and T. Pliakas, K. Nanchahal
Faculty of Public Health and Policy, London School of Hygiene and Tropical Medicine, London WC1E 7HT, UK.

R.J. Silverwood
Faculty of Epidemiology and Population Health, London School of Hygiene & Tropical Medicine, London WC1E 7HT, UK.

C. Sartini and G. Wannamethee
UCL Department of Primary Care & Population Health, UCL Medical School, Rowland Hill Street, London NW3 2PF, UK.

A. Amuzu and J. Atkins
University of Exeter Medical School, Wonford Barrack Road, Exeter EX2 5DW, UK.

S.E. Ramsay
Institute of Health & Society, Newcastle University, Newcastle upon Tyne NE2 4AX, UK.

J.P. Casas
Farr Institute of Health Informatics, Faculty of Population Health Sciences, 222 Euston Road, London NW1 2DA, UK.

R.W. Morris
School of Social and Community Medicine, University of Bristol, Bristol BS8 2PS, UK.

P.H. Whincup
Population Health Research Institute, St George's, University of London, London SW17 0RE, UK.

Karen Lock
Faculty of Public Health and Policy, London School of Hygiene and Tropical Medicine, London WC1E 7HT, UK.
London School of Hygiene & Tropical Medicine, 15-17 Tavistock Place, London, UK.

Deborah F. Tate
Department of Health Behavior, Department of Nutrition, The University of North Carolina at Chapel Hill, Chapel Hill, NC 27599-7440, USA.

Carmina G. Valle
Department of Nutrition, The University of North Carolina at Chapel Hill, Chapel Hill, NC 27599-7294, USA.

Melissa M. Crane
Department of Preventive Medicine, Rush University Medical Center, 1700 W. Van Buren St., Suite 470, Chicago, IL 60612, USA.

Brooke T. Nezami
Lineberger Comprehensive Cancer Center, The University of North Carolina at Chapel Hill, Chapel Hill, NC 27599-7294, USA.

Carmen D. Samuel-Hodge
Department of Nutrition, The University of North Carolina at Chapel Hill, Chapel Hill, NC 27599-7426, USA.

Karen E. Hatley, Molly Diamond and Kristen Polzien
Lineberger Comprehensive Cancer Center, The University of North Carolina at Chapel Hill, Chapel Hill, NC 27599-7294, USA.

Carlos Penilla and Emily J. Ozer
School of Public Health, University of California, Berkeley, 50 University Hall, Berkeley, CA 94720-7360, USA.

Jeanne M. Tschann
Department of Psychiatry, University of California, San Francisco, Box 0848, San Francisco, CA 94143-0848, USA

Emma V. Sanchez-Vaznaugh
Health Education Department, San Francisco State University, 1600 Holloway Ave, San Francisco, CA 94132, USA.

Elena Flores
Department of Counseling, University of San Francisco, 2130 Fulton St., San Francisco, CA 94118, USA.

Michelle Holdsworth, Hibbah Araba Osei-Kwasi and Katie Powell
Public Health Section, School of Health and Related Research-ScHARR, The University of Sheffield, Sheffield, UK.

Mary Nicolaou and Karien Stronks
Academic Medical Centre, University of Amsterdam, Department of Public Health, Amsterdam Public Health research Institute, Amsterdam, The Netherlands.

Lars Jørun Langøien
Department of Physical Education, Norwegian School of Sport Sciences, Oslo, Norway.

Sebastien F. M. Chastin
Institute for Applied Health Research, School of Health and Life Science, Glasgow Caledonian University, Glasgow, UK.

F. Marijn Stok
Department of Psychological Assessment and Health Psychology, University of Konstanz, Constance, Germany.

Laura Capranica
Department of Movement, Human and Health Sciences, University of Rome Foro Italico, Rome, Italy.

Nanna Lien
Department of Nutrition, University of Oslo, Oslo, Norway.

Laura Terragni
Department of Nursing and Health Promotion Faculty of Health Sciences, Oslo and Akershus University College of Applied Sciences, Oslo, Norway.

Pablo Monsivais
UKCRC Centre for Diet and Activity Research, MRC Epidemiology Unit, University of Cambridge School of Clinical Medicine, Box 285, Institute of Metabolic Science, Cambridge Biomedical Campus, Cambridge CB2 0QQ, UK.
Present address: Department of Nutrition and Exercise Physiology, Elson S Floyd College of Medicine, Washington State University, Spokane WA 99210-1495, USA.

Mario Mazzocchi
Department of Public Health, Ghent University, Ghent, Belgium.

Lea Maes
Department of Public Health, Ghent University, Ghent, Belgium.

Gun Roos
Consumption Research Norway SIFO, Oslo and Akershus University College of Applied Sciences, Oslo, Norway.

Caroline Mejean
UMR MOISA, Campus INRA-SupAgro de la Gaillarde, Montpellier, France.

Nomathemba Dube, Sarah Loehr and Paul Veugelers
Department of Public Health Sciences, Population Health Intervention Research Unit, School of Public Health, University of Alberta, 3-50 University Terrace, 8303 112 Street, Edmonton, AB T6G 2T4, Canada

Kaviul Khan
Department of Public Health Sciences, Population Health Intervention Research Unit, School of Public Health, University of Alberta, 3-50 University Terrace, 8303 112 Street, Edmonton, AB T6G 2T4, Canada
Dalla Lana School of Public Health, University of Toronto, Toronto, ON, Canada

Yen Chu
Department of Public Health Sciences, Population Health Intervention Research Unit, School of Public Health, University of Alberta, 3-50 University Terrace, 8303 112 Street, Edmonton, AB T6G 2T4, Canada
Centre for Clinical Epidemiology and Evaluation, University of British Columbia, Vancouver, BC, Canada.

Cut Novianti Rachmi
Discipline of Child & Adolescent Health, The Children's Hospital at Westmead, University of Sydney Clinical School, Locked Bag 4001 Westmead, NSW 2145, Australia

Cynthia Louise Hunter
School of Social and Political Sciences, The University of Sydney, RC Mills Building (A26), Sydney, NSW 2006, Australia
Sydney School of Public Health, The University of Sydney, Edward Ford Building (A27), Fisher Rd, Sydney, NSW 2006, Australia

Mu Li
Sydney School of Public Health, The University of Sydney, Edward Ford Building (A27), Fisher Rd, Sydney, NSW 2006, Australia

Louise Alison Baur
Discipline of Child & Adolescent Health, The Children's Hospital at Westmead, University of Sydney Clinical School, Locked Bag 4001 Westmead, NSW 2145, Australia
Sydney School of Public Health, The University of Sydney, Edward Ford Building (A27), Fisher Rd, Sydney, NSW 2006, Australia

Gareth R. Dutton and Marissa A. Gowey and Cora E. Lewis
Division of Preventive Medicine, Department of Medicine, University of Alabama at Birmingham, Birmingham, AL, USA.

Fei Tan and Dali Zhou
Department of Mathematical Sciences, Indiana University-Purdue University Indianapolis, Indianapolis, IN, USA.

Jamy Ard
Department of Epidemiology and Prevention, Wake Forest University School of Medicine, Winston Salem, NC, USA.

Michael G. Perri
Department of Clinical and Health Psychology, University of Florida, Gainesville, FL, USA.

Teresia M. O'Connor, Sheryl O. Hughes, Tom Baranowski and Truc Pham
USDA/ARS Children's Nutrition Research Center, Baylor College of Medicine, 1100 Bates St, Houston, TX, USA.

Louise C. Mâsse
BC Children's Hospital Research Institute, School of Population and Public Health, University of British Columbia, Vancouver, BC, Canada.

Andrew W. Tu
Child & Family Research Institute, School of Population and Public Health, University of British Columbia, Vancouver, BC, Canada.

Allison W. Watts
Division of Epidemiology and Community Health, School of Public Health, University of Minnesota, Minneapolis, MN, USA.

Mark R. Beauchamp
School of Kinesiology, University of British Columbia, Vancouver, BC, Canada.

Jerica M. Berge
Department of Family Medicine and Community Health, University of Minnesota Medical School, Minnesota, MN, USA.

Barbara Fiese
Family Resilience Center, Department of Human Development and Family Studies, University of Illinois at Urbana-Champaign, Urbana, IL, USA.

Rebecca Golley
Sansom Institute for Health Research (PHRC), School of Pharmacy and Medical Sciences, University of South Australia, Adelaide, Australia.

Melanie Hingle
Department of Nutritional Sciences, College of Agriculture and Life Sciences, University of Arizona, Tucson, AZ, USA.

Stef P. J. Kremers
NUTRIM School of Nutrition and Translational Research in Metabolism, Maastricht University Medical Center, Maastricht, The Netherlands.

Kyung E. Rhee
Department of Pediatrics, University of California, San Diego, CA, USA.

Helen Skouteris
School of Psychology, Deakin University, Melbourne, Australia.

Amber Vaughn
Department of Nutrition, Gillings School of Global Public health, University of North Carolina, Chapel Hill, NC, USA.

Ester F. C. Sleddens, Jessica S. Gubbels, Stef P. J. Kremers and Eline van der Plas
Department of Health Promotion, NUTRIM School of Nutrition and Translational Research in Metabolism, Maastricht University, Maastricht University Medical Center, P.O. Box 616, 6200 MD Maastricht, the Netherlands

Carel Thijs
Department of Epidemiology, Maastricht University, CAPHRI Care and Public Health Research Institute, P.O. Box 616, 6200 MD Maastricht, the Netherlands

Andrea S. Richardson, Wendy M. Troxel, Madhumita Ghosh-Dastidar, Gerald P. Hunter, Robin Beckman, Rebecca L. Collins and Tamara Dubowitz
RAND Corporation, Health Division, 4570 Fifth Avenue, Pittsburgh, PA 15213, USA.

Natalie Colabianchi
University of Michigan, School of Kinesiology, Ann Arbor, MI 48109-2013, USA.

Sarah Mummah
Department of Medicine, Stanford University School of Medicine, Stanford, CA, USA.
Department of Public Health and Primary Care, University of Cambridge, Cambridge, UK.

Thomas N. Robinson
Department of Medicine, Stanford University School of Medicine, Stanford, CA, USA.
Department of Pediatrics, Stanford University School of Medicine, Stanford, CA, USA

Maya Mathur, Sarah Farzinkhou and Christopher D. Gardner
Department of Medicine, Stanford University School of Medicine, Stanford, CA, USA.

Stephen Sutton
Department of Public Health and Primary Care, University of Cambridge, Cambridge, UK.

Jørgen Dejgård Jensen
University of Copenhagen, Department of Food and Resource Economics, Rolighedsvej 25, 1958 Frederiksberg C, Denmark.

Iben Sommer
Danish Cancer Society, Strandboulevarden 49, 4100 København Ø, Copenhagen, Denmark.

Index